# Proceedings of the Twelfth Annual Conference of the British Association for Biological Anthropology and Osteoarchaeology

Department of Archaeology and Anthropology
University of Cambridge 2010

Edited by

Piers D. Mitchell
Jo Buckberry

BAR International Series 2380
2012

Published by

Archaeopress
Publishers of British Archaeological Reports
Gordon House
276 Banbury Road
Oxford OX2 7ED
England
bar@archaeopress.com
www.archaeopress.com

BAR S2380

*Proceedings of the Twelfth Annual Conference of the British Association for Biological Anthropology and Osteoarchaeology. Department of Archaeology and Anthropology University of Cambridge 2010*



ISBN 978 1 4073 0970 5

Printed in England by Information Press, Oxford

All BAR titles are available from:

Hadrian Books Ltd
122 Banbury Road
Oxford
OX2 7BP
England
www.hadrianbooks.co.uk

The current BAR catalogue with details of all titles in print, prices and means of payment is available free from Hadrian Books or may be downloaded from www.archaeopress.com

# Table of Contents

## List of Contributors

Evilena Anastasiou
Department of Archaeology and Anthropology
University of Cambridge
The Henry Wellcome Building
Fitzwilliam Street
Cambridge, CB2 1QH, UK

Jelena Bekvalac
Centre for Human Bioarchaeology
Museum of London
150 London Wall
London, EC2Y 5HN, UK

Gurdyal S. Besra
School of Biosciences
University of Birmingham
Edgbaston
Birmingham, B15 2TT, UK

Heather Bonney
Department of Palaeontology
Natural History Museum
Cromwell Road
London, SW7 5BD, UK

Jo Buckberry
Biological Anthropology Research Centre
Archaeological Sciences
University of Bradford
Bradford, BD7 1DP, UK

Ian D. Bull
Bristol Biogeochemistry Research Centre
School of Chemistry
University of Bristol
Bristol, BS8 1TS, UK

Jonathan Castro
Freelance Archaeologist
Ibiza, Spain

Angela Clark
Department of Anatomy
School of Medical Sciences
University of Otago
Dunedin, New Zealand

Margaret Clegg
Department of Palaeontology
Natural History Museum
Cromwell Road
London, SW7 5BD, UK

Anna F. Clement
Institute of Archaeology
University College London
31-34 Gordon Square
London, WC1H 0PY, UK

Gabrielle Delbarre
Department of Palaeontology
Natural History Museum
Cromwell Road
London, SW7 5BD, UK

Natasha Dodwell
Cambridge Archaeological Unit
Department of Archaeology
University of Cambridge
Downing Street
Cambridge, CB2 3DZ, UK

Helen D. Donoghue
Research Department of Infection
University College
London, W1T 4JF, UK

Alison Freyne
Institute of Archaeology
University College London
31-34 Gordon Square
London, WC1H 0PY, UK

Matthew A. Gasperetti
Phenotypic Adaptability, Variation and Evolution Research Group
Department of Archaeology and Anthropology
University of Cambridge
Pembroke Street
Cambridge CB2 3DZ, UK

Karina Gerdau Radonic
Bournemouth University
School of Applied Sciences,
Christchurch House, Talbot Campus
Fern Barrow, Poole
Dorset, BH12 5BB, UK

Siân Halcrow
Department of Anatomy
School of Medical Sciences
University of Otago
Dunedin, New Zealand

Nigel Jeffries
Museum of London Archaeology
Mortimer Wheeler House
46 Eagle Wharf Road
London, N1 7ED, UK

Elena F. Kranioti
Forensic Anthropology
School of History, Classics and Archaeology
The University of Edinburgh
Edinburgh, UK

Robert Kruszynski
Department of Palaeontology
Natural History Museum
Cromwell Road
London, SW7 5BD, UK

Xenia-Paula Kyriakou
Forensic Anthropology
School of History, Classics and Archaeology
The University of Edinburgh
Edinburgh, UK

Helen Langstaff
Forensic Anthropology
School of History, Classics and Archaeology
The University of Edinburgh
Edinburgh, UK

Oona Y-C. Lee
School of Biosciences
University of Birmingham
Edgbaston
Birmingham, B15 2TT, UK

Antonia Marcsik
Department of Anthropology
University of Szeged
H-6701 Szeged, Hungary

Nicholas Márquez-Grant
Cellmark Forensic Services
Abingdon, UK

Simon Mays
English Heritage
Fort Cumberland, Eastney
Portsmouth, PO4 9LD, UK

David E. Minnikin
School of Biosciences
University of Birmingham
Edgbaston
Birmingham, B15 2TT, UK

Piers D Mitchell
Department of Archaeology and Anthropology
University of Cambridge
The Henry Wellcome Building
Fitzwilliam Street
Cambridge, CB2 1QH, UK

Erika Molnár
Department of Anthropology
University of Szeged
H-6701 Szeged, Hungary

Carrie Springs Pacelli
Forensic Anthropology
School of History, Classics and Archaeology
The University of Edinburgh
Edinburgh, UK

György Pálfi
Department of Anthropology
University of Szeged
H-6701 Szeged, Hungary

Paola V. Ponce
Department of Archaeology
Durham University
South Road
Durham, DH1 3LE, UK

Charlotte Roberts
Department of Archaeology
Durham University
South Road
Durham, DH1 3LE, UK

Roland Rodell
Anthropology/Department of Anthropology and Sociology
University of Wisconsin – Rock County
Janesville, WI 53546, USA

Joan Roig
Freelance Archaeologist
Ibiza, Spain

Cara Samuels
Forensic Anthropology
School of History, Classics and Archaeology
The University of Edinburgh
Edinburgh, UK

Richard J. Slater
Bournemouth University
School of Applied Sciences
Christchurch House
Talbot Campus
Fern Barrow, Poole
Dorset, BH12 5BB, UK

Martin J. Smith
Bournemouth University
School of Applied Sciences
Christchurch House
Talbot Campus
Fern Barrow, Poole
Dorset, BH12 5BB, UK

Jay T. Stock
Phenotypic Adaptability, Variation and Evolution Research Group
Department of Archaeology and Anthropology
University of Cambridge
Pembroke Street
Cambridge CB2 3DZ, UK

Norman C. Sullivan
Anthropology/Department of Social and Cultural Sciences
Marquette University
Milwaukee, WI 53233, USA

Nancy Tayles
Department of Anatomy
School of Medical Sciences
University of Otago
Dunedin, New Zealand

Katrien Van de Vijver
Physical Anthropologist, St. Rumbold Cemetery
City Council of Mechelen
Department of Archaeology
Pitzemburgstraat 8
2800 Mechelen, Belgium

# Introduction: Biological Anthropology

Piers D Mitchell[1] and Jo Buckberry[2]

[1]Department of Archaeology and Anthropology
University of Cambridge
The Henry Wellcome Building
Fitzwilliam Street
Cambridge, CB2 1QH, UK

[2]Biological Anthropology Research Centre
Archaeological Sciences
University of Bradford
Bradford BD7 1DP, UK

Email for correspondence: pdm39@cam.ac.uk

Biological anthropology is a broad field that explores all aspects of the physical development of humans. This includes human evolution, primatology, comparative anatomy, human behavioural ecology, human genetics, palaeopathology, forensic anthropology, evolutionary medicine, nutrition and modern health, among others. Each year at the conference of the British Association for Biological Anthropology and Osteoarchaeology (BABAO) we hold sessions dedicated to different branches of biological anthropology. This has the aim of ensuring research from all aspects of the field is presented to the association, so broadening its audience and maintaining the all-inclusive nature of the organisation. BABAO has over 500 members currently, so there is a good deal of research being undertaken in this field. Each year the topic of these sessions will vary, but over time the yearly volumes in this series combine to provide a useful archive of research and education on all aspects of biological anthropology, for both students and professionals alike.

The articles published in the volume are all based upon research presented at the 12th annual BABAO conference, which was held at the University of Cambridge by Piers Mitchell in September 2010. Every paper has passed through a vigorous peer review process, so that only the best submissions were accepted for inclusion here. The volume has been divided into five sections to reflect the nature of their content.

*Human Evolution to the Dawn of Agriculture* groups together papers that explore how early humans developed as hunter gatherers to the point that they started to farm particular crops. The impact of the material, cultural and dietary changes upon human anatomy, group population size, material culture and health are all important areas that intrigue researchers.

*Palaeopathology* brings together papers that investigate health in past populations. Findings from the excavation of ancient sites from across the world are presented. There is a mixture of approaches including the study of human skeletal remains for lesions caused by disease, biomolecular analysis of proteins of those infectious diseases that caused illness in past societies, and microscopic study of coprolites from latrine soils to identify the eggs of human intestinal parasitic worms.

*Museums, Curation and Data Recording* highlights the importance of museums and their curators in preserving, recording, imaging and displaying material that helps us to understand biological anthropology better. The expertise of the Natural History Museum and the Museum of London is highlighted with these papers. Skeletal collections where the age at death, sex, and racial background are known are rare, but are of key importance for many aspects of biological anthropology research. The creation of such a collection at the NHM is clearly of great research interest.

*Methods of Analysis* highlights how new techniques can lead to new discoveries, but also that techniques currently in use can often be improved, or their accuracy clarified to highlight those that are not quite as helpful as many of us presume. Papers in this group include both those based upon laboratory research, and also practical experiments in the field that have been undertaken in order to understand how burials from the past came to take the form we find today at excavation.

*Interpreting Burials in Past Populations* completes the volume, with a group of papers that investigate burials in order to understand what people in the past thought was appropriate to do to the bodies of those who died in their societies. Such investigations help us to understand the thought processes and religious beliefs of people long since disappeared, and so allows us to see how our own modern beliefs fit in the others of our species over time and space.

This volume brings together a fabulous collection of high quality biological anthropology research into one place. This helps us to appreciate how the different research areas within the field interact and overlap. This reinforces why we believe all aspects of this broad field should remain under the distinct label of biological anthropology, and why it benefits from an umbrella organisation such as BABAO.

# Human Evolution after the Origin of our Species: Bridging the Gap between Palaeoanthropology and Bioarchaeology

Jay T. Stock

Phenotypic Adaptability, Variation and Evolution Research Group
Department of Archaeology and Anthropology
University of Cambridge
Pembroke Street
Cambridge CB2 3DZ, UK

Email for correspondence: jts34@cam.ac.uk

**Abstract**
The study of evolution within our species has had a problematic past, which has led to an artificial divide between palaeoanthropological approaches which focus on adaptation among fossil hominins, and biocultural approaches which focus on understanding variation among modern humans. The contrast between research on the Upper Palaeolithic and Neolithic is where this shift in approach has tended to occur, largely due to the assumption that human control over the environment associated with the origins of agriculture is associated with a buffering of environmental stress and natural selection.

The evolution of cultural and physiological mechanisms to buffer environmental stress is central to our success as a species, allowing us to colonize a wide range of niches. However the common assumption that environmental buffering relaxes natural selection can no longer be fully supported. Recent research demonstrates a complex system of feedback between cultural and biological evolution which continues to influence variation within our species. Plasticity in biological systems is central to understanding the relationship between culture and genes, and beginning to disentangle their various influences on the human phenotype. This paper attempts to bridge the divide between evolutionary and biocultural approaches by suggesting areas where bioarchaeologists can contribute to our understanding of the mechanisms which shape phenotypic diversity, and continuing morphological change within our species. A review of recent evidence for relationships between cultural evolution, plasticity and genetic adaptation demonstrates the benefits of a more integrated approach to understanding our own species.

**Keywords:** Skeletal Morphology, Adaptation, Functional Morphology, Plasticity, Phenotype

## Introduction

In this paper I would like to address a number of issues, both theoretical and practical, which relate to how we interpret skeletal variation within our species. For many years there has been an artificial divide between palaeoanthropology and bioarchaeology, with the former focusing on inter-specific variation, and the latter focusing on variation within populations through time. These different approaches differ with respect to their views on the role of evolution in shaping human diversity. In bioarchaeology, comparisons between populations have often been considered methodologically flawed at best, and at worst, inappropriate due to the legacy of scientific racism. This criticism can easily be countered by the general observation that the study of phenotypic variation is only inappropriate when social values are imposed upon the variation. The importance of cultural relativism in anthropology has also had a major impact on how we view modern human diversity. Much of this stems from the work of Franz Boas who demonstrated tremendous plasticity in the human phenotype, and argued that the comparison of human populations is either too difficult or irrelevant. The theme of the plasticity of the human phenotype is prevalent throughout the work of Boas. In Race, Language and Culture, he argued that "change due to environment that occur under our eyes, such as minute changes in size and proportion of the body, are probably not hereditary, but merely expressions of the reaction of the body to external conditions and subject to new adjustments under new conditions" (Boas 1940: 246). While the true implications of Boas' classic migrant studies have been debated it is clear that the human phenotype is influenced by both plasticity within the lifespan, and intergenerational population history through genetics.

In contrast to the issue of plasticity within the lifespan, our understanding of the influence of evolution by natural selection on the human phenotype is quite limited. The majority of introductory textbooks in biological anthropology feature chapters on human evolution which end with modern human dispersals. At this point it is generally considered that the human evolutionary career is over, and we have told the story of the evolution of our species (cf. Klein 2009). A major factor in this perspective is the importance of technology in modern human dispersals. It is clear that the adaptive radiation of *Homo sapiens* out of Africa was culturally dependent, involving such technologies as fire, housing, watercraft, microlithic technologies, marine resource exploitation, symbolism, language, and artistic expression. It is often assumed that since culture is such a strong adaptive mechanism, capable of very rapid horizontal transmission between individuals, that it not only becomes our primary means of adaptation but that it effectively brings our biological evolution to an end (Dyson 2007). If the shift in mechanisms from biological to cultural evolution is not seen to be complete with the origin and dispersal of our species, then agriculture is often seen as the final component of this process. Agricultural subsistence can feed 100 times as many people as foraging for the same area of land, it leads to sedentism, food storage, rapid demographic growth, task specialized duration of individuals, and a runaway technological evolution. In this context agriculture provides the basis for the development of civilizations, the Industrial Revolution, trade, and the global economy. The most important implication of this is that this technological development is often seen as a mechanism of cultural buffering, which allows for rapid adaptation to environmental change without needing to resort to the slow process of biological evolution (Stock 2008).

When we consider human variation, we initially note the great phenotypic diversity found within our species. This diversity is generally continuous in nature, and clinally distributed, often in relation to geography or environmental variation. This tremendous diversity can be contrasted with our relative genetic homogeneity. There is evidence to suggest that there is considerably more genetic variation amongst individual populations of chimpanzees or gorillas than there is within our entire species (Kaessmann *et al.* 2001). This is largely a reflection of our recent common African origin, but it also suggests that at least some of the tremendous phenotypic diversity in our species is related to biological plasticity in response to environmental variation or other non adaptive mechanisms.

In order to bring together the apparent gap between palaeoanthropology and bioarchaeology, we must consider models of how evolution may function relative to cultural developments in the Holocene. Clearly evolution by natural selection is the central theory of evolutionary biology and as such will be relevant to understanding recent human diversity. However more recent perspectives may be highly relevant to understanding evolution after the Pleistocene. Dual inheritance theory, or gene culture co-evolution, suggests that we have both genetic and cultural systems of inheritance which are each subject to natural selection (Richerson and Boyd 2005). In this context, these systems are not only mechanisms of adaptation themselves, but they influence one another, or co-evolve. A further level of complexity may be added to this, if we consider the role of adaptive networks which involve a developmental component, or an Evo-Devo approach.

The general assumption that adaptation by natural selection has ended with agriculture has been overturned using mathematical methods for detecting signatures of natural selection in the genome (Sabetti *et al.* 2006), and evidence for a number of genes which demonstrate signatures of selection across the genome (cf. Voight *et al.* 2006; Sabeti *et al.* 2007). Recently, it has been noted that when we consider the function of many of these genes, their recent selection may relate to cultural change within recent human prehistory. In this case, rather than buffering the genome from selective pressure, culture is largely driving the evolution of biological systems in humans (Laland *et al.* 2010; Richerson *et al.* 2010). This can be viewed as not only the coming of age of dual inheritance theory, or gene culture co-evolution, but it also suggests that we need to revisit the central issue that has plagued the study of human variation since the beginning of anthropology, that of genetic versus environmentally plastic influences on the phenotype in light of the relationship between cultural change and human adaptability.

## What Factors Control Human Phenotypic Variation?

In order to investigate the factors which influence phenotypic variation, a simple phenotypic character to consider, due to the ease of quantification, is stature. Twin studies demonstrate that there is between 60 and 90% heritability in height, which implicates underlying genetic mechanisms as the determinants of stature. In twin studies, whatever proportion of variation cannot be attributed to shared genes by heritability estimates, is generally attributed to environmental variation. Thus far, stature has been associated with approximately 180 specific genes, each contributing a very small effect (Allen *et al.* 2010; Lanktree *et al.* 2011). These were recently thought to account for as little as 5% of the variation in adult stature (Weedon *et al.* 2008; Lettre *et al.* 2008; Gudbjarsson *et al.* 2008), however a recent study has demonstrated that approximately 40% of variation may be controlled deeper within the genome (Yang *et al.* 2010). There remains promise that more variation may be found within the genome, perhaps related to: a) unknown genetic variants which will be revealed by genome wide association studies; b) copy number variations in specific genes; or c) currently undetectable networks of genes. However it is also possible that heritability estimates from twin studies are artificially inflated due to the common foetal environment, similarities in genetic regulation during development in response to similar environmental conditions, or epigenetic effects and other intergenerational mechanisms of phenotypic control (Wells and Stock 2011). These complications illustrate that the human phenotype is a continuum between plasticity and genetic canalization, and that some environmental effects may actually artificially inflate our heritability estimates.

When we consider the expression of morphological variation in the phenotype, we can contrast traits which are canalized from those that are plastic. Canalized traits are developmentally stable, showing minimal variation in different environmental conditions. Traits that appear to be highly canalized include brain size and dental morphology, as they are self righting in the face of environmental variation, and hence likely to be under very close genetic regulation during development. Plastic traits vary in relation to environmental conditions are particularly flexible in early life, allowing for modification of the phenotype during the lifespan, and allow for more rapid adaptation than is possible through intergenerational genetic change.

In a recent paper, we argued that a biological emphasis on mechanisms of plasticity is a central feature of our species which contributes toward adaptive success in different environments (Wells and Stock 2007). In this paper we identified a variety of levels of plasticity which can be seen as intermediate biological mechanisms which serve to buffer the genome from the necessity to commit to adaptation, or selective sweeps in response to environmental stress. At the top level are cultural mechanisms of plasticity, what we can consider the extended phenotype including technology, cultural learning, sociality, and individual level behaviour. These generally correspond with the cultural component of dual inheritance theory. Beyond these, there are a number of mechanisms of physiology and biology which can be manipulated through changes in life history. These include body size and physique, energy stores, variation in the developmental schedule, and other mechanisms of metabolic plasticity. These mechanisms may be essential in modifying the phenotype to fit local environmental conditions, without risky commitment to genetic adaptation. Genetic adaptation in this context would commit an individual or population to phenotypic characteristics which would be slow to respond to future environmental variation. Plastic mechanisms however, can allow adaptation of phenotype within the lifespan and particularly during development, and perhaps more importantly, can allow for relatively rapid return to 'ancestral' morphological states.

If we consider plasticity as an additional adaptive system which, by nature of the speed of its adaptive response exists between culture and technology and genetic adaptation, then we could consider humans to have a three level, hierarchical adaptive system (Fig. 1). In this case, plasticity itself can be divided into different mechanisms which function on a fast to slow continuum from physiological plasticity, through developmental plasticity, to transgenerational epigenetic inheritance. Each of these has the capacity to change the phenotype without underlying genetic adaptation.

## Variation in the Skeletal System

If we consider the issue of the relationship between Bioarchaeology and Palaeoanthropology within the context of a multi-level hierarchy of adaptive systems, we may gain insight into understanding the skeletal phenotype. There is considerable evidence that phenotypic diversity among humans correlates with environmental variation, despite cultural buffering mechanisms, however in most cases we do not yet know whether variation is caused by plasticity or long-term genetic adaptation. Additional variation seems to correspond only with geographic distance, suggesting random factors of demography and population history may be more important than selection (Betti *et al.* 2010). Resolving these issues is central to improving our interpretations of the fossil record, and to investigating whether adaptation by natural selection is still occurring within the Holocene.

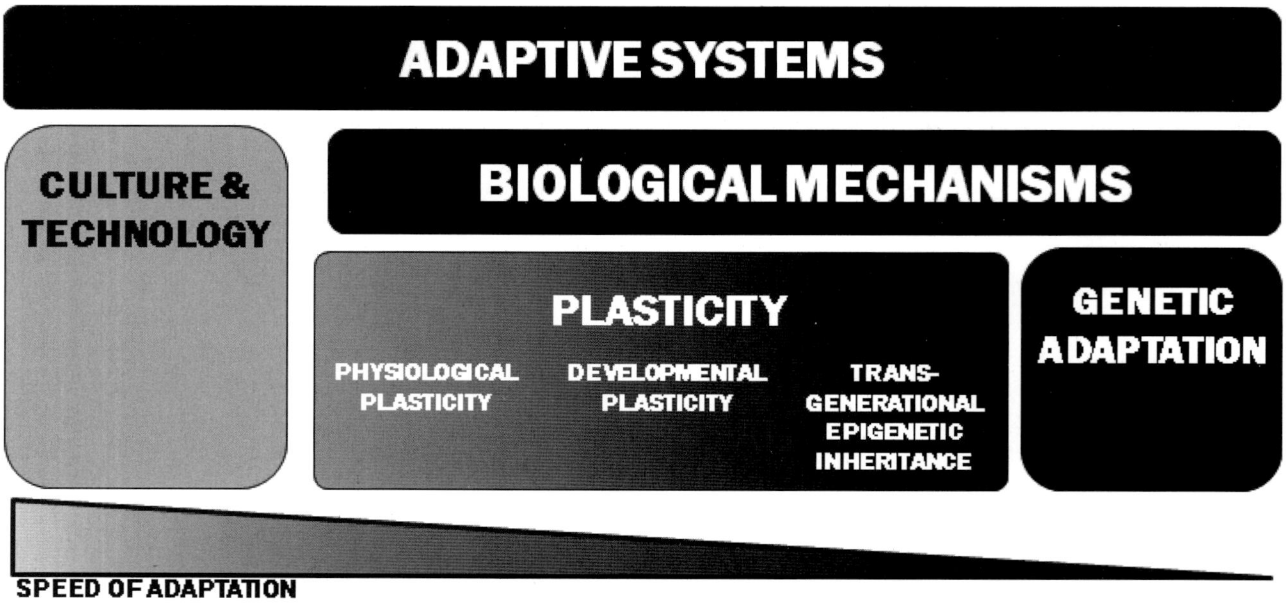


**Figure 1:** Cultural and biological adaptive systems and their relative speed.

A consideration of skeletal variation within this broad context of adaptive systems outlined in Figure 1, we can see that a variety of mechanisms can influence skeletal morphology from genetic variation, to the range of mechanisms of biological plasticity, and to cultural mechanisms which could influence any of the biological mechanisms directly. This lies in contrast to many common implicit assumptions made in palaeoanthropology, when studying the fossil record:

- skeletal variation represents genetic variation in the population or species level
- morphological traits are adaptive, in other words they are particulate rather than integrated
- derived characteristics are independent, and have equal relevance in cladistic approaches to taxonomy
- any modern human skeletons are sufficient for interspecific comparisons to the fossil record

Modern human cranial variation provides an interesting example of how skeletal morphology is at once influenced by many different factors. Figure 2 represents the output of canonical variates analysis of over 7000 modern human crania from around the world (Stock *et al.* 2007). It illustrates several important factors about the nature of human variation, that: a) it is continuous, with no discrete subsets; b) there is a geographic patterning or clinal distribution to human variation; and perhaps most importantly, c) morphometric variation represents both human geography and the chronology of human dispersals out of Africa. African variation is central, with variation outside of Africa ranging in a continuum from Australia to Europe, with all populations showing divergence from the African centroid. Human cranial variation supports a recent African origin of our species (Howells 1978; Lahr 1996), which suggests that it is highly canalised by genes. It is a fairly common assumption that variation which is tightly controlled by genes must also illustrate adaptation. This is not likely to be the case for human cranial variation. While Howells data was used to illustrate the recent African origin of modern humans, it has more recently been re-analyzed in association with molecular data to investigate whether there is evidence for natural selection acting upon modern human cranial form (Roseman 2004). The results of the study suggested that the majority of cranial variation in humans could be attributed to random genetic drift associated with the migration of small populations of hunter gatherers in the Pleistocene, a conclusion that has been supported with larger datasets (Betti *et al.* 2010). Evidence for selection in cranial phenotype appeared only in size and shape of the cranial vault among the native populations of Siberia suggesting that random factors may be largely responsible for the variation we see among human populations. The interpretation of Siberian morphology as adaptation demonstrates that the author considers cranial morphology to be more tightly controlled by genes than plasticity. However, as this study points only to strong directional morphological change in one population, the analysis is insufficient to determine whether this is caused by natural selection or extreme phenotypic plasticity. There is evidence for some degree of plasticity within the human skull. In general, some morphological characteristics previously thought to have illustrated multiregional continuity among fossil and modern human populations, such as cranial robusticity, may be related to developmental plasticity in response to biomechanical loading (Lahr and Wright 1996). The best example of this may be the prevalence of sagittal keeling among Australian aboriginal crania, which illustrates that this size and shape of the human skull is driven by a combination of natural selection, genetic drift and founder of fact, and aspects of habitual behaviour through biomechanics and plasticity which may driven by cultural and environmental variation.

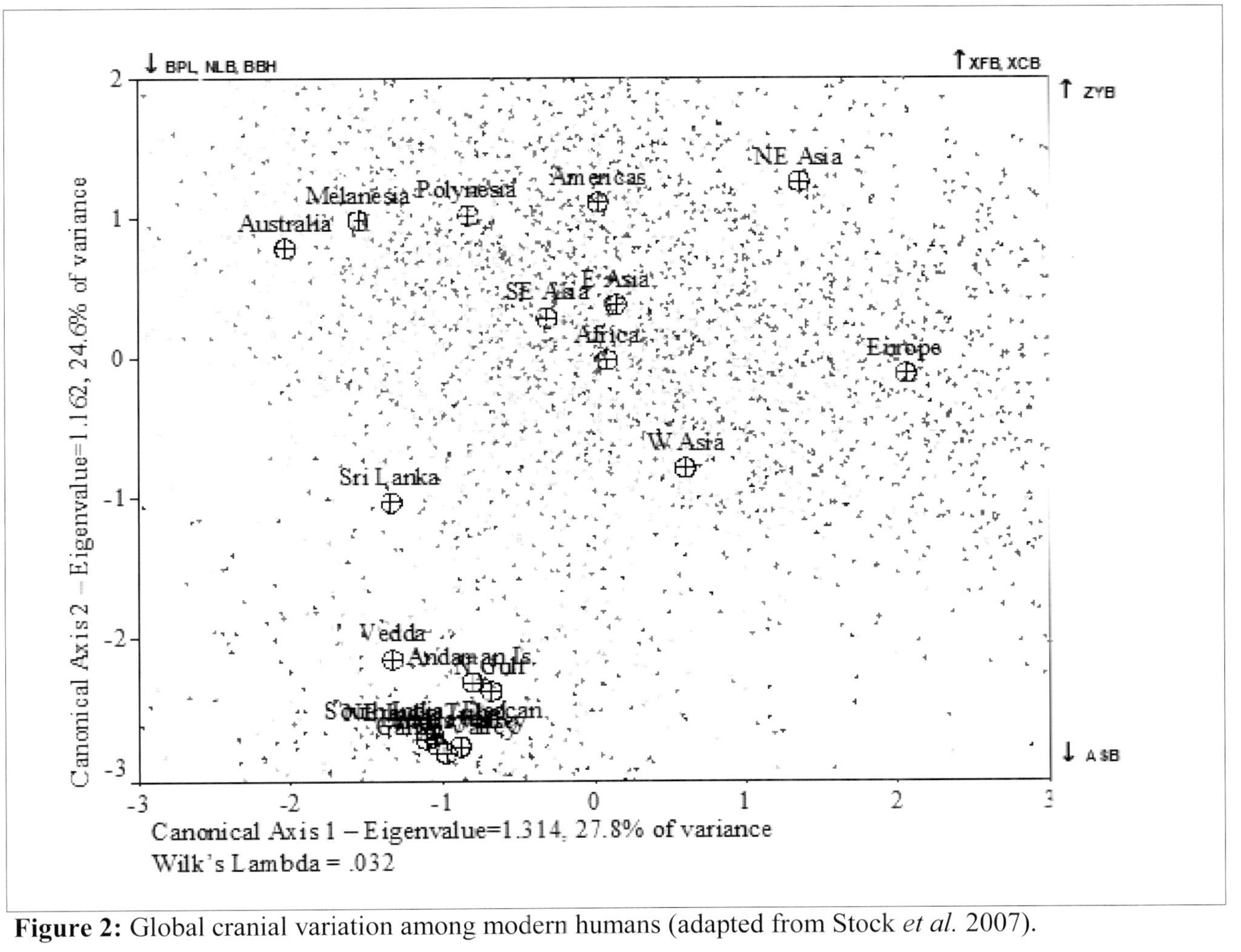


**Figure 2:** Global cranial variation among modern humans (adapted from Stock *et al.* 2007).

### Phenotypic Variation: Adaptation or Plasticity?

The mechanisms of phenotypic or developmental plasticity are poorly understood in humans, on account of our long generation times and comparatively short research projects, however numerous examples of plasticity can be found among nonhuman species. One of the best examples is the regulation of the Himalayan gene among Siamese cats in response to environmental variation (Searle 1968). The gene results in temperature sensitive albinism, which causes variation in pigmentation of the coat relative to temperature producing the distinctive dark patches of fur on the snout, ears, paws, and tail of the cat. Siamese cats raised in warm environments have much lighter coloration in these regions. Similar systems of developmental plasticity can influence the phenotype both soft tissues and the skeleton.

The most classic examples of skeletal phenotypic adaptation relative to environmental conditions are Bergmann's and Allen's rules. Bergman's rule suggests that individuals of the species who inhabit cold climates will have increased body mass when compared to tropically living members of the same species, while Allen's rule suggests that limb lengths will be longer in individuals who inhabit tropical regions and shorter in colder climates. Clinal variation in mammalian physique fits the expectations of Bergmann's and Allen's rules, and there is considerable evidence that human variation also corresponds with these expectations (Roberts 1953; 1978). Bergman's rule has been tested using skeletal estimates of stature and body mass as estimated by bone lengths and bi-iliac breadth or femoral head diameter. Similarly, Allen's rule has been tested using crural indices (the ratio of tibial length to bicondylar femoral length). Trinkaus (1981) demonstrated that modern human crural indices fit a pattern of climatic adaptation expected of Allen's rule, with the lowest values found amongst Eskimos and Scandinavian Lapps. When Neanderthals are interpreted in this context, they fall at the very low end of the spectrum, suggesting long-term adaptation to cold stress. In contrast, Holliday (1997) demonstrated at the earliest upper Palaeolithic humans in Europe had very long lower limbs and distal limb segments, a morphological pattern that would be expected with adaptation to the hotter environments of Africa or the Near East. Holliday also noted that later upper Palaeolithic and Mesolithic Europeans had shorter tibiae than the earliest upper Palaeolithic people in Europe, which suggests that over thousands of years Europeans became more cold-adapted in response to colder environments. These studies both make the assumption, and indeed provide some support for, the interpretation that body proportions are largely genetically controlled, with very low selective rates and evidence for long-term adaptation by natural selection. This research seemingly contradicts evidence for phenotypic plasticity in limb proportions that we might expect on the basis of the pig studies. Despite the strong evidence that human phenotypic variation generally corresponds with Bergmann's and Allen's rules, the pattern of human variation in body mass and limb proportions may be more complicated than this. Katzmarzyk and Leonard (1998) demonstrated that the strength of this relationship between physique and climate decreased after 1950, perhaps due to the homogenization of the human diet related to global cultural processes. If human limb proportions can change relatively dramatically over a short period of time, it suggests that there may be some mechanism of phenotypic plasticity acting within our species as well.

In the 1960's, a macaque colony from Honshu, Japan (35°N Latitude) was transferred to research stations in Beaverton, Oregon (45°N) and southern Texas (28°N), creating a natural experiment of environmental influence on physique. After 20 years, the Oregon group showed higher body mass, shorter limb segments, and greater subcutaneous fat (Paterson 1996). While this demonstrates climatic adaptability among macaques, it does not demonstrate whether it is achieved through developmental plasticity (genetic regulation) or underlying genetic (base pair) differences. Classic experiments on pigs have demonstrated developmental plasticity in a variety of phenotypic traits, as more body hair, greater body mass, shorter limbs, and shorter tails and ears were features of pigs raised in colder environments (Weaver and Ingram 1969). In contrast, exposure to warm environments during development led to opposite phenotypic expression, with pigs raised in intermediate environmental conditions showing morphology that was intermediate between the two extremes. Subsequent research has shown a daily heat production among pigs raised in cold environments is reduced at low temperatures, but there is an increased amount of dorsal fat which leads to greater retention of body heat (Demo *et al.* 1995).

These differences in limb proportions noted in the pig studies demonstrate developmental plasticity of the skeleton in response to temperature. Another example of skeletal adaptation illustrates how the environmental conditions may be influenced by behaviour. An interesting paper investigating size variation in the skull of the rock hyrax, *Procavia capensis,* (Yom-Tov 1993) suggests that cranial morphology is influenced by temperature extremes in southern Africa. Studies of geographic variation in the hyrax skull suggest that it is particularly sensitive to heat stress rather than cold temperatures. In this case it was hypothesized that cold stress was mediated through behavioural adaptations and the use of caves to buffer from thermal stress. If this interpretation is correct, it illustrates the relationship between behavioural buffering and skeletal variation in phenotype in a nonhuman species. In this context we may expect that humans would show similar variation relative to a much broader range of cultural environments used to buffer environmental stress (Stock 2008).

Recent experimental research on mice has proposed a mechanism for the developmental plasticity of limb proportions. Serrat *et al.* (2008) tested the effect of ambient temperature during growth on the phenotype, including blood flow and the size and morphology of skeletal elements. They found that mice raised in cold environments had less blood flow to peripheral tissues, which resulted in decreased linear growth in the tail and ear. Based upon this evidence, they measured blood flow to the femur and tibia relative to the thoracic spine, and identified a critical window early in development between 4 1/2 in 6 1/2 weeks, when blood flow to the limb is particularly susceptible to low environmental temperatures. They then studied metatarsal growth in vitro, using antimeres of the same individual, and demonstrated that warm temperatures led to greater growth than metatarsals grown in cold conditions. Histological analysis showed cartilage proliferation in the growth plate of the 'warm' samples, which suggested that a physiological regulation of blood flow in response to environmental stress influences cartilage development and bone growth. This provides the first direct test of a mechanism of developmental plasticity in limb lengths in response to thermal stress. This contrast, between features that are at once genetically conservative and canalised, but which also demonstrate some level of plasticity, can be identified in studies of the postcranial skeleton as well. The research of Trinkaus (1981), Holiday (1997), and Ruff (2002) generally interprets post-cranial variation as heritable characteristics which represent long term adaptation by natural selection among species. In contrast, there is strong evidence for considerable plasticity in limb proportions of migrants to the United States, which occurs within a single generation (Bogin *et al.* 2002). This apparent contradiction is not at odds with the work of Trinkaus and Ruff, if we consider them to represent interspecific rather than intraspecific comparisons, but they do seem to contradict Holliday's results (1997) which suggest that limb proportions of early modern humans evolved over thousands of years as an adaptation to the colder European environments.

The contradictions raised when we consider evidence for variation in human and animal body mass and limb lengths highlights the we know very little about the mechanisms which drive variation in the human and hominin skeleton. It is likely that human limbs may respond to environmental variation during development using the same physiological mechanisms as mice and pigs, which suggests considerable plasticity. However, this does not explain why there is a time-lag of thousands of years before modern humans in Europe show more cold-adapted phenotypes. This apparent conflict between evidence for canalization or plasticity exists throughout the history of studies of human phenotypic variation.

Early craniometric studies emphasized the heritability of craniofacial morphology, and racial typology, but these were largely rejected based on the demonstration of plasticity in cranial morphology of migrants to the New World work by Franz Boas (Boas 1911). Thus much of the artificial divide between palaeoanthropology and Bioarchaeology is based upon general assumptions held within anthropology for much of the past century, that interspecific differences were largely genetic, while intraspecific variation within our species was thought to be highly plastic in response to environmental and cultural variation. In the 1970s through 1990s, the work of Howells (1978), Pietrusewsky (1990), Hanihara (1992) and Lahr (1996) brought renewed focus on the heritability of cranial morphology, and its utility in determining modern human population history. This work clearly demonstrated the recent African origin of modern humans before it was supported by genetic evidence, which later reinforced our assumptions of a high heritability to cranial morphology. Boas' demonstration of cranial plasticity does not seem to fit with our current understanding of the canalization and heritability of cranial morphology A reanalysis of Boas' original data by Sparks and Jantz (2002), suggests that he overlooked evidence or greater heritability of cranial morphology within his sample. A further reanalysis by Gravlee *et al.* (2003) demonstrates that the Boas' dataset illustrates both high heritability of cranial features, and some degree of plasticity among migrants. In this context, Boas was correct in noting plasticity in the human phenotype, he may have simply emphasized this more than the evidence for morphological similarity which his data also show.

At present there is contradictory evidence for both canalization and plasticity of the phenotype of both human cranial and post-cranial skeletons. The weight of evidence suggests that cranial variation is more highly conserved and canalized, while aspects of post-cranial variation (particularly bone lengths and diaphyseal strengths) are influenced by plasticity during the lifespan in response to nutrition, health and habitual activity. This demonstrates perhaps the most significant area where Bioarchaeology and Palaeoanthropology need to engage, by placing more effort in understanding the mechanisms underlying phenotypic variation within our species and the fossil record. In this context, a number of fundamental questions are poorly understood: How is variability distributed throughout the skeleton? Which areas of the skeleton are canalized or plastic? What factors (genetic, biomechanic, energetic etc) contribute to the phenotypic variation that we observe? How do these different factors interact, and is there morphological integration across regions of the skeleton? It is not possible to disentangle these fundamental issues of bone biology using the fossil record. The answer to these questions will need to be addressed through focussed research in Bioarchaeology, and skeletal biology using animal models and the study of skeletal variation among living humans (Shaw and Stock 2009a; 2009b). Through very focussed studies which aim to address some of these issues we can gain a better understanding of the continuum between canalization and plasticity, and provide better means of interpreting the variation we see in the fossil record. For example, regions of the skeleton which are highly canalized will particularly useful in the interpretation of phylogenetic relationships, while variation in regions which are plastic provide a means of interpreting biomechanical and adaptive aspects of morphology which relate to the environmental and behavioural context of growth and development.

The influence of habitual activity on long-bone robusticity has been one of the best documented aspects of skeletal plasticity. It is based on the principal that bone responds to biomechanical loading by stimulating bone deposition in areas of high strain. When this strain is repetitive, it is thought to causing hypertrophy of trabecular and cortical bone which counteracts the loading (see Ruff *et al.* 2006 for review). Studies of professional tennis players provide strong evidence for adaptive bone remodelling in humans, as they demonstrate that high levels of humeral bilateral asymmetry correspond with the duration of their competitive participation in the sport (Jones *et al.* 1977). The general correspondence between long bone diaphyses and habitual activity has been supported by studies of cricketers, swimmers, distance runners and field hockey players (Shaw and Stock 2009a; 2009b). While mechanically induced plasticity clearly influences cross-sectional geometry of long bone diaphyses, there is also evidence that habitual activity may cause systemic differences in skeletal morphology in other regions of the skeleton such as the skull (Lieberman 1996).

**How can Anthropological Research Contribute to Our Understanding of Human Adaptability?**

One way of understanding the broad patterns of humans adaptability is through adoption of a systems approach. Systems biology is an approach which builds upon our understanding of genotype-phenotype interactions to incorporate environmental effects and developmental pathways into analyses (Klingenberg 2008). In this way, the phenotype is viewed as a series of modular systems which relate to one another through a series of developmental, energetic and physiological relationships. The phenotypic characters of an individual, or species, will thus be the result of a series of mechanisms and biological processes influencing the process of tissue development and maintenance. Thus, the morphology of any particular character may be influenced by developmental, genetic or functional constraints or which integrate the development and/or performance of the phenotype. These function of these 'modules' may be balanced by natural selection, remodelling of tissues, or developmental modification through heterochrony, or differences in developmental timing. The greatest challenge in trying to understand modular integration and development in determining the human phenotype is the complexity of interactions involved. However we try to understand these systems, we are likely to be oversimplifying the complexity of interactions. We should not be discouraged if our models are overly simplistic, as long as they begin to account for the complexity of different factors and systems which may be driving morphological variation.

Diaphyseal robusticity is an example of a simple skeletal characteristic which is influenced by multiple factors, modules, or adaptive systems. It is easily quantified through cross-sectional geometric properties of cortical bone distribution (Ruff *et al.* 2006). Our understanding of the factors which determine the strength of a long bone diaphysis, reveal tremendous complexity. Genetic mechanisms clearly influence bone mineral density and bone mechanical properties, as over 350 quantitative trait loci (QTLs) have been correlated with these in the mouse genome (Jepsen 2009). Despite the strong genetic component, decades of biomechanical research demonstrate a clear adaptive response of bone tissue to mechanical strain, demonstrating that habitual loading during lifetime does influence the morphology and strength of skeletal tissue, with higher strains stimulating bone deposition and greater bone strength (see Ruff *et al.* 2006 for review). These two seemingly conflicting influences on morphology can be brought together through model of phenotypic integration where the genotype of an individual is mediated throughout a lifetime by terms of growth and functional trait interactions to produce the expressed phenotype (Jepsen 2009). In this case we can already view the adult phenotype as a complex interaction of biological adaptive systems ranging from genes to plasticity. These mechanisms however, may be highly influenced by environmental variation. The hyper-robust skeletons of Neanderthals for example, have long been hypothesized to be related to a combination of adaptation to cold climates, and high levels of habitual activity (Trinkaus 1997). Subsequent research has tried to disentangle the competing influences of climate and habitual activity on the skeleton, and is demonstrated at the influences of these factors vary depending upon the region of the body under consideration. Amongst hunter gatherers for example, the robusticity of limb bones appears to be highly correlated with patterns of habitual mobility, but they are confounded by climatic influences on robusticity closer to the trunk (Stock 2006). These influences are driven by morphological integration with body breadth, which is itself an adaptation to climatic variation. As a result, behavioural signatures within long bones may be stronger and more distal locations within the limbs. This provides a very simple model of how we can begin to understand the complexity of mechanisms driving skeletal variation. By adding a developmental component to this, we can further disentangle the mechanisms which influence observable variation.

Critics of the biomechanical approach to interpreting behaviour from the skeleton have often argued the cross-sectional geometry is determined by developmental mechanisms, genetics, or morphological integration with other features, rather than habitual activity during life (for review see Pearson and Lieberman 2004). However, like the previous debates about human cranial morphology, skeletal robusticity is at once determined by development, genetics, morphological integration and activity during life. Depending on where we look in the skeleton, robusticity may correlate to a greater or lesser extent with any of these mechanisms. Thus it is not a case of which model is correct, but whether we are getting a strong enough signal of any one of these mechanisms in order to use it as a basis for interpretation of morphology in the past.

The previous example dealt specifically with the issue of skeletal robusticity and how we may interpret it. It may be worthwhile to explore broader patterns of adaptation within human populations, to try to investigate whether our adaptability is primarily focused on the adaptive system of cultural variation, plasticity, or the genome. The Inuit provide an excellent model for understanding human adaptation under extreme environmental conditions. It is certain that technological capacity is a central adaptation which allowed the Inuit to colonize the high Arctic thousands of years ago. Animal skin clothing and watercraft, as well as dwellings made of ice and animal skins, and advanced hunting technologies were all essential components of Inuit adaptability in this harsh environment. The recent sequencing of an ancient human genome of a prehistoric Inuit man from Greenland, demonstrated a number of single nucleotide polymorphisms associated with possible adaptations to cold, including genes that have been linked to vasoconstriction, high body mass index, and the leptin thermogenic pathway (Rasmussen *et al.* 2010). These two perspectives alone could be considered to be an excellent example of dual inheritance theory, with two parallel mechanisms of adaptation to the natural environment. However, there is also evidence for human adaptation through physiological mechanisms. The Inuit show a high prevalence of cold induced vasodilation, a physiological mechanism which periodically dilates the blood vessels which allows for warming of the extremities. We may be tempted to consider this as a genetic adaptation to cold, however the characteristic is shared with North Sea fisherman who develop a CIVD response in response to lifetime exposure rather than their genetic makeup. Similarly, body mass and body fat distribution is both highly influenced by genes and plastic during the lifespan, allowing for an added level of plastic adaptability to environmental stress. There is now growing evidence that limb proportions may be developmentally stable, suggesting that their development is canalised and as such under genetic control (Eleazer and Cowgill 2010). This seems in contrast to what we know about plasticity and limb growth among mice and pigs from the experimental research. The examples of Inuit adaptations to the environment emphasize how a multi-level model of adaptive systems may be useful to interpreting human variation. Future studies of skeletal development may play a crucial role in understanding whether developmental mechanisms and plasticity are responsible for the considerable variation in the adult phenotype.

## Conclusion

There are a number of ways in which bioarchaeology can contribute to the study of human evolution. First and foremost, there is no reason to distinguish between the Pleistocene and Holocene in evolutionary analyses. There is considerable evidence that evolution continues after the origins of agriculture, but that it may be primarily driven by cultural stresses rather than those found in the natural environment. Secondly, skeletal morphology is still our primary means of understanding the phenotype in evolutionary adaptations of recent humans and fossil species. Thirdly, questions of the factors which control the skeletal phenotype are inherently multivariate and multidisciplinary, and bioarchaeological approaches can be used to begin to disentangle the complexity of the phenotype. It is clear that future research needs to focus on our understanding of the mechanisms which produce skeletal variation, and continuing patterns of human adaptation relative to Holocene natural and cultural environments.

With a multi-level model of adaptive systems, focussing on culture, plasticity and genes, carefully designed research on skeletal morphology can contribute to our understanding of the mechanisms which produce variation in the human phenotype. To start, we need to have a better understanding of the relationship between plastic and canalized traits or regions of the skeleton (Stock and Buck 2010). Studies of ontogenetic variation will be of central importance to understanding both the timing of susceptibility of the human phenotype to environmental variation, and also regions of the skeleton which are particularly canalized sharing development. Renewed emphasis should also be placed on the simple study of morphological integration, which provides a means of understanding the modularity of systems which influenced phenotype, regardless of their aetiology. Our growing understanding of genotype phenotype interactions coming from genetics and genome wide association studies may also contribute to our understanding of the mechanisms controlling skeletal morphology. For example, as we identify the function of many of the genes which correlate with stature, we may discover that individually these influence the morphology of particular regions of the skeleton which correlate with adult stature, rather than simply stature in isolation. Continued studies of bone biomechanics and the remodelling process, will help us to understand the role of mechanical plasticity in influencing skeletal morphology during development and in relation to adult activity. Finally, research on human variation in the Holocene can give is crucial insights into the relationship between cultural change in morphological change, whether it be ultimately related to plasticity during life or genetic adaptation.

## Acknowledgements

I would like to thank J.C.K. Wells for stimulating conversations on the relationship between genes, plasticity and the human phenotype. While the contents of this paper represent a review of recent perspectives, I would like to acknowledge generous research funding from NERC, and the AHRC, U.K. which has supported my research for the past 7 years.

## Literature Cited

Allen H,L,. Estrada K., Lettre G., Berndt S.I., Weedon, M.N., Rivadeneira, F., Willer, C.J., Jackson, A.U., Vedantam, S., Raychaudhuri, S., *et al*. 2010. Hundreds of variants clustered in genomic loci and biological pathways affect human height. *Nature*. 467: 832-838.

Betti, L., Balloux, F., Hanihara, T., and Manica, A. 2010. The relative role of drift and selection in shaping the human skull. *American Journal of Physical Anthropology* 141: 76-82.

Boas, F. 1911. *Changes in the bodily form of descendants of immigrants*. Government Printing Office: Washington.

Boas, F. 1940. *Race, language and culture*. New York: MacMillan

Bogin, B., Smith, P.K., Orden, A.B., Varela Silva, M.I., and Loucky, J. 2002. Rapid change in height and body proportions of Maya American children. *American Journal of Human Biology* 14: 753-761.

Demo, M., Jentsch, W., and Hoffman, L. 1995. Effect of long term exposure to different environmental temperatures on heat production of growing pigs. *Livestock Production Science*. 43(2): 149-152.

Dyson, F. 2007. The era of Darwinian evolution is over. *New Perspect Q* 24: 58–59

Eleazer, C.D. and Cowgill, L.W. 2010. Variation in human body proportions during ontogeny. *American Journal of Physical Anthropology Supplement.* 141(s50): 82.

Gravlee, C.C., Bernard, H.R., and Leonard, W.R. 2003. Heredity, environment, and cranial form: a re-analysis of Boas's immigrant data. *American Anthropologist* 105 (1): 125-38.

Gudbjartsson D.F., Walters, G.B., Thorleifsson, G., Stefansson, H., Halldorsson, B.V., Zusmanovich, P., Sulem, P., Thorlacius, S., Gylfason, A., Steinberg, S., *et al.* 2008. Many sequence variants affecting diversity of adult human height. *Nature Genetics* 40(5): 609-15

Hanihara T. 1992. Dental and cranial affinities among populations of East-Asia and the Pacific – the basic populations in East-Asia. *American Journal of Physical Anthropology* 88(2): 163-182.

Holliday, T.W. 1997. Body proportions in late Pleistocene Europe and modern human origins. *Journal of Human Evolution* 32: 423-447.

Howells, W.W. 1978. *Cranial variation in man: a study by multivariate analysis of patterns of difference among recent human populations.* Harvard University Press: Cambridge.

Jepsen, K.J. 2009. Systems analysis of bone. *WIREs Systems Biology and Medicine* 1(1): 73-88.

Jones, H.H., Preist, J.D., Hayes, W.C., Tichenor, C.C., and Nagel, D.A. 1977. Humeral hypertrophy in response to exercise. *Journal of Bone and Joint Surgery* 59-A: 204-208.

Kaessmann, H., Wiebe, V., Weiss, G. and Pääbo, S. 2001. Great ape DNA sequences reveal a reduced diversity and an expansion in humans. *Nature Genetics* 27: 155-156.

Katzmarzyk, P.T., and Leonard, W.R. 1998. Climatic influences on human body size and proportions: ecological adaptations and secular trends. *American Journal Physical Anthropology* 106: 483-503.

Klein, R.G. 2009. *The human career: human biological and cultural origins.* University of Chicago Press: Chicago.

Klingenberg, C.P. 2008. Morphological integration and developmental modularity. *Annual Review of Ecology, Evolution, and Systematics* 39: 115–32.

Lahr, M.M. 1996. *The evolution of modern human cranial diversity: a study in cranial variation.* Cambridge University Press: Cambridge.

Lahr, M.M. and Wright, R.S.V. 1996. The question of robusticity and the relationship between cranial size and shape in Homo sapiens. *Journal of Human Evolution* 31: 157-191.

Laland, K.N., Odling-Smee, J. and Myles, S. 2010. How culture shaped the human genome: bringing genetics and the human sciences together. *Nature Reviews Genetics* 11 (2): 137-148.

Lanktree, M.B., Guo, Y., Murtaza, M., Glessner, J.T., Bailey, S.D., Onland-Moret, N.C., Lettre, G., Ongen, H., Rajagopalan, R., Johnson, T. *et al.* 2011. Meta-analysis of dense genecentric association studies reveals common and uncommon variants associated with height. *The American Journal of Human Genetics* 88(1): 6-18

Lettre, G., Jackson, A.U., Gieger, C., Schumacher, F.R., Berndt, S.I., Sanna, S., Eyheramendy, S., Voight, B.F., Butler, J.L., Guiducci, C., et al. 2008. Identification of ten loci associated with height highlights new biological pathways in human growth. *Nature Genetics* 40(5): 584-91.

Lieberman, D.E. 1996. How and why humans grow thin skulls: experimental evidence for systemic cortical robusticity. *American Journal of Physical Anthropology* 101: 217-236.

Patterson, J.D. 1996. Coming to America: acclimation in macaque body structures and Bergmann's rule. *International Journal of Primatology* 17(4): 585-611.

Pearson, O.M. and Lieberman, D.E. 2004. The aging of Wolff's "law": ontogeny and responses to mechanical loading cortical bone. *American Journal of Physical Anthropology* 47: 63-99.

Pietrusewsky, M. 1990. Craniofacial variation in Australasian and Pacific populations. *American Journal of Physical Anthropology* 82: 319-340.

Rasmussen, M., Li, Y., Lindgreen, S., Pedersen, J.S., Albrechtsen, A., Moltke, I., Metspalu, M., Metspalu, E., Kivisild, T., Gupta, R., et. al. 2010. Ancient human genome sequence of an extinct Palaeo-Eskimo. *Nature* 463: 757-762.

Richerson, P.J. and Boyd, R. 2005. *Not by genes alone: how culture transformed human evolution*. University of Chicago Press: Chicago.

Richerson, P. J., Boyd, R. and Henrich, J. 2010. Gene-culture coevolution in the age of genomics. *Proceedings of the National Academy of Sciences* 107: 8985–8992.

Roberts, D.F. 1953. Body weight, race and climate. *American Journal of Physical Anthropology* 11: 533–558.

Roberts, D.F. 1978. *Climate and human variability*. Cummings: Menlo Park.

Roseman, C.C. 2004. Detecting interregionally diversifying natural selection on modern human cranial form by using matched molecular and morphometric data. *Proceedings of the National Academy of Sciences* 101(35): 12824–12829.

Ruff, C.B. 2002 Variation in human body size and shape. *Annual Review of Anthropology*. 31: 211-232.

Ruff, C.B., Holt, B. and Trinkaus, E. 2006. "Wolff's Law" and bone functional adaptation. *American Journal of Physical Anthropology* 129: 484-498.

Sabeti, P.C., Schaffner, S.F., Fry, B., Lohmueller, J., Varilly, P., Shamovsky, O., Palma, A., Mikkelsen, T.S., Altshuler, D. and Lander, E.S. 2006. Positive natural selection in the human lineage. *Science* 312(5780): 1614-1620.

Sabeti, P.C., Varilly, P., Fry, B., Lohmueller, J., Hostetter, E., Cotsapas, C., Xie, X., Byrne, E.H., McCarroll, S.A., Gaudet, R., *et al*. 2007. Genome-wide detection and characterization of positive selection in human populations. *Nature* 449: 913–918.

Searle, A.G. 1968. *Comparative genetics of coat colour in mammals*. Academic Press, Inc.: New York.

Shaw, C.N. and Stock, J.T. 2009a. Intensity, repetitiveness, and directionality of habitual adolescent mobility patterns influence the tibial diaphysis morphology in athletes. *American Journal of Physical Anthropology* 140: 149-159.

Shaw, C.N. and Stock, J.T. 2009b. Habitual throwing and swimming correspond with upper limb diaphyseal strength and shape in modern human athletes. *American Journal of Physical Anthropology* 140: 160-172.

Sparks, C.S. and Jantz, R.L. 2002. A Reassessment of human cranial plasticity: Boas revisited. *Proceedings of the National Academy of Sciences* 99 (23): 14636-14639.

Stock, J.T. 2006. Hunter-gatherer postcranial robusticity relative to patterns of mobility, climatic adaptation, and selection for tissue economy. *American Journal of Physical Anthropology* 131(2): 194-204.

Stock, J.T. 2008. Are humans still evolving? In: Moore, A. (ed.) *The future of our species. EMBO Reports. Science and Society Special Issue*. 9: S51-S54.

Stock, J.T., Mirazón-Lahr, M. and Kulatilake, S. 2007. Cranial diversity in South Asia relative to human dispersals and global patterns of human variation. In: Petraglia, M.D. and Allchin, B. (eds.) *The evolution and history of human populations in South Asia: interdiscipinary studies in archaeology, biological anthropology, linguistics and genetics*. Springer/Kluwer: Dordrecht. 245-268.

Stock, J.T. and Buck, L. 2010. Canalization and plasticity in humans and primates: implications for interpreting the fossil record. In: Perote Alejandre, A., and Mateos Cachorro, A. (eds.) *150 años después de Darwin: evolución, future o crisis? Lecciones sobre evolución humana*. Instituto Tomás Pascual Sanz / Centro Nacional de Investigación sobre la Evolución Humana: Madrid. 91-101.

Serrat, M.A., King, D., Lovejoy, C.O. 2008. Temperature regulates limb length in homeotherms by directly modulating cartilage growth. *Proceedings of the National Academy of Sciences* 105(49): 19348-19353.

Trinkaus, E. 1981. Neanderthal limb proportions and cold adaptation. In: Stringer, C.B. (ed.) *Aspects of human evolution*. Taylor and Francis: London. 187-224.

Trinkaus, E. 1997. Appendicular robusticity and the paleobiology of modern human emergence. *Proceedings of the National Academy of Sciences* 94(24): 13367-13373.

Voight, B.F., Kudaravalli, S., Wen, X. and Pritchard, J.K. 2006. A map of recent positive selection in the human genome. *PLoS Biology* 4(3): e72. doi:10.1371/journal.pbio.0040072

Weaver, M.E. and Ingram, D.L. 1969. Morphological changes in swine associated with environmental temperature. *Ecology* 50: 710-713.

Weedon, M.N., Lango, H., Lindgren, C.M., Wallace, C., Evans, D.M., Mangino, M., Freathy, R.M., Perry, J.R., Stevens, S., Hall, A.S., et al. 2008. Genome-wide association analysis identifies 20 loci that influence adult height. *Nature Genetics* 40(5): 575-83.

Wells, J,C.K. and Stock, J.T. 2007. The biology of the colonizing ape. *Yearbook of Physical Anthropology* 50:191-222.

Wells, J.C.K. and Stock, J.T. 2011. Re-examining heritability: genetics, life history and plasticity. *Trends in Endrocrinology and Metabolism* 22(10): 421-428.

Yang, J., Benyamin, B., McEvoy, B.P., Gordon, S., Henders, A.K., Nyholt, D.R Nyholt, D.R., Madden, P.A., Heath, A.C., Martin, N.G., Montgomery, G.W., Goddard, M.E., and Visscher, P.M. 2010. Common SNPs explain a large proportion of the heritability for human height. *Nature Genetics* 42(7): 565-569.

Yom-Tov, Y. 1993. Does the rock hyrax, Procavia capensis, conform with Bergmann's rule? *Zoological Journal of the Linnean Society* 108: 171-177.

# Sexual Dimorphism in Adult Skeletal Remains at Ban Non Wat, Thailand, during the Intensification of Agriculture in Early Prehistoric Southeast Asia

Angela Clark,* Nancy Tayles and Siân Halcrow

Department of Anatomy
School of Medical Sciences
University of Otago
Dunedin
New Zealand

*Email for correspondence: angela.clark@anatomy.otago.ac.nz

**Abstract**
Sexual dimorphism, the size and shape differences between males and females, is a useful measure of human biocultural adaptation. A decrease in population sexual dimorphism is generally associated with a shift to intensified subsistence practices. The extent to which the intensification of rice-based agriculture influenced the level of sexual dimorphism in Southeast Asia has received little attention.

The large sample (N = 637) from Ban Non Wat, Thailand spans the period of the intensification of rice agriculture. This study aimed to use osteometric evidence to quantify the level of sexual dimorphism in this prehistoric community. This paper presents initial results from the earliest phases, the Neolithic and Early Bronze Age. Sixteen bilateral long bone dimensions were collected and stature estimated for male (n = 18) and female (n = 23) adult individuals. Sexual dimorphism was calculated and statistically compared across time periods. Results indicated a general increase in long bone dimensions and stature from the Neolithic to Early Bronze Age. A reduction in sexual dimorphism was a result of an increase in female body size. Contrary to previous research, these results did not support the hypothesis that males are more sensitive to environmental changes than females. These results are possibly an indication of a difference in nutritional status between males and females, improvement in female socio-cultural status, and/or female migration. Further stages of this research will incorporate a larger sample size and independent indicators of health status, to better understand the human biological adaptations of a rice-based agricultural community.

**Keywords**: Sex, Agriculture, Health Status, Thailand, Bronze Age, Neolithic

## Introduction

Previous studies have suggested that the intensification of agriculture had a dramatic effect on the skeletal biology of past populations, mainly resulting from changes in diet (Goodman *et al.* 1984; Larsen 1995; 2002). The onset of agriculture and consequential effects on health and social organisation are of significant interest in human history. Human skeletal remains are an excellent resource for understanding how past populations adapted to changing environmental and cultural situations (Schutkowski 2008). Humans modify their surrounding natural and cultural environments resulting in a variety of human biological responses (Schutkowski 2006). Growth and development are significantly influenced by environmental factors, including socioeconomic status, nutrition, health, sexual division of labour, and parental investment (Malina 1979; Bogin 1999; Loesch *et al.* 2000; Stinson 2000; Giannecchini and Moggi-Cecchi 2008). As a result, final adult body size and shape differs within and between populations, both past and present. The level of sexual dimorphism is a measure of the morphological differences between females and males in a population. When examined over time it can be a good overall indicator of the biocultural aspects of a population (Tobias 1975; Brock and Ruff 1988; Gaulin and Boster 1992; Holden and Mace 1999; Schweich 2005).

Males are on average larger than females in a population. Females generally have greater amounts of oestrogenic hormones that accelerate epiphyseal closure compared with the anabolic steroid testosterone, mainly found in males, which sustains continued growth (Tanner 1978; Stini 1985; Mays 1998). Male long bone growth therefore continues for a longer period of time resulting in greater stature and general body size compared with females (Stini 1985). Stature sexual dimorphism is often used in ethnographic and archaeological literature to reflect adaptation to the environment during growth and development (Stini 1969; Eveleth 1975; Valenzuela *et al.* 1978; Cole 2007; Giannecchini and Moggi-Cecchi 2008). Previous research suggests that low levels of sexual dimorphism indicate adverse conditions for growth and development and consequently low health status (Jantz and Jantz 1999; Schweich and Knüsel 2004). Such factors are associated with agricultural development and the resulting social, cultural and economic changes (Cohen and Armelagos 1984; Steckel *et al.* 2002; Cohen 2007; Lukacs 2008; Barker 2009). These past studies have based their interpretations on the female genetic buffering hypothesis, assuming that males are more sensitive to changes in environmental conditions than females (Stini 1975). Therefore, when environmental conditions become less favourable, males will not reach their genetic potential for growth and as a result have a smaller body size, thus reducing the degree of sexual dimorphism in the population.

It is generally accepted that a decline in health occurred in Western populations with sedentism and the intensification of agriculture (Steckel *et al.* 2002; Lukacs 2008; Barker 2009). It is suggested that a reduction in dietary quality had a significant effect on the health of prehistoric populations (Larsen 2002). However, current research in Southeast Asia suggests that this trend is not universal (Nelsen 1999; Tayles *et al.* 2000; Domett 2001; Pietrusewsky and Douglas 2002). It is suggested that prehistoric Southeast Asian populations enjoyed a relatively varied diet during and after the adoption of rice agriculture (Tayles and Oxenham 2006). Consequently, there is as of yet no evidence for the diachronic decline in health as experienced in Western populations. The large sample (N = 637) from the prehistoric community of Ban Non Wat, Thailand, provides an opportunity to test this assertion on a single population. A biocultural approach (Goodman *et al.* 1988; Larsen 2002; Schutkowski 2008) will be used to fully investigate how the prehistoric people adapted to agricultural intensification and socio-economic change over a period greater than two thousand years from 3750 to 1500 BP (Higham and Higham 2009). The Ban Non Wat population is ideal for a diachronic study as not only is a large number of adult individuals available from a single site, but isotopic evidence also suggests minimal immigration (Cox 2009). This paper presents the findings from an initial study conducted on a sample of 41 individuals, reflecting approximately 20 per cent of the final adult sample with sex estimates (n = 190). It therefore is borne in mind that any non-significant differences demonstrated might be a result of the small sample size. Here, we test the hypothesis that contrary to the general model of sexual dimorphism change with agricultural development in other regions of the world, the degree of sexual dimorphism increases as rice agriculture develops and intensifies. This would result from a more nutrious diet and more beneifical environmental factors associated with the intensification of rice agriculture where males can grow and develop to their genetic potential.

Epiphyseal dimensions show higher levels of sexual dimorphism than stature estimates or long bone lengths (Hamilton 1982; Clark 2007; Charisi *et al.* 2010), although an assessment of sexual dimorphism and diachronic changes of these measurements have seldom been undertaken (cf. Hamilton 1982; Clark 2007). The dimensions at the articular surfaces on the long bones examined in this paper do not reflect robusticity and are therefore less affected than long bone length dimensions by factors of adult life, such as occupation, and provide a more sensitive indicator of biocultural factors during growth and development. The main focus of this novel research is to investigate the level of sexual dimorphism in stature and skeletal dimensions during the intensification of rice agriculture in a single prehistoric Southeast Asian population over a long chrononology in the same geographical area. In addition to the primary aim of determining whether changes in the level of sexual dimorphism in the Ban Non Wat sample reflects current theories and hypotheses based on deteriorating nutrition in Western populations, this paper assesses whether or not sexual dimorphism in stature shows consistent patterns with changes in other osteometric dimensions of the long bones. The research presented in this paper is part of a larger project that is the first to undertake an in-depth analysis of sexual dimorphism in a prehistoric Southeast Asian population; consequently, there is a heavy reliance on literature based on Western populations. To date there is no published research in English, which discusses the levels of sexual dimorphism in Southeast Asian human remains.

## Materials

Ban Non Wat is a village located in the Mun River valley, Nakhon Ratchasima Province in Northeast Thailand (Fig. 1). Radiocarbon dates have placed the earliest occupation of the site at around 3750 BP with continued occupation throughout the Bronze and Iron Ages, until 1500 BP (Higham and Higham 2009). The site is located on a mound, which is elevated several metres above the surrounding rice fields and the area is still being used today as a farming village. Excavations first began in December 2001 and continued as part of the 'Origins of Angkor' project until December 2007, uncovering a total area of 906m$^2$ and 637 human burials (Higham and Kijngam 2009). This is the largest skeletal sample to date from prehistoric mainland Southeast Asia and is one of the few sites in the region that spans from the Neolithic to the end of prehistory. Archaeological evidence from the site suggests a change in social structure and increased agricultural dependence between the Neolithic and early Iron Age (Higham and Kijngam 2009). The number of burials and temporal depth provide opportunities for research and interpretations of prehistoric life in the Mun River Valley and Northeast Thailand.

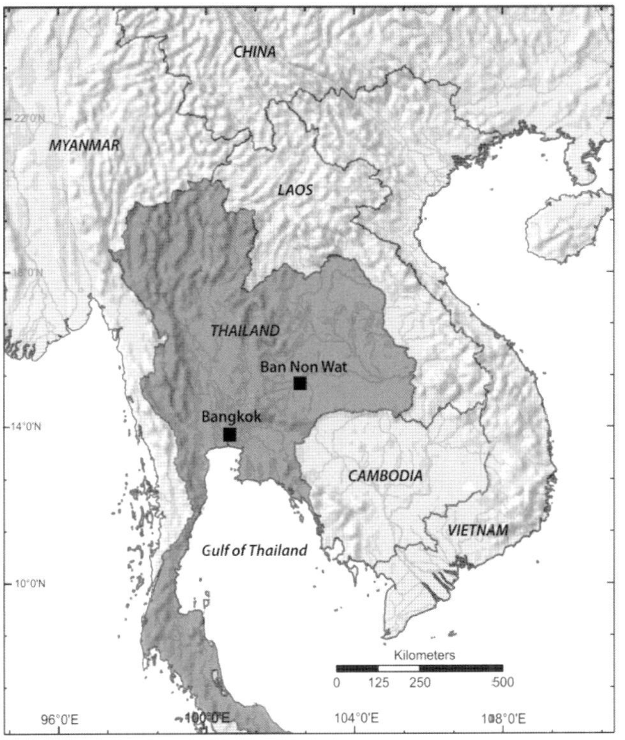


**Figure 1:** Map of the terrain and river network in mainland Southeast Asia, the site of Ban Non Wat highlighted and current political boundaries demarcated. Modified from original images courtesy of Kate Domett.

This paper presents data on a total sample of 41 individuals (18 males and 23 females) from the Neolithic (n = 23) and Early Bronze Age (n = 18). Neolithic occupation at the site lasted around 700 years, from 3750 BP to 3050 BP (Higham and Higham 2009). In total, 54 adult individuals were excavated during the Neolithic. However due to the preservation of the remains only 14 females and 9 males could be included in this investigation. The Bronze Age at Ban Non Wat is divided into five different phases based on mortuary evidence (Higham and Kijngam 2009). This paper investigates the early Bronze Age occupation, from around 3050 BP to 2300 BP (Higham and Higham 2009). In total, 19 adult individuals were excavated in this phase, including 9 females and 9 males and one individual whose remains were too fragmentary for an accurate sex assessment.

## Methods

To evaluate the level of sexual dimorphism, the sex of the individuals represented in this study must be established. Sex assessment was based on the morphology of the bony pelvis using standard guidelines (Phenice 1969; Buikstra and Ubelaker 1994). Wherever practical, high reliance was placed on features of the *os pubis* for the final sex assessment. However, this bone is often damaged in archaeological situations due to its position in the ground and fragile nature (Walker 2005). Therefore, other features of the bony pelvis based on well-known and documented methodologies (Buikstra and Ubelaker 1994) were also taken into consideration.

Sixteen long bone dimensions were recorded. Long bone lengths were measured according to Buikstra and Ubelaker (1994) with a standard osteometric board and rounded to the nearest half millimetre. Mitutoyo® digital sliding calipers (0.010 mm precision) were used to measure all the other dimensions at the epiphyses. To minimise measurement error, measurements were repeated three times on both the left and right sides and the mean for each side was used in the analysis. The following measurements were taken using standard methods (Olivier 1969; Buikstra and Ubelaker 1994):

1) Humeral epicondylar breadth (HEB): the distance between the most laterally projecting points on the lateral and medial epicondyles of the distal epiphyses
2) Vertical humeral head diameter (HHD): the direct distance between the most superior and inferior points on the border of the proximal articular surface
3) Antero-posterior proximal ulna breadth (APUB): the maximum distance between the

most anterior and posterior points of the diaphysis directly below the radial notch

4) Transverse proximal ulna breadth (TPUB): the maximum distance between the most laterally projecting points of the diaphysis directly below the radial notch
5) Coronoid process breadth (CPB): the maximum distance between the proximal posterior shaft and the most anterior aspect of the articular rim of the coronoid process
6) Antero-posterior radial head diameter (APHD): the maximum distance between the most anterior and posterior points of the radial head
7) Medio-lateral radial head diameter (MLHD): the maximum distance between the most medial and lateral points of the radial head
8) Distal radial epicondylar breadth (DRB): the maximum distance between the most laterally projecting points on the distal epicondyle
9) Maximum femoral head diameter (FHD): the maximum diameter of the direct distance between two points on the border of the proximal articular surface
10) Supero-inferior femoral neck diameter (SID): the minimum distance between the most superior and inferior points of the femoral neck
11) Femoral epicondylar breadth (FEB): the distance between the most laterally projecting points on the lateral and medial epicondyles of the distal epiphyses
12) Proximal tibial breadth (PTB): the maximum distance between the most laterally projecting points on the medial and lateral condyles of the proximal epiphysis
13) Distal tibial epicondylar breadth (DTB): the maximum distance between the two most laterally projecting points on the medial malleolus and the lateral surface of the distal epiphyses inside the fibular notch
14) Maximum femoral length (MFL): the distance from the most superior part of the femoral head to the most inferior point on the distal condyles
15) Maximum tibia length (MTL): the distance from the superior articular surface of the lateral condyle of the tibia to the tip of the medial malleolus
16) Maximum fibula length (MFiL): the maximum distance between the most superior point of the head of the fibula to the most inferior point on the lateral malleolus

All statistical analyses were performed using STATA 11.0, with the statistical significance defined at 5% ($p \leq .050$). Stature was estimated using lower limb bone sex-specific equations established by Sangvichien (1985) that were based on individuals of Thai and Chinese ancestry. The sexual dimorphism index (Tobias 1975) is a simple and practical way to quantify the difference in size between males and females within a population (Equation 1). The index clearly shows a quantitative expression of size sexual dimorphism as the relationship between the mean values of the males and females within a population. Although the validity of such a ratio equation has been questioned (see Smith 1999), this simple equation is essential for an accurate representation of the relationship between the mean values of the two sexes (Smith 1999). This equation can be written as:

$$\frac{\bar{X}_m - \bar{X}_f}{\bar{X}_m} \times 100$$

**Equation 1:** The degree of sexual dimorphism is used to establish the percentage difference between the mean male measurements and the mean female measurements, equation after Tobias (1975).

Student's t-tests were conducted to evaluate the univariate differences in the degree of sexual dimorphism between the Neolithic period and Early Bronze Age following Greene (1989). The Student's t-tests for equal variances were accompanied by Bonferroni correction for the multiple pairwise comparisons of means in order to evaluate whether statistically significant results may have occurred by chance.

## Results

The data is normally distributed for both periods (Kolmogorov-Smirnov test, $p > .050$) and very few statistically significant differences were apparent between the left and right sides (Table 1). In all four cases of significant asymmetry, the left side was smaller than the right. As only four out of 59 paired measurements demonstrated significant asymmetry, with none of these being highly statistically significant ($p = .025$ to $.050$), data for the two sides has been pooled and the consequent mean used for further analysis. Descriptive statistics for each measurement is shown in table 2, including the mean value, standard deviation, the range, the number of individuals analysed and the degree of sexual dimorphism. As expected, males have higher values than females in all dimensions investigated and these differences are statistically significant (Student's t-test, $p \leq .050$), therefore validating an investigation of sexual dimorphism in this sample.

**Table 1:** Paired sample Student's t-tests for Ban Non Wat individuals for the Neolithic and Early Bronze Age periods, including the number of individuals (n), mean difference between the left and right measurements (Mean Diff), standard deviation (SD), and p value. Statistically significant differences highlighted in bold font.

| Variable[a] | Neolithic | | | | | | | | Early Bronze Age | | | | | | | |
|---|---|---|---|---|---|---|---|---|---|---|---|---|---|---|---|---|
| | Males | | | | Females | | | | Males | | | | Females | | | |
| | n | Mean Diff (mm) | SD | p | n | Mean Diff (mm) | SD | p | n | Mean Diff (mm) | SD | p | n | Mean Diff (mm) | SD | p |
| HEB | 1 | -1.75 | . | . | 7 | -0.02 | 1.76 | 0.977 | 7 | -0.77 | 0.95 | 0.076 | 2 | -0.26 | 0.13 | 0.222 |
| HHD | 4 | 0.63 | 1.02 | 0.302 | 6 | -0.73 | 0.66 | **<0.050** | 5 | 0.25 | 1.13 | 0.651 | 2 | 0.46 | 1.12 | 0.666 |
| APUB | 5 | 0.49 | 0.98 | 0.327 | 8 | 0.31 | 1.39 | 0.544 | 7 | -0.54 | 1.64 | 0.420 | 4 | -0.48 | 1.19 | 0.477 |
| TPUB | 5 | -0.67 | 1.09 | 0.243 | 7 | 0.50 | 0.86 | 0.176 | 7 | -0.20 | 1.49 | 0.731 | 4 | -0.93 | 0.88 | 0.124 |
| CPB | 4 | -1.41 | 1.26 | 0.110 | 7 | -1.07 | 1.29 | 0.071 | 6 | -0.40 | 1.67 | 0.578 | 3 | -0.10 | 0.41 | 0.711 |
| APHD | 3 | 0.34 | 1.14 | 0.657 | 6 | 0.68 | 1.75 | 0.387 | 5 | 0.19 | 0.90 | 0.670 | 3 | -0.74 | 1.03 | 0.339 |
| MLHD | 2 | 0.15 | 0.15 | 0.409 | 6 | 1.88 | 3.84 | 0.285 | 6 | -0.08 | 0.57 | 0.736 | 3 | -0.49 | 0.99 | 0.483 |
| DRB | 3 | -0.27 | 1.79 | 0.817 | 4 | -0.15 | 1.24 | 0.828 | 4 | -0.93 | 1.19 | 0.217 | 2 | -2.55 | 2.93 | 0.434 |
| FHD | 5 | -0.56 | 0.37 | **<0.050** | 7 | 0.11 | 0.84 | 0.743 | 7 | -0.59 | 0.53 | **<0.050** | 4 | -0.67 | 0.50 | 0.076 |
| SID | 4 | 0.13 | 1.20 | 0.840 | 7 | 0.25 | 0.88 | 0.487 | 7 | -0.12 | 1.41 | 0.836 | 5 | -0.04 | 0.68 | 0.890 |
| FEB | 2 | -0.74 | 0.47 | 0.270 | 5 | 0.24 | 0.88 | 0.572 | 3 | -0.74 | 1.56 | 0.497 | 1 | -2.02 | . | . |
| PTB | 4 | 1.03 | 3.76 | 0.621 | 4 | -0.06 | 1.94 | 0.956 | 2 | -0.81 | 1.66 | 0.616 | 2 | 1.38 | 2.20 | 0.539 |
| DTB | 5 | 1.52 | 2.18 | 0.195 | 6 | -2.01 | 1.92 | **0.050** | 4 | -0.20 | 0.96 | 0.704 | 4 | 2.99 | 2.57 | 0.103 |
| MFL | 3 | 0.00 | 0.00 | . | 4 | 0.00 | 0.00 | . | 4 | 0.00 | 0.00 | . | 3 | 0.00 | 0.00 | . |
| MTL | 5 | 0.00 | 0.00 | . | 4 | 0.00 | 0.00 | . | 1 | 0.00 | . | . | 2 | 0.00 | 0.00 | . |
| MFiL | 3 | 3.33 | 2.67 | 0.163 | 1 | -4.50 | . | . | 2 | -0.75 | 1.77 | 0.656 | 1 | 5.00 | . | . |

[a] HEB, humeral epicondylar breadth; HHD, vertical humeral head diameter; APUB, antero-posterior proximal ulna breadth; TPUB, transverse proximal ulna breadth; CPB, coronoid process breadth; APHD, antero-posterior radial head diameter; MLHD, medio-lateral radial head diameter; DRB, distal radial epicondylar breadth; FHD, maximum femoral head diameter; SID, supero-inferior femoral neck diameter; FEB, femoral epicondylar breadth; PTB, proximal tibial breadth; DTB, distal tibial epicondylar breadth; MFL, maximum femoral length; MTL, maximum tibia length; MFiL, maximum fibula length.

**Table 2**: Descriptive statistics for the Ban Non Wat individuals for the Neolithic and Early Bronze Age periods, including the mean, standard deviation (SD), number of individuals (n), range of values and summary information for sexual dimorphism; percentage dimorphism (D%), Student's t-test value (t), degrees of freedom (df) and p value. Statistically significant differences highlighted in bold font.

| Period | Variable[a] | Males | | | | | Females | | | | | Sexual Dimorphism | | | |
|---|---|---|---|---|---|---|---|---|---|---|---|---|---|---|---|
| | | n | Mean (mm) | SD | Min (mm) | Max (mm) | n | Mean (mm) | SD | Min (mm) | Max (mm) | D% | t | df | p |
| Neolithic | HEB | 6 | 65.09 | 2.61 | 60.52 | 67.72 | 10 | 55.46 | 1.48 | 52.58 | 57.76 | 17.36 | 9.50 | 14 | **≤0.001** |
| Bronze Age | | 7 | 65.23 | 1.91 | 63.31 | 68.00 | 9 | 57.64 | 1.77 | 54.24 | 60.33 | 13.17 | 8.24 | 14 | **0.001** |
| Neolithic | HHD | 6 | 45.93 | 1.68 | 44.32 | 48.39 | 8 | 39.08 | 1.62 | 35.83 | 41.07 | 17.53 | 7.72 | 12 | **0.001** |
| Bronze Age | | 5 | 46.21 | 1.59 | 44.38 | 48.76 | 7 | 39.88 | 0.85 | 38.49 | 40.90 | 15.88 | 8.97 | 10 | **0.001** |
| Neolithic | APUB | 7 | 26.32 | 3.10 | 22.32 | 31.36 | 11 | 22.01 | 1.61 | 18.97 | 24.86 | 19.59 | 3.90 | 16 | **<0.001** |
| Bronze Age | | 8 | 24.88 | 1.90 | 20.78 | 27.49 | 8 | 22.96 | 1.73 | 20.94 | 25.88 | 8.36 | 2.12 | 14 | **<0.050** |
| Neolithic | TPUB | 7 | 20.95 | 1.78 | 19.15 | 24.30 | 12 | 17.71 | 2.29 | 13.33 | 21.14 | 18.30 | 3.21 | 17 | **<0.010** |
| Bronze Age | | 8 | 21.09 | 1.95 | 19.15 | 24.29 | 8 | 18.79 | 1.68 | 16.55 | 21.41 | 12.24 | 2.52 | 14 | **<0.050** |
| Neolithic | CPB | 6 | 35.74 | 1.47 | 33.69 | 38.26 | 11 | 31.46 | 1.39 | 29.72 | 34.60 | 13.61 | 5.95 | 15 | **0.001** |
| Bronze Age | | 7 | 36.49 | 1.34 | 35.12 | 38.49 | 7 | 32.78 | 1.78 | 30.31 | 35.58 | 11.34 | 4.41 | 12 | **0.001** |
| Neolithic | APHD | 8 | 23.47 | 1.38 | 21.89 | 26.02 | 11 | 19.87 | 1.36 | 17.21 | 21.51 | 18.12 | 5.67 | 17 | **0.001** |
| Bronze Age | | 6 | 21.96 | 0.74 | 20.94 | 22.91 | 9 | 19.60 | 0.93 | 18.54 | 20.83 | 12.04 | 5.18 | 13 | **0.001** |
| Neolithic | MLHD | 7 | 23.31 | 0.98 | 22.19 | 24.75 | 12 | 20.39 | 1.66 | 17.60 | 24.06 | 14.36 | 4.23 | 17 | **≤0.001** |
| Bronze Age | | 8 | 22.37 | 0.69 | 21.28 | 23.24 | 9 | 20.16 | 0.92 | 18.68 | 21.15 | 10.96 | 5.55 | 15 | **0.001** |
| Neolithic | DRB | 7 | 33.28 | 1.35 | 32.01 | 36.09 | 9 | 29.19 | 1.51 | 26.38 | 30.72 | 14.02 | 5.64 | 14 | **0.001** |
| Bronze Age | | 8 | 34.11 | 2.44 | 31.45 | 39.48 | 6 | 29.74 | 1.04 | 28.28 | 31.19 | 14.68 | 4.08 | 12 | **0.001** |
| Neolithic | FHD | 7 | 47.13 | 2.22 | 43.27 | 49.79 | 10 | 40.55 | 1.37 | 38.01 | 43.02 | 16.23 | 7.60 | 15 | **0.001** |
| Bronze Age | | 8 | 47.88 | 2.33 | 44.20 | 50.18 | 8 | 42.07 | 0.83 | 41.11 | 43.44 | 13.80 | 6.64 | 14 | **0.001** |
| Neolithic | SID | 8 | 31.94 | 1.72 | 28.91 | 34.48 | 8 | 27.51 | 1.21 | 25.33 | 29.17 | 16.10 | 5.96 | 14 | **≤0.001** |
| Bronze Age | | 7 | 33.01 | 3.01 | 29.34 | 37.55 | 7 | 28.88 | 1.83 | 26.63 | 31.28 | 14.30 | 3.11 | 12 | **<0.010** |
| Neolithic | FEB | 6 | 76.67 | 6.39 | 64.83 | 81.33 | 5 | 70.57 | 1.35 | 68.74 | 72.15 | 8.65 | 2.08 | 9 | **<0.010** |
| Bronze Age | | 5 | 80.83 | 2.35 | 78.57 | 84.46 | 5 | 73.57 | 3.11 | 70.22 | 78.22 | 9.86 | 4.17 | 8 | **<0.010** |
| Neolithic | PTB | 5 | 74.96 | 2.15 | 71.98 | 77.58 | 6 | 66.82 | 3.41 | 61.23 | 71.18 | 12.18 | 4.61 | 9 | **0.001** |
| Bronze Age | | 5 | 74.54 | 3.01 | 70.13 | 76.76 | 5 | 67.78 | 1.36 | 66.39 | 69.55 | 9.98 | 4.58 | 8 | **0.001** |
| Neolithic | DTB | 7 | 46.46 | 3.04 | 41.48 | 50.31 | 7 | 38.88 | 0.87 | 37.59 | 39.91 | 19.51 | 6.35 | 12 | **0.001** |
| Bronze Age | | 7 | 49.56 | 2.29 | 47.08 | 53.84 | 6 | 43.41 | 1.59 | 41.27 | 45.36 | 14.16 | 5.52 | 11 | **0.001** |
| Neolithic | Stature | 7 | 1652.93 | 4.82 | 1597.95 | 1728.37 | 5 | 1498.91 | 1.73 | 1471.75 | 1512.99 | 10.28 | 6.76 | 10 | **0.001** |
| Bronze Age | | 8 | 1688.23 | 4.77 | 1640.31 | 1783.51 | 5 | 1606.02 | 1.76 | 1589.55 | 1633.60 | 5.12 | 3.65 | 11 | **<0.010** |

[a] For measurement abbreviations, see Table 1.

Stature estimates could be calculated for twelve Neolithic and thirteen Early Bronze Age individuals. In the Neolithic period mean male stature is 165 cm, and this does not change significantly (p = 0.178) in the Early Bronze Age males, whose average stature is 169 cm (Table 3). Female stature changed significantly over time (p < .001), from an average of 150 cm in the Neolithic period to 161 cm in the Early Bronze Age (Table 3). The level of sexual dimorphism in stature is 10% in the Neolithic compared with 5% in the Early Bronze Age (Table 2). As a result of the increase in stature in Early Bronze Age females, the degree of stature sexual dimorphism declines significantly (p < .050) between the two time periods (Table 4). The degree of sexual dimorphism in stature estimates is almost always lower than the percentage values for the epiphyseal dimensions, especially when the level of stature sexual dimorphism is low in the Early Bronze Age (Table 2).

**Table 3:** The diachronic trends in each measurement from the Neolithic to the Early Bronze Age. Male and female values were assessed separately; the data shown includes the Student's t-test value (t), degrees of freedom (df) and p value (following Bonferroni correction). Significant differences highlighted in bold font.

| Variable[a] | Males | | | Females | | |
|---|---|---|---|---|---|---|
| | t | df | p | t | df | p |
| HEB | -0.11 | 11 | 0.911 | -2.92 | 17 | **<0.010** |
| HHD | -0.28 | 9 | 0.784 | -1.17 | 13 | 0.264 |
| APUB | 1.10 | 13 | 0.292 | -1.24 | 17 | 0.231 |
| TPUB | -0.14 | 13 | 0.893 | -1.14 | 18 | 0.271 |
| CPB | -0.97 | 11 | 0.353 | -1.76 | 16 | 0.098 |
| APHD | 2.42 | 12 | **<0.050** | 0.51 | 18 | 0.618 |
| MLHD | 2.19 | 13 | **<0.050** | 0.37 | 19 | 0.716 |
| DRB | -0.79 | 13 | 0.442 | -0.78 | 13 | 0.449 |
| FHD | -0.63 | 13 | 0.538 | -2.75 | 16 | **<0.010** |
| SID | -0.85 | 13 | 0.405 | -1.73 | 13 | 0.107 |
| FEB | -1.37 | 9 | 0.204 | -1.98 | 8 | 0.083 |
| PTB | 0.25 | 8 | 0.805 | -0.59 | 9 | 0.572 |
| DTB | -2.15 | 12 | **<0.050** | -6.54 | 11 | **0.001** |
| Stature | -1.42 | 13 | 0.178 | -9.69 | 8 | **0.001** |

[a] HEB, humeral epicondylar breadth; HHD, vertical humeral head diameter; APUB, antero-posterior proximal ulna breadth; TPUB, transverse proximal ulna breadth; CPB, coronoid process breadth; APHD, antero-posterior radial head diameter; MLHD, medio-lateral radial head diameter; DRB, distal radial epicondylar breadth; FHD, maximum femoral head diameter; SID, supero-inferior femoral neck diameter; FEB, femoral epicondylar breadth; PTB, proximal tibia breadth; DTB, distal tibial epicondylar breadth.

The mean female measurements of the upper limb do not change significantly between the two periods, with the exception of the HEB (p < .010), where the dimension increases in the Early Bronze Age (Table 3). For male upper limb measurements, the two dimensions of the radial head, the APHD (p < .050) and the MLHD (p < .050) decrease significantly (Table 3). The highest level of sexual dimorphism in the upper limb is seen in the APUB (20%) in the Neolithic period and HHD (16%) in the Early Bronze Age (Table 2). Although the degree of sexual dimorphism observed in all upper limb measurements, with the exception of the DRB, decrease from the Neolithic to the Early Bronze Age (Table 2); these changes are not statistically significant (Table 4).

The measurements of the lower limb also demonstrate few significant changes through time. For female measurements, FHD (p < .010) and DTB (p < .001) increase significantly from the Neolithic to Early Bronze Age (Table 3). The male DTB also increases significantly over time (p < .050), although no significant changes are seen in the other dimensions (Table 3). With the exception of the FEB, the degree of sexual dimorphism decreases through time in the lower limb (Table 2); however, these changes are not significant (Table 4).

**Table 4:** Greene (1989) Student's t-test ($t_g$) to evaluate the univariate differences in the degree of sexual dimorphism between the Neolithic period and Early Bronze Age, including degrees of freedom (df) and p value (following Bonferroni correction). Significant difference highlighted in bold font.

| Variable[a] | $t_g$ | df | p |
|---|---|---|---|
| HEB | 1.49 | 28 | 0.148 |
| HHD | 0.45 | 22 | 0.660 |
| APUB | 1.66 | 30 | 0.108 |
| TPUB | 0.68 | 31 | 0.499 |
| CPB | 0.51 | 27 | 0.611 |
| APHD | 1.50 | 30 | 0.144 |
| MLHD | 0.88 | 32 | 0.386 |
| DRB | -0.22 | 26 | 0.831 |
| FHD | 0.63 | 29 | 0.534 |
| SID | 0.20 | 26 | 0.840 |
| FEB | -0.33 | 17 | 0.746 |
| PTB | 0.59 | 17 | 0.561 |
| DTB | 0.88 | 23 | 0.390 |
| Stature | 2.24 | 21 | **<0.050** |

[a] HEB, humeral epicondylar breadth; HHD, vertical humeral head diameter; APUB, antero-posterior proximal ulna breadth; TPUB, transverse proximal ulna breadth; CPB, coronoid process breadth; APHD, antero-posterior radial head diameter; MLHD, medio-lateral radial head diameter; DRB, distal radial epicondylar breadth; FHD, maximum femoral head diameter; SID, supero-inferior femoral neck diameter; FEB, femoral epicondylar breadth; PTB, proximal tibial breadth; DTB, distal tibial epicondylar breadth.

## Discussion

This investigation has provided evidence that the level of sexual dimorphism in stature declined with the intensification of agriculture in the small Neolithic and Early Bronze Age samples from the site of Ban Non Wat. Based on current theories and hypotheses on the relationship between health status and sexual dimorphism developed from Western populations, this may be interpreted as deterioration in health, resulting in poor growth and development in the people in the Early Bronze Age compared with the Neolithic period. However, the results indicate that stature increases over time for both males and females, with the increase in female stature being statistically significant. An increase in stature is usually an indicator of an increasingly favourable environment (Steckel 1995; Bogin *et al.* 2002; Cole 2003). This increase is not unexpected as previous work conducted on Southeast Asian populations reveals that the standard of living and quality of life does not deteriorate as severely with the intensification of agriculture (Tayles *et al.* 2000; Domett 2001; Pietrusewsky and Douglas 2002; Oxenham *et al.* 2005; Tayles and Oxenham 2006). A reduction in the level of sexual dimorphism and increase in stature in the prehistoric people from Ban Non Wat appears to conflict with the general bioarchaeological model of health change with agricultural intensification based on research mainly in the Americans and Europe. Such studies posit that there was a general decline in health with the intensification of agriculture (Larsen 1995; Steckel *et al.* 2002; Larsen 2006), whereas in this prehistoric population, a decreasing level of sexual dimorphism and improved health status are associated with the intensification of agriculture.

As expected, the levels of sexual dimorphism in the long bone epiphyseal dimensions are generally much greater than those of stature estimates (see Hamilton 1982; Clark 2007; Charisi *et al.* 2010). However, there are no statistically significant changes in the level of sexual dimorphism in epiphyseal dimensions between the Neolithic and Early Bronze Age, suggesting that environmental pressures remained constant over time. Factors, such as parental investment, socio-economic status, adaptation to new foods, availability of food, quality of diet, different food preparation methods, and socio-political circumstances, may have had an effect on the level of sexual dimorphism within a population during agricultural development (Hall 1978; Stinson 1985). Alternatively the lack of statistically significant diachronic changes in the degree of sexual dimorphism in epiphyseal measurements could be explained by sampling error due to a small sample size.

In addition to diachronic changes in stature estimates, there are other statistically significant temporal changes for long bone epiphyseal dimensions. Although only three of thirteen epiphyseal measurements yielded statistically significant differences for both sexes, the female values were always more highly statistically significant than the males values. The two mean measurements for males of the radial head decrease significantly from the Neolithic to the early Bronze Age. In isolation, this trend supports the female genetic buffering hypothesis based on the reduced male size during the intensification of agriculture. However, there are greater statistically significant values in female dimensions, along with stature estimates between the Neolithic and Early Bronze Age, which do not support the female genetic buffering hypothesis. Although previous studies have found support for the hypothesis (e.g. Greulich 1951; Stini 1969; 1975; Bielicki and Charzewski 1977) there are also many studies that have not found support or provide contradictory conclusions (e.g. Brundtland *et al.* 1980; Silventoinen *et al.* 2001).

The statistically significant difference in stature estimates may be a result of differing environmental factors between the two periods that are specific to females. These increases in body size and shape may be an indicator of change in treatment of females, perhaps allowing more equal access to nutritional resources for males and females, and/or improvement in female socio-cultural status. This result may also be a consequence of female immigration, although there was little immigration to the prehistoric population of Ban Non Wat, preliminary isotopic analysis on a small sample has indicated that a group of females migrated to Ban Non Wat from other regions in Southeast Asia in the Early Bronze Age (Cox 2009). This group of females may have had better conditions for growth in their childhood environment and were therefore taller than the Neolithic inhabitants, or perhaps they were from a gene pool that had greater genetic potential for stature/body size. Due to the complex interacting factors influencing growth and development within the population and small sample size in this investigation, it is difficult to isolate any one possible causative factor at this stage.

It is generally agreed that during the early phases of occupation in prehistoric Southeast Asia there was a retention of a hunting-gathering-cultivating economy, whereby people were not only harvesting natural resources, such as fish and small animals, they were also breeding domestic animals (Pietrusewsky and Douglas 2002). Evidence of hunting has been found during this period of a wide range of animals, including water buffalo, wild deer, rhinoceros, tigers, hares and rats (Thosarat in press). Evidence of domesticated cattle, pigs, dogs and possibly chickens has also been unearthed from the Neolithic period at Ban Non Wat (Kijngam in press; Thosarat in press). The prehistoric wetland landscape situated on the edge of woodlands and forests clearly made the area of Ban Non Wat an attractive food, water and salt source for both humans and animals alike.

This bioarchaeological investigation suggests that with the introduction of bronze, the quality, quantity, and variety of subsistence base has become more favourable and therefore increases in body size are observed with the intensification of rice agriculture at the site of Ban Non Wat. Pietrusewsky and Douglas (2002) suggest that prehistoric populations in mainland Southeast Asia had an increased emphasis but not a dependence on rice; they maintained hunting and gathering in addition to cultivating in a very rich tropical environment, resulting in a broad spectrum, varied diet and overall better quality of life. The results presented here support the hypothesis of an increasingly favourable environment from the Neolithic to the Early Bronze Age, but they clearly do not support the hypothesis that the degree of sexual dimorphism increases as rice agriculture develops and intensifies.

## Conclusion

A decreasing level of stature sexual dimorphism from the Neolithic to Early Bronze Age period is associated with the intensification of rice agriculture in the prehistoric population of Ban Non Wat, Thailand. This lower degree of dimorphism is a result of the statistically significant increase in female body size and not therefore associated with detrimental environmental conditions. This increase in the Early Bronze Age may be a factor of an increasingly favourable natural and cultural environment or a possible immigration of females. These results suggest that the decline in health associated with the intensification of agriculture cannot be applied universally as previously proposed. The more highly statistically significant differences in female stature and epiphyseal dimensions compared to males do not indicate that males are more sensitive to changes in the environment; therefore this research does not support the female genetic buffering hypothesis. Although the degree of sexual dimorphism decreases significantly in stature, no statistically significant changes in dimorphism are found in the epiphyseal dimensions over time. It must be considered that this may be a result of the small sample size in this preliminary investigation.

This research has demonstrated that sexual dimorphism is a useful measure of human cultural and biological adaptation. However, it is not yet possible to attribute these changes to any single factor. Continuing this research into the later periods of the Bronze and Iron Ages is necessary to observe temporal trends throughout prehistoric occupation at Ban Non Wat. Further stages of this project will incorporate independent indicators of health status and stress to further comprehend the human biological adaptations of a rice-based agricultural community.

**Acknowledgements**

The authors would like to thank the directors of the Origins of Angkor Project (2001-2007) Charles Higham and Rachanie Thosarat, in addition to the Thai Fine Arts Department, the National Research Council and the Kingdom of Thailand for the opportunity to work on the prehistoric people of Ban Non Wat. Thanks also go to the Otago Branch of the New Zealand Federation for Graduate Women and the Department of Anatomy, University of Otago who provided funding that enabled AC to present an oral version of this paper at the 2010 BABAO Conference in Cambridge. Robbie McPhee is thanked for his assistance with the figures. This study forms part of a larger research project by AC funded by a University of Otago Doctoral Scholarship. The authors are also very grateful to the two anonymous reviewers for their constructive comments.

**Literature Cited**

Barker, G. 2009. *The agricultural revolution in Prehistory: why did foragers become farmers?* Oxford University Press: Oxford.

Bielicki, T. and Charzewski, J. 1977. Sex differences in the magnitude of statural gains of offspring over parents. *Human Biology* 49: 265-277.

Bogin, B. 1999. *Patterns of human growth.* Cambridge University Press: Cambridge.

Bogin, B., Smith, P., Orden, A. and Varela Silva, M. 2002. Rapid change in height and body proportions of Maya American children. *American Journal of Human Biology* 14(6): 753-761.

Brock, S. and Ruff, C. 1988. Diachronic patterns of change in structural properties of the femur in the Prehistoric American Southwest. *American Journal Physical Anthropology* 75(1): 113-127.

Brundtland, G., Liestøl, K. and Walløe, L. 1980. Height, weight and menarcheal age of Oslo schoolchildren during the last 60 years. *Annals of Human Biology* 7(4): 307-322.

Buikstra, J. and Ubelaker, D. 1994. *Standards for data collection from human skeletal remains.* Arkansas Archaeological Survey Research Series. Arkansas Archaeological Survey: Fayetteville.

Charisi, D., Eliopoulos, C., Vanna, V., Koilias, C. and Manolis, S. 2010. Sexual dimorphism of the arm bones in a modern Greek population. *Journal of Forensic Sciences* 56(1): 10-18.

Clark, A. 2007. *Investigating the effects of secular change on metric sexing techniqures in British skeletal populations.* Unpublished MSc Thesis. University of Bradford.

Cohen, M. 2007. Feed or feedback: Agriculture population dynamics and the state of the planet. *Human Ecology* 35(2): 255-256.

Cohen, M. and Armelagos, G. 1984. *Paleopathology at the origins of agriculture.* Academic Press: Orlando.

Cole, T. 2003. The secular trend in human physical growth: a biological view. *Economics and Human Biology* 1(2): 161-168.

Cole, T. 2007. Secular trends in growth. *Proceedings of the Nutrition Society* 59(2): 317-324.

Cox, K. 2009. *Human migration in Prehistoric Northeast Thailand.* Unpublished PhD Thesis. University of Otago.

Domett, K. 2001. *Health in late Prehistoric Thailand.* BAR International Series No. 946. Archaeopress: Oxford.

Eveleth, P. 1975. Differences between ethnic groups in sex dimorphism of adult height. *Annals of Human Biology* 2(1): 35-39.

Gaulin, S. and Boster, J. 1992. Human marriage systems and sexual dimorphism in stature. *American Journal Physical Anthropology* 89(4): 467-475.

Giannecchini, M. and Moggi-Cecchi, J. 2008. Stature in archeological samples from central Italy: methodological issues and diachronic changes. *American Journal Physical Anthropology* 135(3): 284-292.

Goodman, A., Lallo, L., Armelagos, G. and Rose, J. 1984. Health changes at Dickson Mounds, Illinois (A.D. 950-1300). In: Cohen, M. and Armelagos, G. (eds.) *Paleopathology at the origins of agriculture*. Academic Press: New York. 271-301.

Goodman, A., Brooke Thomas, R., Swedlund, A. and Armelagos, G. 1988. Biocultural perspectives on stress in prehistoric, historical, and contemporary population research. *Yearbook of Physical Anthropology* 31: 169-202.

Greene, D. 1989. Comparison of t-tests for differences in sexual dimorphism between populations. *American Journal of Physical Anthropology* 79(1): 121-125.

Greulich, W. 1951. The growth and development status of Guamanian school children in 1947. *American Journal of Physical Anthropology* 9: 55-70.

Hall, R. 1978. Sexual dimorphism for size in seven nineteenth century Northwest coast populations. *Human Biology* 50: 159-171.

Hamilton, M. 1982. Sexual dimorphism in skeletal samples. In: Hall, R. (ed.) *Sexual dimorphism in Homo sapiens: a question of size*. Praeger: New York. 107-149.

Higham, C. and Higham, T. 2009. A new chronological framework for prehistoric Southeast Asia, based on a Bayesian model from Ban Non Wat. *Antiquity* 83(319): 125-144.

Higham, C. and Kijngam, A. 2009. *The origins of the civilization of Angkor. Volume III - the excavation of Ban Non Wat: introduction.* Fine Arts Department of Thailand: Bangkok.

Holden, C. and Mace, R. 1999. Sexual dimorphism in stature and women's work: a phylogenetic cross-cultural analysis. *American Journal of Physical Anthropology* 110(1): 27-45.

Jantz, L. and Jantz, R. 1999. Secular change in long bone length and proportion in the United States, 1800-1970. *American Journal of Physical Anthropology* 110(1): 57-67.

Kijngam. in press. The mammalian fauna. In: Higham, C. and Kijngam, A. (eds.) *The origins of the civilization of Angkor, volume 4 - the excavation of Ban Non Wat. Part II: the Neolithic occupation.* Fine Arts Department of Thailand: Bangkok. 199-207.

Larsen, C. 1995. Biological changes in human populations with agriculture. *Annual Review of Anthropology* 24(1): 185-213.

Larsen, C. 2002. Bioarchaeology: the lives and lifestyles of past people. *Journal of Archaeological Research* 10(2): 119-166.

Larsen, C. 2006. The agricultural revolution as environmental catastrophe: implications for health and lifestyle in the Holocene. *Quaternary International* 150(1): 12-20.

Loesch, D., Stokes, K. and Huggins, R. 2000. Secular trend in body height and weight of Australian children and adolescents. *American Journal of Physical Anthropology* 111(4): 545-556.

Lukacs, J. 2008. Fertility and agriculture accentuate sex differences in dental caries rates. *Current Anthropology* 49(5): 901-914.

Malina, R. 1979. Secular changes in size and maturity: causes and effects. *Monographs of the Society for Research in Child Development* 44(3/4): 59-102.

Mays, S. 1998. *The archaeology of human bones.* Routledge: London.

Nelsen, K. 1999. *Dental health of the people from Noen U-Loke, a prehistoric Iron Age site in northeast Thailand.* Unpublished MSc Thesis. University of Otago.

Olivier, G. 1969. *Practical Anthropology.* Charles C Thomas: Springfield, Illinois.

Oxenham, M., Thuy, N. and Cuong, N. 2005. Skeletal evidence for the emergence of infectious disease in bronze and iron age northern Vietnam. *American Journal Physical Anthropology* 126(4): 359-376.

Phenice, T. 1969. A newly developed visual method of sexing the os pubis. *American Journal Physical Anthropology* 30(2): 297-302.

Pietrusewsky, M. and Douglas, M. 2002. Intensification of agriculture at Ban Chiang: is there evidence from the skeletons? *Asian Perspectives* 40(2): 157-178.

Sangvichien, S. 1985. Estimation of stature of Thai and Chinese from the length of femur, tibia and fibula. *Siriraj Hospital Gazette* 37: 215-218.

Schutkowski, H. 2006. *Human ecology: biocultural adaptations in human communities.* Ecological Studies 182. Springer-Verlag: Berlin.

Schutkowski, H. 2008. Introduction. In: Schutkowski, H. (ed.) *Between biology and culture.* Cambridge University Press: Cambridge. 1-11.

Schweich, M. 2005. *Diachronic effects of bio-cultural factors on stature and body proportions in British archaeological populations.* Unpublished PhD Thesis. University of Bradford.

Schweich, M. and Knüsel, C. 2004. Physical variation in past populations. In: Bodzsár, E. and Susanne, C. (eds.) *Physique and body composition: variability and sources of variations.* Eötvös University Press: Budapest. 173-181.

Silventoinen, K., Kaprio, J., Lahelma, E., Viken, R. and Rose, R. 2001. Sex differences in genetic and environmental factors contributing to body-height. *Twin Research and Human Genetics* 4(1): 25-29.

Smith, R. 1999. Statistics of sexual size dimorphism. *Journal of Human Evolution* 36(4): 423-458.

Steckel, R. 1995. Stature and the standard of living. *Journal of Economic Literature* 33(4): 1903-1940.

Steckel, R., Rose, J., Larsen, C. and Walker, P. 2002. Skeletal health in the Western Hemisphere from 4000 BC to the present. *Evolutionary Anthropology* 11(4): 142-155.

Stini, W. 1969. Nutritional stress and growth: sex differences in adaptive response. *American Journal Physical Anthropology* 31: 417-426.

Stini, W. 1975. Adaptive strategies of human populations under nutritional stress. In: Watts, E., Johnston, F. and Lasker, G. (eds.) *Biosocial interrelations in population adaptation.*World Anthropology Series. Mouton: The Hague. 19-53.

Stini, W. 1985. Growth rates and sexual dimorphism in evolutionary perspective. In: Gilbert, R. and Mielke, J. (eds.) *The analysis of prehistoric diets.* Academic Press: San Diego. 191-226.

Stinson, S. 1985. Sex differences in environmental sensitivity. *Yearbook of Physical Anthropology* 28: 123-147.

Stinson, S. 2000. Growth variation: biological and cultural factors. In: Stinson, S., Bogin, B., Huss-Ashmore, R. and O'Rourke, D. (eds.) *Human biology: an evolutionary and biocultural perspective.* Wiley-Liss: New York. 425-463.

Tanner, J. 1978. *Fetus into man: physical growth from conception to maturity.* Harvard University Press: Cambridge.

Tayles, N., Domett, K. and Nelsen, K. 2000. Agriculture and dental caries? The case of rice in prehistoric Southeast Asia. *World Archaeology* 32(1): 68-83.

Tayles, N. and Oxenham, M. 2006. Introdution: Southeast Asian bioarchaeology past and present. In: Oxenham, M. and Tayles, N. (eds.) *Bioarchaeology of Southeast Asia.* Cambridge University Press: Cambridge. 1-30.

Thosarat, R. in press. Faunal remains. In: Higham, C. and Kijngam, A. (eds.) *The origins of the civilization of Angkor, volume 4 - The excavation of Ban Non Wat. Part II: the Neolithic occupation.* Fine Arts Department of Thailand: Bangkok. 179-189.

Tobias, P. 1975. Anthropology among disadvantaged peoples: studies in Southern Africa. In: Watts, E., Johnston, F. and Lasker, G. (eds.) *Biosocial interrelations in population adaptation.*World Anthropology Series. Mouton: The Hague. 287-305.

Valenzuela, C., Rothhammer, F. and Chakraborty, R. 1978. Sex dimorphism in adult stature in four Chilean populations. *Annals of Human Biology* 5(6): 533-538.

Walker, P. 2005. Greater sciatic notch morphology: sex, age, and population differences. *American Journal of Physical Anthropology* 127(4): 385-391.

# The Bioarchaeology of Agriculture in the Southern Levant: A Comparative Study of Epipaleolithic Hunter-Gatherers and Bronze Age Agriculturalists

Matthew A. Gasperetti

Phenotypic Adaptation, Variation, and Human Evolution Research Group
Department of Archaeology and Anthropology
University of Cambridge
Pembroke Street
Cambridge, CB2 3DZ

Email for correspondence: mag59@cam.ac.uk

**Abstract**

The shift from hunting-and-gathering in the Pleistocene to agriculturally based subsistence in the Holocene was one of the most important transitions in the history of *Homo sapiens*. Recent research has helped elucidate the origins of agriculture in diverse geographic contexts; however, this transition has not been studied as thoroughly in the southern Levant, one of the first loci of domestication, as in other regions. The current research analyses the interrelationship between diet, health, and behaviour by documenting dental attrition, oral pathology, linear enamel hypoplasia (LEH), and long bone cross-sectional geometry in a population of Bronze Age agriculturalists from Jericho (Early Bronze I–Middle Bronze II; *circa* 5,500–3,650 cal. BP). Results are compared to published and original work documenting the same indicators in populations of Natufian hunter-gatherers from Ain Mallaha, Nahal Oren, and Hayonim (Early Natufian–Late Natufian; *circa* 14,600–11,000 cal. BP). Comparative statistical analyses indicated that attrition was generally lower in the Bronze Age population, whereas oral pathology was higher with the exception of dental caries. This is interpreted to reflect a shift to a broad dietary strategy and less abrasive, cooked foods. Rates of LEH indicated no significant change in health when populations were compared. Finally, analysis of cross-sectional geometry showed that the upper limbs of the Bronze Age population were significantly more robust than the Natufian populations, while both groups had femoral and tibial $I_{max}/I_{min}$ ratios indicating greater bone strength in the anteroposterior plane than the mediolateral plane, which is consistent with high mobility.

**Keywords:** Oral Pathology, Attrition, Linear Enamel Hypoplasia, Agriculture, Natufian, Bronze Age

The shift from hunting-and-gathering in the Pleistocene to agriculture in the Holocene was one of the most important transitions in the history of *Homo sapiens* (Childe 1936). This dramatic change in subsistence reshaped the relationship between human beings and the natural environment, and has been the topic of a plethora of research in the field of biological anthropology (Cohen 1977; Cohen and Armelagos 1984; Larsen 1995, 2006; Steckel and Rose 2002). This research has shown that domestication occurred gradually in at least eight independent loci of prehistoric agriculture (i.e. the Near East, South China, North China, New Guinea, Sub-Saharan Africa, South America, central Mexico, and the eastern United States) (Larsen 2006). The prerequisite knowledge and techniques needed to domesticate plants spread from these centres of agriculture to adjacent areas and allowed hunter-gatherers to develop agricultural subsistence economies on every inhabited continent, with the exception of Australia, during the first 5,000 years of the Holocene (Larsen 1995; Diamond 1997; Diamond and Bellwood 2003).

A large body of scholarship has helped elucidate the origins of agriculture in diverse geographic contexts including the Near East (Peterson 2002; Eshed *et al* 2006; Pinhasi *et al.* 2008), Africa (Allen 1997; Zakrzewski 2003; Starling and Stock 2007), the Americas (Goodman *et al.* 1980; Buikstra 1986; Bridges 1989), Asia and the Pacific (Turner 1979; Lukacs 1992; Bentley *et al.* 2005) and Europe (Pinhasi and Pluciennik 2004; Bocquet-Appel and Naji 2006; Marchi 2008). This research has added to our understanding of the extraordinary changes associated with the shift to agriculturally based subsistence strategies while examining the impact this transition had on prehistoric populations. In antiquity, agriculture allowed sedentism, task specialisation, surplus storage and other socio-cultural and technological innovations and advantages (Diamond and Bellwood 2003; Larsen 2006). These advances provided the foundation of civilization and still underpin the subsistence economies of almost every society in the contemporary world.

Although agriculture is associated with rapid socio-cultural development, economic growth, and technological innovation, reliance on staple crops had many adverse effects on the first farmers (Cohen and Armelagos 1984; Steckel and Rose 2002; Larsen 2006). Research indicates that as communities became more reliant on domesticated plants, there was a decline in the overall quality of nutrition, an increase in the incidence of infection, a decrease in skeletal robusticity, and a general decline in health (Cohen and Armelagos 1984; Larsen 1995; Steckel and Rose 2002). This trend has been documented in many contexts and is thought to be related to over-reliance on a narrow cadre of plants, population density, poor sanitation, exposure to zoonotic disease, and other factors (Armelagos and Dewey 1970; Cohen and Armelagos 1984; Cohen 1989).

The advantages of sedentary agriculture far outweighed the disadvantages, however, which was evidenced by the rapid spread of farming into neighbouring regions: large populations, centralized power, new technologies, surpluses, and resistance to disease (resulting from prolonged exposure to pathogens) offered farmers many adaptive advantages unavailable to their hunter-gatherer counterparts (Diamond 1997; Bellwood 2001; Diamond and Bellwood 2003).

Although bioarchaeological studies of agriculture often report similar trends, it is clear that this transition was not uniform throughout the world and regional and temporal comparisons are needed (cf. Cohen and Armelagos 1984; Larsen 2006; Stock and Pinhasi 2011).

This is especially true when analysing the transition to agriculture in the Near East because unlike populations in other areas that relied almost entirely on single staple crops for their subsistence needs, populations in the Near East began domesticating many species of plants (i.e. diploid einkorn wheat, tetraploid emmer wheat, barley, pea, lentil, chickpea, bitter vetch, and flax) and animals (i.e. cattle, pigs, goats and sheep) as early as the Pre-pottery Neolithic (*circa* 11,500-8,500 cal BP) and orchard crops (i.e. figs, dates and olives) in later periods (Horwitz *et al.* 1999; Gopher *et al.* 2001; Issar and Zohar 2007). It is clear that subsistence regimes in the Near East, or the southern Levant for our purposes, were much different (i.e. more diverse) than in other centres of agriculture that were primarily reliant on single staple crops (e.g. maize in many prehistoric North American populations). This variation undoubtedly had a variety of effects on prehistoric populations in the region.

The current study adds to scholarship on the transition to agriculture in the southern Levant by documenting dental attrition, oral pathology, linear enamel hypoplasia (LEH) and cross-sectional geometry in a population of agriculturalists from Bronze Age Jericho. This data is compared to both published and original data examining the same indicators in Natufian hunter-gatherer populations from Ain Mallaha, Nahal Oren, and Hayonim. Statistical analyses are used to compare diet, health, and behaviour between the two periods in order to examine the biological response of prehistoric populations to sedentary life and agriculture in the southern Levant, while exploring how these changes differentiate the region from other loci of domestication.

## Materials

Skeletal material from Bronze Age Jericho (EB I–MB II; *circa* 5,500–3,650 cal. BP) was examined in the current study. Data were recorded from permanent teeth, adult jaws, and complete adult long bones. Early Bronze Age (EB I–IV) and Middle Bronze Age (MB I–II) material was combined into a single 'Bronze Age' sample, and Early and Late Natufian comparative data from Ain Mallaha, Nahal Oren, and Hayonim Cave and Terrace (Early and Late; *circa* 14,600–11,000 cal. BP) were grouped into a single 'Natufian' sample in order to maximize sample sizes (see Table 1). Although Bronze Age and Natufian populations were separated chronologically by nearly 10,000 years and by vast socio-cultural differences, there is a variety of evidence for genetic continuity in the southern Levant until well after the Middle Bronze Age II (Arensburg *et al.* 1980; Smith 1995; Ullinger *et al.* 2005).

**Table 1:** Chronology of the southern Levant

| Period | Analytical Units | Approx. Dates (cal BP)* |
|---|---|---|
| Terminal Epipaleolithic | Early Natufian and Late Natufian | 14,600–11,500 |
| Pre-Pottery Neolith c | Pre-Pottery Neolithic A, B, and C | 11,500–8,500 |
| Pottery Neolithic | Yarmoukian and Jericho IX | 8,500–7,700 |
| Chalcolithic | Wadi Rabah, Middle Chalcolithic, and Late Chalcolithic | 7,700–5,500 |
| Early Bronze | Early Bronze I, II, III, and IV | 5,500–4,000 |
| Middle Bronze | Middle Bronze I and II | 4,000–3,650 |

* Dates from Aurenche *et al.* 2001; Dever 2003; Banning 2007; and Guerrero *et al.* 2008.

The minimum number of adult individuals (MNI) examined from Bronze Age Jericho was 115, while Eshed and colleagues (2004) reported an MNI of 74 for Ain Mallaha, 31 for Nahal Oren, and 32 for Hayonim. Although the fragmentary nature of the Jericho material made ageing and sexing the remains impossible in most cases, an initial examination of the material was preformed D. R. Hughes (1965) who reported a sex ratio (males/females x 100) of 208 for the Bronze Age skeletons from Jericho and constructed an age distribution for the collection. When compared to data published by Eshed and colleagues (2004), who reported a sex ratio of 216 for Ain Mallaha, Nahal Oren, and Hayonim, Fisher's exact test showed no statistical difference by sex (p=1.00). When age was considered, however, the number of individuals that were aged between 20 and 30 was significantly lower for the Bronze Age population (p=0.001), when compared to the Natufian populations, while the opposite was true for individuals aged between 40 and 50 (p=0.01) (see Table 2).

**Table 2:** Age and sex distributions for the Bronze Age and Jericho Populations

| | Male | | Female | | 20-30 | | 30-40 | | 40-50 | | >50 | |
|---|---|---|---|---|---|---|---|---|---|---|---|---|
| | N | % | N | % | N | % | N | % | N | % | N | % |
| Natufian* | 54 | 68.4 | 25 | 31.6 | 26 | 37.7 | 20 | 29.0 | 19 | 27.5 | 4 | 5.8 |
| Bronze Age | 25 | 67.6 | 12 | 32.4 | 1 | 4.2 | 6 | 25.0 | 14 | 58.3 | 3 | 12.5 |
| p-value | 1.00 | | 1.00 | | **0.001** | | 0.80 | | **0.01** | | 0.37 | |

*Natufian Data from Eshed and colleagues (2004)

A total of 940 Bronze Age teeth and 2,426 Bronze Age dental alveoli were examined. Rates of dental attrition (n=940), dental caries (n=922), periapical lesions (n=3,335), dental calculus (n=895), periodontal disease (n=872), AMTL (n=2,426) and LEH (n=849) were calculated. Complete adult clavicles (n=31), humeri (n=48), ulnae (n=34), femora (n=28) and tibiae (n=29) were also examined. The material from Bronze Age Jericho is curated at the Duckworth Laboratory at the University of Cambridge. Jericho is located to the west of the Jordan River, eight miles north of the Dead Sea, with the mountains of Judah to the west, and floodplains to the east (Fig. 1) (Kenyon 1957). The material analyzed in this study was excavated from Bronze Age tombs dating to Early Bronze I-IV and Middle Bronze I-II (Kenyon 1960). Tombs usually contained multiple interments, were frequently reused, and burials were often commingled (Kenyon 1960).

The Natufian comparative data, incorporated into the current study, were from Ain Mallaha, Nahal Oren, and Hayonim. This material is curated at the Sackler Faculty of Medicine at Tel Aviv University. Dental analyses were preformed and published by Eshed and colleagues (2006), except for analysis of LEH, which was preformed by Hershkovitz and Gopher (2008). The sample examined consisted of 1,160 teeth and 1,753 dental alveoli (Eshed *et al.* 2006). The Natufian osteometric data and cross-sectional moulds used in the current study were collected by Jay Stock (University of Cambridge) and prepared and analyzed by the author in order to reduce inter-observer error. Data were recorded from complete clavicles (n=19), humeri (n=25), ulnae (n=19), femora (n=17) and tibiae (n=11).

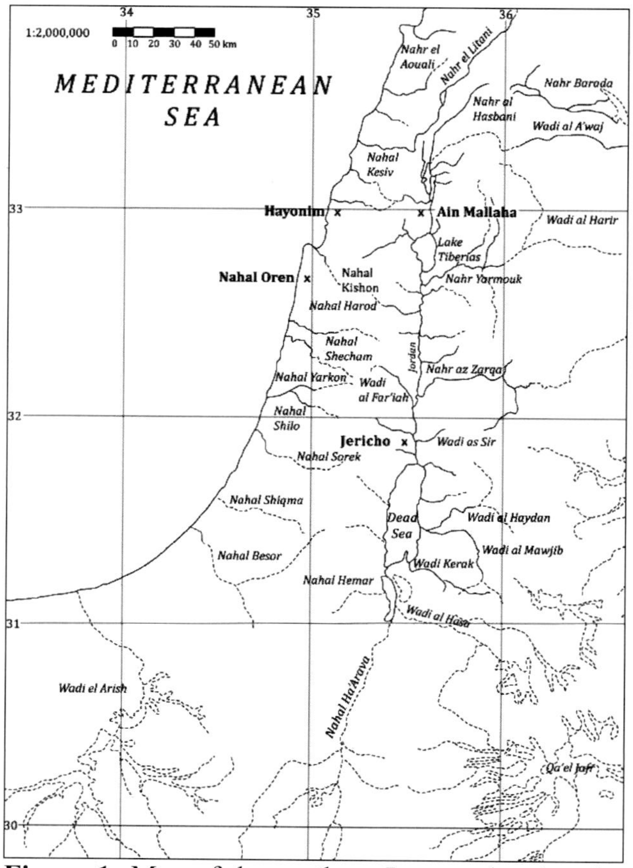


**Figure 1:** Map of the southern Levant showing the location of the Bronze Age and Natufian sites studied.

Ain Mallaha, Nahal Oren, and Hayonim are in northern Israel. Ain Mallaha is located on the shore of Lake Hulah in the northern Jordan Valley, Nahal Oren is to the west along the western ridge of Mount Carmel and Hayonim is in western Galilee (Fig. 1) (Perrot 1960; Stekelis and Yizraely 1963; Belfer-Cohen 1988). Individuals at Ain Mallaha were typically inhumed in collective burials of three individuals with two of these individuals buried face-to-face in flexed positions. (Perrot 1960). At Nahal Oren, the dead were usually inhumed in individual graves marked with limestone mortars, in flexed positions, with their heads oriented north (Stekelis and Yizraely 1963). The graves at Hayonim contained both group and individual burials, and, in rare cases, were paved with stones or limestone slabs (Belfer-Cohen 1988).

## Methods

### *Dental Analyses*

All permanent teeth, or adult alveoli, from the sample from Bronze Age Jericho were examined macroscopically and dental attrition, dental caries, periapical lesions, dental calculus, periodontal disease, AMTL and LEH were scored. Dental attrition and oral pathology were scored following the criteria used by Eshed and colleagues (2006). This approach was selected in order to reduce inter-observer error and in order to help establish a consistent methodological approach for research in the southern Levant.

Teeth with the occlusal surface intact were examined for evidence dental attrition. Dental attrition was scored from one (unworn) to 10 (no enamel) based on degree of occlusal wear (Littleton and Frohlich 1993) (Fig. 2). Dental caries were scored from one ('pinprick-sized' lesion) to four (complete destruction of tooth) (Metress and Conway 1975), and location was recorded as 'occlusal', 'smooth surface', 'cervical' or 'root' (Powell 1985). Periapical lesions were scored as 'present' or 'absent' for all dental alveoli based on the presence or absence of a smooth, rounded lesion at the apex of a tooth root, which would have allowed the lesion to drain through the bone of the jaw or into the maxillary sinus (Lukacs 1989). Dental calculus was scored as 'slight', 'moderate' or 'severe' for all teeth with the buccal/lingual surface intact according to Brothwell's (1981) criteria. Periodontal disease was scored as 'present' or 'absent' based on the distance between the cemento-enamel junction (CEJ) and the alveolar crest. If the distance between the CEJ and alveolar crest was greater than 2mm and the corresponding alveolar bone showed evidence of lipping or porosity, periodontal was scored as 'present' (Tal 1985; Clarke *et al.* 1986). AMTL was scored as 'present' or 'absent' based on the presence or absence of alveolar resorption within dental alveoli (Ortner and Putschar 1985; Frayer 1989). Finally, LEH was scored as 'present' if the width of an enamel defect was of greater diameter than adjacent perikymata (Guatelli-Steinberg 2003). Fisher's exact test was used to identify statistically significant differences between rates of oral pathology and LEH in the Bronze Age sample and the Natufian comparative samples.

### *Cross-Sectional Geometry*

Cross-sectional geometry can be used to quantify skeletal robusticity and to interpret and contextualize aspects of the mechanical environment that have influenced the morphology of a given skeletal element (Martin *et al.* 1998). The current study employed a latex moulding method in order to examine the cross-sectional properties of clavicles, humeri, ulnae, femora and tibiae (cf. Stock 2002). Moulds were taken at 50% length for all long bones with the exception of humeral moulds, which were taken at 35% (Stock and Pfeiffer 2004; Stock 2006). Changes in habitual behaviour were studied by calculating total subperiosteal area (TA), maximum and minimum second moments of area ($I_{max}$ and $I_{min}$), polar second moments of area ($J$) and $I_{max}/I_{min}$ ratios using ImageJ 1.42q.

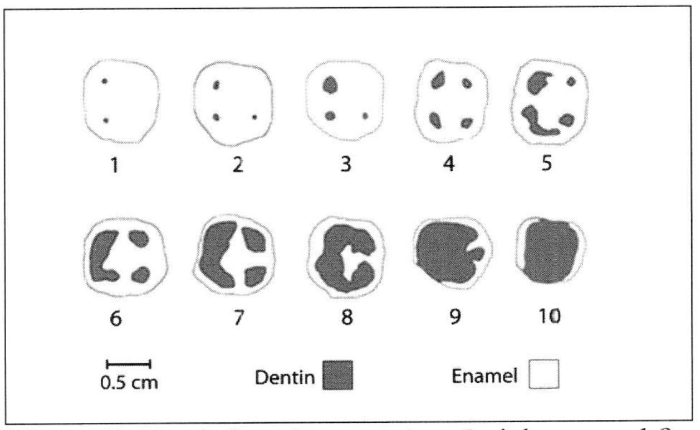


**Figure 2:** Teeth from Bronze Age Jericho scored for dental attrition, from 1-10, based on criteria established by Littleton and Frohlich (1993).

Second moments of area were calculated in order to assess maximum ($I_{max}$) and minimum ($I_{min}$) bending strength. Polar second moments of area ($J$) were calculated in order to quantify torsional strength, and $I_{max}/I_{min}$ was calculated in order to study diaphyseal shape. Research indicates that femoral and tibial $I_{max}/I_{min}$ ratios greater than one indicate greater hypertrophy in the anteroposterior plane than the mediolateral plane and can be used as a mobility index in Holocene populations (Ruff 1987; Larsen 1996; Ruff 1999). Polar moments of area and second moments of area were standardized by length$^2$, rather than by body mass because the commingled nature of the collection made standardisation by body mass impractical (Ruff 1984). Student's t-test was used to test for statistically significant differences between Bronze Age and Natufian samples.

## Results

### *Dental Attrition*

The average rate of dental attrition was 4.0 for the Bronze Age teeth examined (n=913). The rate of dental attrition was 3.9 on average for the Bronze Age maxillary teeth (n=345) compared to 4.1 for the mandibular teeth (n=568). When Bronze Age rates of attrition were compared to Natufian data published by Eshed and colleagues (2006), attrition was found to be higher in both Natufian jaws and in all Natufian teeth except $P_4$, $M_3$, $M^2$, and $M^3$ (Fig. 3). Statistical analyses were not possible because the appropriate Natufian data were unavailable.

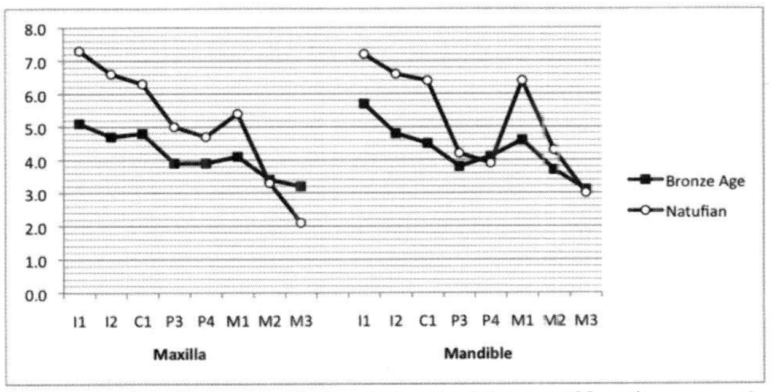


**Figure 3:** Rates of dental attrition affecting teeth from Bronze Age Jericho and Natufian Ain Mallaha, Nahal Oren, and Hayonim. Natufian data from Eshed and colleagues (2006).

### *Dental Caries*

Dental caries were scored as present for 6.1% of the Bronze Age teeth examined (n=56/922). The rate of caries for maxillary teeth (n=13/353) was 3.7%, whereas the rate of caries for mandibular teeth (n=43/569) was 7.6%. When compared to Natufian data published by Eshed and colleagues (2006), the Bronze Age sample showed a higher rate of caries for $I_1$, $C_1$, $P_3$, $P_4$, and $M_1$ in addition to $I^1$, $C^1$, and $P^4$. Fisher's exact test returned no statistical difference when Bronze Age and Natufian rates of caries were compared (p=0.79) and when rates of caries for mandibular teeth were compared (p=0.08). Fisher's exact test did, however, report a statistically significant difference when rates of caries affecting maxillary teeth were compared (p=0.009). When individual teeth were considered, the rate of caries affecting $M_1$ was found to be significantly higher for the Bronze Age sample than for the Natufian sample (p=0.02), while the opposite was true for $M^1$ (p=0.004) and $M^2$ (p=0.02) (see Table 3).

### *Periapical Lesions*

Of the Bronze Age dental alveoli examined (n=29/3,335), 0.9% showed evidence of a pericapical lesion. The rate of affection was 0.4% for the Bronze Age maxillary alveoli (n=7/1,627) and 1.3% for mandibular alveoli (n=22/1,708). When compared to rates reported for the Natufian populations published by Eshed and colleagues (2006), Fisher's exact test reported no statistically significant differences for total rates of affection (p=0.12), mandibular rates of affection (p=0.69), or maxillary rates of affection (p=0.23). The only statistical difference noted was for $M_1$, which showed a higher rate of periapical infection in the Bronze Age sample (p=0.03) (see Table 4).

**Table 3:** Rates of dental caries and P-values comparing Bronze Age and Natufian samples.

| | Bronze Age | | Natufian* | | | | Bronze Age | | Natufian* | | |
|---|---|---|---|---|---|---|---|---|---|---|---|
| **Tooth** | **n/N** | **%** | **n/N** | **%** | **P** | **Tooth** | **n/N** | **%** | **n/N** | **%** | **p** |
| $I_1$ | 1/22 | 4.5 | 0/53 | 0.0 | 0.29 | $I^1$ | 1/16 | 6.3 | 0/34 | 0.0 | 0.32 |
| $I_2$ | 0/29 | 0.0 | 0/64 | 0.0 | 1.00 | $I^2$ | 0/29 | 0.0 | 0/35 | 0.0 | 1.00 |
| $C_1$ | 2/51 | 3.9 | 0/86 | 0.0 | 0.14 | $C^1$ | 1/31 | 3.2 | 1/62 | 0.0 | 1.00 |
| $P_3$ | 3/64 | 4.7 | 1/89 | 1.1 | 0.31 | $P^3$ | 3/52 | 5.2 | 0/69 | 1.1 | 0.08 |
| $P_4$ | 4/74 | 5.4 | 3/85 | 3.5 | 0.71 | $P^4$ | 0/63 | 0.0 | 1/77 | 3.5 | 1.00 |
| $M_1$ | 14/122 | 11.5 | 3/102 | 2.9 | **0.02** | $M^1$ | 3/74 | 4.1 | 6/82 | 2.9 | 0.50 |
| $M_2$ | 13/125 | 10.4 | 13/108 | 12.0 | 0.84 | $M^2$ | 4/67 | 6.0 | 18/74 | 12.0 | **0.004** |
| $M_3$ | 6/82 | 7.3 | 14/82 | 17.1 | 0.09 | $M^3$ | 1/32 | 3.1 | 14/58 | 17.1 | **0.02** |
| Sum | 43/569 | 7.6 | 34/669 | 5.0 | 0.08 | Sum | 13/353 | 3.7 | 40/491 | 8.1 | **0.009** |

*Natufian Data from Eshed and colleagues (2006)

**Table 4:** Rates of periapical abscessing and p-values comparing Bronze Age and Natufian samples.

| | Bronze Age | | Natufian* | | | | Bronze Age | | Natufian* | | |
|---|---|---|---|---|---|---|---|---|---|---|---|
| **Tooth** | **n/N** | **%** | **n/N** | **%** | **p** | **Tooth** | **n/N** | **%** | **n/N** | **%** | **p** |
| $I_1$ | 2/274 | 0.7 | 0/137 | 0.0 | 0.54 | $I^1$ | 0/297 | 0.0 | 0/85 | 0.0 | 1.00 |
| $I_2$ | 1/273 | 0.4 | 0/136 | 0.0 | 1.00 | $I^2$ | 0/274 | 0.0 | 0/90 | 0.0 | 1.00 |
| $C_1$ | 4/223 | 1.7 | 0/136 | 0.0 | 0.30 | $C^1$ | 1/215 | 0.9 | 0/90 | 0.0 | 1.00 |
| $P_3$ | 2/159 | 1.3 | 0/133 | 0.0 | 0.50 | $P^3$ | 1/220 | 0.5 | 3/89 | 3.4 | 0.07 |
| $P_4$ | 1/154 | 0.6 | 1/131 | 0.8 | 1.00 | $P^4$ | 0/206 | 3.3 | 0/91 | 0.0 | 1.00 |
| $M_1$ | 12/176 | 6.8 | 2/130 | 1.5 | **0.03** | $M^1$ | 5/150 | 0.0 | 0/90 | 0.0 | 0.16 |
| $M_2$ | 0/207 | 0.0 | 0/127 | 0.0 | 1.00 | $M^2$ | 0/116 | 0.0 | 3/88 | 3.4 | 0.08 |
| $M_3$ | 0/213 | 0.0 | 0/115 | 0.0 | 1.00 | $M^3$ | 0/148 | 0.0 | 0/85 | 0.0 | 1.00 |
| Sum | 22/1708 | 1.3 | 3/1045 | 0.3 | 0.69 | Sum | 7/1,627 | 0.4 | 6/708 | 0.9 | 0.23 |

*Natufian Data from Eshed and colleagues (2006)

### *Calculus*

Calculus was noted in 36.1% of the Bronze Age teeth examined (n=323/895). Calculus formation was scored as 'slight' for 34.0% of teeth (n=304/895), scored as 'moderate' for 1.5% of teeth (n=13/895), and scored as 'severe' for 0.6% of teeth (n=6/895) examined. When compared to Natufian data published by Eshed and colleagues (2006), Fisher's exact test showed that calculus was statistically more common for Bronze Age teeth (p<0.001) as well as maxillary (p<0.001) and mandibular teeth (p<0.001) when compared independently. Calculus affected $P^4$ (p=0.004), $M^2$ (p=0.003), $M^3$ (p<0.001), $P_4$ (p=0.003), $M_2$ (p=0.009), and $M_3$ (p<0.001) with a significantly higher frequency in the Bronze Age sample (see Table 5).

### *Periodontal Disease*

Periodontal disease was scored as present for 55.0% of Bronze Age teeth analyzed (n=480/872). The rate of periodontal disease was 58.6% for maxillary teeth (n=188/321) and 53.0% for Bronze Age mandibular teeth (n=292/551). When compared to Natufian data published by Eshed and colleagues (2006), Fisher's exact test showed that periodontal disease was statistically more common in Bronze Age dentitions (p<0.001) and in the upper (p<0.001) and lower (p<0.001) Bronze Age jaws. Periodontal disease affected $P^3$ (p=0.015), $P^4$ (p=0.003), $M^2$ (p=0.009) $M^3$ (p<0.001), $P_4$ (p=0.004), $M_2$ (p=0.003), and $M_3$ (p<0.001) with a statistically higher frequency in the Bronze Age population (see Table 6).

**Table 5:** Rates of ante-mortem tooth loss (AMTL) and p-values comparing Bronze Age and Natufian samples.

| | Bronze Age | | Natufian* | | | | Bronze Age | | Natufian* | | |
|---|---|---|---|---|---|---|---|---|---|---|---|
| Tooth | n/N | % | n/N | % | p | Tooth | n/N | % | n/N | % | p |
| $I_1$ | 8/280 | 2.9 | 6/137 | 4.4 | 0.40 | $I^1$ | 1/248 | 0.4 | 3/85 | 3.5 | 0.05 |
| $I_2$ | 7/255 | 2.7 | 4/136 | 2.9 | 1.00 | $I^2$ | 2/241 | 0.8 | 0/90 | 0.0 | 1.00 |
| $C_1$ | 3/180 | 1.7 | 0/136 | 0.0 | 0.26 | $C^1$ | 1/159 | 0.6 | 1/90 | 1.1 | 1.00 |
| $P_3$ | 8/165 | 4.8 | 0/133 | 0.0 | **0.01** | $P^3$ | 5/145 | 3.4 | 1/89 | 1.1 | 0.41 |
| $P_4$ | 10/144 | 6.9 | 6/131 | 4.6 | 0.45 | $P^4$ | 6/105 | 5.7 | 1/91 | 1.1 | 0.13 |
| $M_1$ | 32/69 | 46.4 | 8/130 | 6.2 | **<0.001** | $M^1$ | 21/52 | 40.1 | 3/90 | 3.3 | **<0.001** |
| $M_2$ | 18/50 | 36.0 | 7/127 | 5.5 | **<0.001** | $M^2$ | 17/83 | 20.5 | 3/88 | 3.4 | **0.001** |
| $M_3$ | 15/116 | 12.9 | 8/115 | 7.0 | 0.19 | $M^3$ | 18/133 | 13.5 | 2/85 | 2.4 | **0.007** |
| Sum | 101/1260 | 8.0 | 39/1045 | 3.7 | **<0.001** | Sum | 71/1166 | 6.1 | 14/708 | 2.0 | **<0.001** |

*Natufian Data from Eshed and colleagues (2006)

**Table 6:** Frequency of periodontal disease in Bronze Age and Natufian samples and the results of Fisher's Exact test.

| | Bronze Age | | Natufian* | | | | Bronze Age | | Natufian* | | |
|---|---|---|---|---|---|---|---|---|---|---|---|
| Tooth | n/N | % | n/N | % | p | Tooth | n/N | % | n/N | % | p |
| $I_1$ | 13/23 | 56.5 | 20/53 | 37.7 | 0.14 | $I^1$ | 9/16 | 56.3 | 0/34 | 0.0 | 0.22 |
| $I_2$ | 12/28 | 42.9 | 24/64 | 37.5 | 0.65 | $I^2$ | 11/18 | 61.1 | 0/35 | 0.0 | 0.25 |
| $C_1$ | 26/48 | 54.2 | 43/86 | 50.0 | 0.72 | $C^1$ | 14/29 | 48.3 | 1/62 | 0.0 | 0.25 |
| $P_3$ | 34/63 | 54.0 | 42/89 | 1.1 | 0.51 | $P^3$ | 30/50 | 60.0 | 0/69 | 1.1 | 0.11 |
| $P_4$ | 46/73 | 63.0 | 33/85 | 3.5 | **0.004** | $P^4$ | 35/59 | 59.3 | 1/77 | 3.5 | **0.003** |
| $M_1$ | 58/117 | 49.6 | 43/102 | 2.9 | 0.28 | $M^1$ | 44/77 | 57.1 | 6/82 | 2.9 | 0.15 |
| $M_2$ | 61/121 | 50.4 | 33/108 | 12.0 | **0.003** | $M^2$ | 23/39 | 59.0 | 18/74 | 12.0 | **0.009** |
| $M_3$ | 42/78 | 53.8 | 16/82 | 17.1 | **<0.001** | $M^3$ | 22/33 | 66.7 | 14/58 | 17.1 | **<0.001** |
| Sum | 292/551 | 53.0 | 254/669 | 5.0 | **<0.001** | Sum | 188/321 | 58.6 | 40/491 | 8.1 | **<0.001** |

*Natufian Data from Eshed and colleagues (2006)

### *Ante-Mortem Tooth Loss*

AMTL was present in 39.4% of individual dentitions analyzed (n=63/160). In addition to assessing the rate of AMTL in individual dentitions, rates of AMTL were assessed by dental alveoli, which yielded a 7.2% rate of tooth loss (n=172/2,426) for the Bronze Age sample. The rate of AMTL was 6.0% for Bronze Age maxillary alveoli (n=71/1,166) and 8.0% for Bronze Age mandibular alveoli (n=101/1,260). When compared to the data published by Eshed and colleagues (2006), Fisher's exact test showed that the total rate of AMTL ($p<0.001$) and the maxillary ($p<0.001$) and mandibular ($p<0.001$) rates of AMTL were significantly higher in the Bronze Age sample. When individual alveoli were compared, Fisher's exact test showed that AMTL affected $M^1$ ($p<0.001$), $M^2$ ($p=0.001$), and $M^3$ ($p=0.007$) with a statistically higher frequency in the Bronze Age dentitions (see Table 7).

### *Linear Enamel Hypoplasia*

LEH was scored as 'present' in 33.9% of dentitions analyzed (n=39/115). When individual teeth were considered, LEH was scored as 'present' for 25.4% of the Bronze Age teeth examined (n=216/849). The total rate of LEH for all Bronze Age maxillary teeth was 26.1% (n=87/333), and the total rate of LEH was 25.0% for mandibular teeth (n=129/516). When compared to data published by Hershkovitz and Gopher (2008), Fisher's exact test did not show a statistically significant difference for rates of LEH per individual ($p=0.22$).

*Cross-Sectional Geometry*

Cross-sectional properties were calculated for Bronze Age and Natufian clavicles, humeri, ulnae, femora, and tibiae. Length, Total area (TA), $I_{max}$, $I_{min}$, $J$, and $I_{max}/I_{min}$ ratios are reported for Bronze Age and Natufian upper limbs in Table 8, and for the Bronze Age and Natufian lower limbs in Table 9. Fisher's exact test reported a number of statistically significant differences when long bone cross-sectional properties were compared. P-values are reported in Tables 8 and 9.

**Table 7:** Frequency of dental calculus in Bronze Age and Natufian populations and the results of Fisher's exact test.

| | BA Mandibles | | N Mandibles | | | BA Maxillae | | N Maxillae | | |
|---|---|---|---|---|---|---|---|---|---|---|
| | n/522 | % | n/669 | % | p | n/343 | % | n/491 | % | p |
| Slight | 221 | 40 | 70 | 12.6 | **<0.001** | 83 | 24.2 | 64 | 10.5 | **<0.001** |
| Moderate | 10 | 1.8 | 20 | 2.9 | 0.20 | 4 | 0.9 | 14 | 3.0 | 0.14 |
| Severe | 4 | 0.7 | 6 | 0.4 | 0.76 | 2 | 0.6 | 2 | 0.9 | 1.00 |
| Sum | 235 | 42.6 | 96 | 19.6 | **<0.001** | 88 | 25.7 | 78 | 11.7 | **<0.001** |

Natufian Data from Eshed and colleagues (2006). BA, Bronze Age; N, Natufian

**Table 8:** Mean cross-sectional properties from Bronze Age and Natufian upper limbs and the results of Student's t-test.

| | Clavicles | | | Humeri | | | Ulnae | | |
|---|---|---|---|---|---|---|---|---|---|
| | BA | N | p | BA | N | p | BA | N | p |
| Sample (*N*) | 27 | 19 | - | 47 | 25 | - | 33 | 19 | - |
| Length (mm) | 143.1 | 141.7 | 0.59 | 303.6 | 299.9 | 0.47 | 249.8 | 253.3 | 0.49 |
| *TA* | 0.62 | 0.58 | 0.25 | 0.83 | 0.76 | **0.02** | 0.47 | 0.42 | **0.009** |
| *Imax* | 6.21 | 4.83 | **0.05** | 19.43 | 15.98 | **0.009** | 6.15 | 4.42 | **0.002** |
| *Imin* | 3.50 | 3.30 | 0.62 | 15.38 | 13.27 | 0.08 | 3.84 | 3.26 | 0.09 |
| *J* | 9.71 | 8.13 | 0.14 | 34.82 | 19.25 | **0.02** | 10.00 | 7.68 | **0.008** |
| *Imax/Imax* | 1.80 | 1.48 | **0.001** | 1.27 | 1.23 | 0.15 | 1.63 | 1.37 | **0.002** |

BA, Bronze Age; N, Natufian

**Table 9:** Mean cross-sectional properties from Bronze Age and Natufian lower limbs and the results of Student's t-test.

| | Femora | | | Tibiae | | |
|---|---|---|---|---|---|---|
| | BA | N | p | BA | N | p |
| Sample (*N*) | 28 | 17 | - | 29 | 11 | - |
| Length (mm) | 421.9 | 438.1 | 0.05 | 355.9 | 359.4 | 0.43 |
| *TA* | 1.21 | 1.16 | 0.41 | 1.15 | 1.18 | 0.63 |
| *Imax* | 62.19 | 58.87 | 0.62 | 60.28 | 66.32 | 0.50 |
| *Imin* | 43.78 | 40.61 | 0.39 | 25.83 | 27.61 | 0.60 |
| *J* | 105.97 | 99.48 | 0.53 | 87.01 | 93.93 | 0.52 |
| *Imax/Imax* | 1.38 | 1.44 | 0.36 | 2.33 | 2.49 | 0.38 |

BA, Bronze Age; N, Natufian

## Discussion

Although comparative population studies provide anthropologists with a valuable tool to study diachronic change in antiquity, there are many limitations to this type of research. For example, unless differences in sex ratios and age are acknowledged, results can be skewed by differences in paleodemography, and when comparative data collected by two different researchers is incorporated into a study, results can be skewed by inter-observer error. In order to minimize these problems, age and sex profiles were compared for the Bronze Age and Natufian populations, the same methodology was used to score dental attrition and oral pathology, and all cross-sectional moulds were processed and analyzed by the author. It should be noted, however, that the accuracy of the age and sex profiles for both the Natufian and Bronze Age populations are uncertain at best because of the fragmentary nature of the material, inter-observer inconsistencies, and problems inherent to paleodemographic reconstruction (cf. Wood *et al.* 1992), which may have introduced error. Although the results of any study of commingled remains should be viewed cautiously, valuable information can still be gained through careful analysis and consideration of these limitations while interpreting results.

### *Dental Attrition*

The Bronze Age population examined in the current study showed much lower rates of attrition than the Natufian populations studied by Eshed and colleagues (2006), which suggests that although the Bronze Age population generally lived longer, and teeth were exposed to attrition for a longer period of time on average, this was outweighed by environmental factors. The results documented indicate that the population from Jericho was consuming a much less abrasive diet than the Natufian population. This is most likely to be related to the consumption of softer foods in addition to technological innovations such as ceramic crockery, which allowed food to be cooked in water and effectively softened (Smith 1984; Powell 1985; Molleson *et al.* 1993).

### *Oral Pathology*

Rates of oral pathology were generally higher in the Jericho population than in the comparative Natufian populations studied by Eshed and colleagues (2006). Rates of dental calculus, periodontal disease, and AMTL were found to be statistically higher in the Bronze Age dentitions, while periapical lesions were more common but not to a significant degree. Counter-intuitively, however, dental caries, the pathological process most commonly associated with high carbohydrate dietary strategies (Cohen and Armelagos 1984; Steckel and Rose 2002; Larsen 2006), was lower in the Bronze Age population examined than the comparative Natufian populations.

The statistically higher rates of dental calculus, periodontal disease, and AMTL documented for the Bronze Age populations is likely the result of heavy reliance on domesticated plants high in carbohydrates, reliance on animal products high in protein, and if Hughes's (1965) age profile is accurate, longer exposure to environmental conditions that would have been conducive to the development of oral pathology. These findings are consistent with archaeological and paleobotanical evidence indicating that agriculturalist populations in the southern Levant consumed a variety of grains, fruits, vegetables, and animal products (Horwitz *et al.* 1999; Gopher *et al.* 2001; Issar and Zohar 2007). In fact, broad, protein-rich diets differentiate the southern Levant from other loci of domestication where prehistoric agriculturalists were primarily reliant on single staple crops.

These subsistence differences may explain rates of oral pathology documented in the population from Bronze Age Jericho. For example, although tentative, a positive correlation has been established between protein consumption and high rates of dental calculus (cf. Lieverse 1999). This is especially important to the current study, because high rates of dental calculus appear to be the key to understanding the oral pathology profile at Bronze Age Jericho: a high rate of dental calculus would be expected to be associated with a high rate of periodontal disease and AMTL because dental calculus is the primary pathological agent for periodontal disease and periodontal disease is the primary cause of AMTL (Lukacs 1989; Hillson 1996; Lieverse 1999). Furthermore, dental calculus (a mineralization process) has been documented to show an inverse relationship to dental caries (a demineralization process) at the population level, which may explain the low rate of caries in the Bronze Age population (Manji *et al.* 1989; Hillson 1996, 2001).

It should be noted, however, that the epidemiology of the pathological conditions studied are complex. For example the aetiology of dental calculus is not fully understood, and although there is evidence that protein rich diets show a correlation with high rates of dental calculus and calculus can show an inverse relationship to caries, these relationships are far from straightforward (cf. Lieverse 1999). Natural processes are also often difficult to differentiate from pathological processes. For example, dental eruption secondary to apical tooth wear may have led to an overestimate of periodontal disease, especially for the Natufian populations, which showed high rates of attrition (cf. Dean *et al.* 1992). Finally, because some individuals are predisposed to developing various oral pathologies, heterogeneity in risk is also an inherent problem (cf. Wood *et al.* 1992).

*Linear Enamel Hypoplasia*

The lack of a statistical difference in rates of LEH signifies that there is no evidence that health was markedly worse at Bronze Age Jericho than in the Natufian populations studied by Hershkovitz and Gopher (2008) as would have been expected (cf. Steckel and Rose 2002). Could the broad dietary strategy at Jericho also explain the lack of a statistically significant difference between Bronze Age and Natufian rates of LEH? It is possible that the broad dietary strategy at Bronze Age Jericho led to a reduction in the cases of LEH related to nutritional deficiency, while LEH resulting from infectious disease was not prevalent enough to cause a significant increase in the rate of LEH.

It should be acknowledged, however, that the results of the current study could be skewed by inter-observer inconsistencies as well as heterogeneity in risk and selective mortality (cf. Wood *et al.* 1992). Even so, the results presented here suggest that the transition to agriculture in the southern Levant may have effected health differently than other loci of domestication. Further research will be needed determine the validity of this interpretation.

*Cross-Sectional Geometry*

Analysis of cross-sectional geometry indicates that the Bronze Age population from Jericho had significantly stronger clavicles, humeri, and ulnae than the Natufian populations studied. The higher rates of hypertrophy noted in the bones of the Bronze Age population indicate that patterns of habitual behaviour at Jericho placed significantly more strain on the upper limbs than behavioural regimes at Natufian Ain Mallaha, Hayonim, and Nahal Oren. The cross-sectional properties of the Bronze Age and Natufian femora and tibia examined were not statistically different. Both the Natufian hunter-gatherers and the Bronze Age agriculturalists showed higher hypertrophy in the anteroposterior plane than the mediolateral plane, indicating that both populations were highly mobile.

When considered within an archaeological context, it is not surprising that the upper limbs of the agriculturalists from Bronze Age Jericho were significantly more robust than the Natufian populations studied. During the Early Bronze Age and again in the Middle Bronze Age, Jericho underwent periods of urban expansion and abandonment, which corresponded with periods of intensive agricultural production (Kenyon 1960; Joffe 1993; Marchetti 2000). The activities required to expand, fortify, and support an urban centre, undoubtedly required a huge investment of labour from the population and significantly higher mechanical demand on the upper limbs than would have been required from a population of Natufian hunter-gatherers.

Although it is not surprising that the populations of hunter-gatherers from Ain Mallaha, Nahal Oren, and Hayonim, were highly mobile, these results suggest that the population from Bronze Age Jericho was much more active than agriculturalists in other loci of domestication (cf. Larsen 1981; cf. Ruff *et al.* 1984); however, as Bridges' (1989) study indicates, this trend is not universal. The cross-sectional properties of femora and tibiae from Bronze Age Jericho indicate that agricultural production, the expansion and fortification of Jericho, and other activities required a significant investment of labour and a highly mobile population that exploited resources far beyond the walls of Jericho.

## Conclusions

Analysis of dental wear indicated that attrition was less severe in the Bronze Age populations than in the Natufian comparative populations. This is attributed to the consumption of less abrasive foods and the use of ceramic crockery, which allowed food to be cooked in water and softened.

Analysis of oral pathology indicated that rates of calculus, periodontal disease and AMTL were statistically higher in the Bronze Age population than the comparative Natufian populations. Periapical lesions were more common during the Early Bronze Age, but not to a significant degree, and surprisingly, rates of caries were lower in the Bronze Age sample. The high rates of pathology are attributed to a carbohydrate rich, high protein dietary strategy. The high rate of calculus likely increased the incidence of periodontal disease and AMTL, and also may have reduced rates of dental caries at the population level.

Analysis of LEH provided no indication that systematic stress was more common in the Bronze Age population than the Natufian populations. This is tentatively attributed to a broad dietary strategy leading to a reduction in nutritional stress.

Analysis of the cross-sectional properties of Bronze Age and Natufian clavicles, humeri, and ulnae indicated that the upper limbs of the inhabitants of the Bronze Age population were significantly more robust than the upper limbs of the Natufian populations. The expansion and fortification of Jericho as well as the diverse activities associated with supporting a large Bronze Age urban centre undoubtedly required a great deal of mechanical demand and account for this difference.

The cross-sectional properties of Bronze Age and Natufian femora and tibiae indicated that both populations were highly mobile. This is not surprising for hunter-gathers; however, it is somewhat atypical for agriculturalists. These results indicate that sedentary agriculture did not necessarily lead to a marked decline in ambulatory activities.

### Acknowledgements

This research was conducted with support from the Council for British Research in the Levant (CBRL), the American Center for Oriental Research (ACOR) and the Darwin College Travel Fund. I would like to thank my supervisor Dr. Jay Stock for the use of his Natufian data and for his help at every stage of this project. I also owe a debt of gratitude to Dr. Lisa Maher and Dr. Chris Knüsel for their help with this research and for their insightful comments. Finally, I would like to thank the curatorial staff at the Duckworth Laboratory (University of Cambridge) for allowing me to examine the material from Bronze Age Jericho, and ACOR for the use of their resources and library.

### Literature Cited

Allen, R.C. 1997. Agriculture and the origins of the state in Ancient Egypt. *Explorations in economic history* 34: 135-154.

Armelagos, G.J. and Dewey, J. 1970. Evolutionary response to human infectious disease. *Bioscience* 20: 271-275.

Arensburg, B., Goldstein, M.S., Nathan, H. and Rak, Y. 1980. Skeletal remains of Jews from the Hellenistic, Roman, and Byzantine periods in Israel. *Bulletins et Mem. de la Société Anatomique de Paris* 7: 175-186.

Aurenche, O., Galet, P., Regagnon-Caroline, E., and Evin, J. 2001. Proto-Neolithic and Neolithic cultures in the Middle East – The birth of agriculture, livestock raising, and ceramics: a calibrated 14C chronology 12,500-5500 cal BC. *Radiocarbon* 43: 1191-1202.

Banning, E.B. 2007. Late Prehistory in Wadi Ziqlab, al-Kura, Jordan: from sedentism to olive oil factories. In: Levy, T.E., Daviau, P.M.M., Younker, R.W. and Shaer, M. (eds.) *Crossing Jordan: North American contributions to the archaeology of Jordan*. Equinox Publishing Ltd., London. 219-223.

Belfer-Cohen, A. 1988. The Natufian graveyard in Hayonim Cave. *Paleorient* 14: 297-308.

Bentley, R., Pietrusewsky, M., Douglas, M. and Atkinson, T. 2005. Matrilocality during the prehistoric transition to agriculture in Thailand? *Antiquity* 79: 865-881.

Bellwood, P. 2001. Early agriculturalist population diasporas? Farming, languages, and genes. *Annual Review Anthropology* 30: 181-207.

Bocquet-Appel, J.-P. and Naji, S. 2006. Testing the hypothesis of a worldwide Neolithic demographic transition. *Current Anthropology* 47: 341-365.

Bridges, P. 1989. Changes in activities with the shift to agriculture in the Southeastern United States *Current Anthropology* 30: 385-394.

Brothwell, D.R. 1981. *Digging up bones: the excavation, treatment and study of human skeletal remains*. 3rd ed. Cornell University Press: Ithaca.

Buikstra, J., Konigsberg, L. and Bullington, J. 1986. Fertility and the development of agriculture in the Prehistoric Midwest. *American Antiquity* 51: 528-546.

Childe, V. 1936. *Man makes himself*. Watts and Co.: London.

Clarke, N.G., Carey, S.E., Srikandi, W., Hirsch, R.S. and Leppard, P.I. 1986. Periodontal disease in ancient populations. *American Journal of Physical Anthropology* 71: 173-183.

Cohen, M. 1977. *The food crisis in Prehistory: overpopulation and the origins of agriculture*. Yale University Press: New Haven.

Cohen, M.N. 1989. *Health and the rise of civilization*. Yale University Press: New Haven.

Cohen, M. and Armelagos, G. 1984. *Paleopathology at the origins of agriculture*. Academic Press: Orlando.

Dean, M.C., Jones, M.E. and Pilley, J.R. 1992. The natural history of tooth wear, continuous eruption and periodontal disease in wild shot Great Apes. *Journal of Human Evolution* 22: 23-39.

Dever, W.G. 2003. Chronology of the Southern Levant. In: Richard, S. (ed.) *Near Eastern Archaeology*. Eisenbrauns, Winona Lake, IN. 82-87.

Diamond, J. 1997. Location, location, location: the first farmers. *Science* 278: 1243-1244.

Diamond, J. and Bellwood, P. 2003. Farmers and their languages: the first expansions. *Science* 300: 597-603.

Eshed, V., Gopher, A., Gage, T.B. and Hershkovitz, I. 2004. Has the transition to agriculture reshaped the demographic structure of prehistoric populations? New evidence from the Levant. *American Journal of Phyical Anthropology* 124(4): 315-329.

Eshed, V., Gopher, A. and Hershkovitz, I. 2006. Tooth wear and dental pathology at the advent of agriculture: new evidence from the Levant. *American Journal of Physical Anthropology* 130: 145-159.

Frayer, D.W. 1989. Oral pathologies in the European upper Palaeolithic and Mesolithic. In: Hershkovitz, I. (ed.) *People and culture in change*. British Archaeological Reports: Oxford. BAR International Series (508i). 255–281.

Goodman, A.H., Armelagos, G.J. and Rose, J.C. 1980. Enamel hypoplasias as indicators of stress in three prehistoric populations from Illinois. *Human Biology* 52: 515-528.

Gopher, A., Abbo, S. and Lev-Yadun, S. 2001. The "when," "where," and "why" of the Neolithic revolution in the Levant. *Documenta Praehistorica XXVIII Neolithic Studies* 8: 49-62.

Guatelli-Steinberg, D.J. 2003. Macroscopic and microscopic analyses of linear enamel hypoplasia in Plio-Pleistocene South African hominins with respect to aspects of enamel development and morphology. *American Journal of Physical Anthropology* 120: 309-322.

Guerrero, E., Naji, S., and Bocquet-Appel, J-P. 2008. The signal of the Neolithic demographic transition in the Levant. In: Bocquet-Appel, J-P. and Bar-Yosef, O. (eds.) *The Neolithic demographic transition and its consequences*. Springer, New York. 57-80.

Hershkovitz, I. and Gopher, A. 2008. Demographic, biological and cultural aspects of the Neolithic revolution: a view from the Southern Levant. In: Bocquet-Appel, J. and Bar-Yosef, O. (eds.) *The Neolithic demographic transition and its consequences*. Springer: New York. 441-479.

Hillson, S. 1996. *Dental anthropology*. Cambridge University Press: Cambridge.

Hillson, S. 2001. Recording dental caries in archaeological human remains. *International Journal of Human Osteology* 11: 249-286.

Horwitz, L., Tchernov, E., Ducos, P., Becker, C., von den Driesch, A., Martin, L. and Garrard, A. 1999. Animal domestication in the Southern Levant. *Paleorient* 25: 63-80.

Hughes, D.R. 1965. Human bones: report on metrical and non-metrical aspects of E.B.-M.B. and middle Bronze Age human remains from Jericho (1957-8 excavations). In: Kenyon, K.M. (ed.) *Excavations at Jericho,* 2, Appendix H, British Schools of Archaeology in Jerusalem: London. 644-685.

Issar, A. and Zohar, M. 2007. *Climate change, environment, and history of the Near East.* 2nd Ed. Springer: New York.

Joffe, A.H. 1993. *Settlement and society in the early Bronze Age I and II, Southern Levant*. Sheffield: Sheffield Academic Press.

Kenyon, K. 1957. *Digging up Jericho*. Benn: London.

Kenyon, K. 1960. Excavations at Jericho, 1957-58. *Palestine Exploration Quarterly* 92: 88-108.

Larsen, C.S. 1981. Skeletal and dental adaptations to the shift to agriculture on the Georgia Bight. *Current Anthropology* 22: 422-423.

Larsen, C.S. 1995. Biological changes in human populations with agriculture. *Annual Review of Anthropology* 24: 185-213.

Larsen, C.S. 2006. The agricultural revolution as environmental catastrophe: implications for health and lifestyle in the Holocene. *Quaternary International* 150: 12-20.

Lieverse, A.R. 1999. Diet and aetiology of dental calculus. *International Journal of Osteoarchaeology* 9: 219-232.

Littleton, J. and Frolich, B. 1993. Fish-eaters and farmers: dental pathology in the Arabian Gulf. *American Journal of Physical Anthropology* 92: 427-447.

Lukacs, J.R. 1992. Dental paleopathology and agricultural intensification in South Asia: new evidence from Bronze Age Harappa. *American Journal of Physical Anthropology* 87: 133-150.

Lukacs, J. 1989. Dental paleopathology: methods of reconstructing dietary patterns. In: Iscan, M. and Kennedy, K. (eds.) *Reconstruction of life from the skeleton*. A.R. Liss: New York. 261-286.

Manji, F., Fejerskov, O., Baelum, V. and Nagelkerke, N. 1989. Dental calculus and caries experience in 14–65 year olds with no access to dental care. In: Ten Cate, J.M. (ed.) *Recent advances in the study of dental calculus*. IRL Press at Oxford University Press: Oxford. 223–234.

Marchetti, N. 2000. A middle Bronze II public building and residential quarter in the lower town. In: Marchetti, N. and Nigro, L. (eds.) *Excavations at Jericho, 1998: preliminary report on the second season of archaeological excavations and surveys at Tell es-Sultan, Palestine*. Eisenbrauns Winona Lake, IN. 193-281.

Marchi, D. 2008. Relationships between lower limb cross-sectional geometry and mobility: the case of a Neolithic sample from Italy. *American Journal of Physical Anthropology* 137: 188-200.

Martin, B., Burr, D.R. and Sharkley N. 1998. *Skeletal tissue mechanics*. Springer: New York.

Metress, J.F. and Conway, T. 1975. Standardised system for recording dental caries in prehistoric skeletons. *Journal of Dental Research* 54: 908.

Molleson, T., Jones, K. and Jones, S. 1993. Dietary change and the effects of food preparation on microwear patterns in the late Neolithic of Abu Hureyra, Northern Syria. *Journal of Human Evolution* 24: 455-468.

Ortner, D.J. and Putschar, W.G. 1981. *Identification of pathological conditions in human skeletal remains*. Academic Press: Amsterdam. Smithsonian Contributions to Anthropology 28.

Perrot, J. 1960. Excavations at "Eynan ("Ein Mallaha) preliminary report on the 1959 season. *Israeli Exploration Journal* 10: 14-22.

Peterson, J. 2002. *Sexual revolutions: gender and labor at the dawn of agriculture*. Altamira Press: Walnut Creek.

Pinhasi, R. and Pluciennik, M. 2004. A regional biological approach to the spread of farming in Europe. *Current Anthropology* 45: 59-82.

Pinhasi, R., Eshed, V. and Shaw, P. 2008. Evolutionary changes in the masticatory complex following the transition to farming in the Southern Levant. *American Journal of Physical Anthropology* 135: 136-148.

Powell, M.L. 1985. The analysis of dental wear and caries for dietary reconstruction. In: Gilbert, R.I. and Mielke, J.H. (eds.) *The analysis of prehistoric diets*. Academic Press: Orlando. 307-338.

Ruff, C.B. 1984. Allometry between length and cross-sectional dimensions of the femur and tibia in *Homo sapien sapiens*. *American Journal of Physical Anthropology* 65: 347-358.

Ruff, C.B. 1987.Sexual dimorphism in human lower limb bone structure: relationship to subsistence strategy and sexual division of labor. *Journal of Human Evolution* 16: 391-416.

Ruff, C.B. 1999. Skeletal structure and behavioral patterns of prehistoric Great Basin populations. In Hemphill, B.E. and Larsen, C.S. (eds.) *Understanding prehistoric lifeways in the Great Basin wetlands: bioarchaeological reconstruction and interpretation*. University of Utah Press: Salt Lake City. 290-320.

Ruff, C.B., Larsen, C.S. and Hayes, W.C. 1984. Structural changes in the femur with the transition to agriculture on the Georgia Coast. *American Journal of Physical Anthropology* 64: 125-136.

Smith, B.D. 1984. Patterns of molar wear in hunter-gatherers and agriculturalists. *American Journal of Physical Anthropology* 63: 39-56.

Smith, P. 1995. People of the Holy Land from prehistory to the recent past. In: Levy, T.E. (ed.) *The archaeology of society in the Holy Land*. Leicester University Press: London. 58-74.

Starling, A.P. and Stock, J.T. 2007. Dental indicators of health and stress in early Egyptian and Nubian agriculturalists: a difficult transition and gradual recovery. *American Journal of Physical Anthropology* 134: 520-528.

Steckel, R.H. and Rose, J.C. 2002. *The backbone of history, health and nutrition in the Western Hemisphere*. Cambridge University Press: Cambridge.

Stekelis, M. and Yizraely, T. 1963. Excavations at Nahal Oren: preliminary report. *Israel Exploration Journal* 13: 1-12.

Stock, J.T. 2002. A test of two methods of radiographically deriving long bone cross-sectional properties compared to direct sectioning of the diaphysis. *International Journal of Osteoarchaeology* 12: 335-342.

Stock, J.T. 2006. Hunter-gatherer postcranial robusticity relative to patterns of mobility, climatic adaptation, and selection for tissue economy. *American Journal of Physical Anthropology* 131: 194-204.

Stock, J.T. and Pfeiffer, S.K. 2004. Long bone robusticity and subsistence behaviour among later Stone Age foragers of the forest and Fynbos Biomes of South Africa. *Journal of Archaeological Science* 31: 999-1013.

Stock, J.T. and Pinhasi, R. 2011. Introduction: changing paradigms in our understanding of the transition to agriculture: human bioarchaeology, behaviour and adaptation. In: Pinhasi, R. and Stock, J.T. (eds.) *Human bioarchaeology of the transition to agriculture*. John Wiley & Sons, Ltd: Chichester. 1-13.

Tal, H. 1985. Periodontal bone loss in the dry mandibles of South African Blacks: a biometric study. *Journal of Dental Research* 6: 925-929.

Turner II, C.G. 1979. Dental anthropological indications of agriculture among the Jomon people of central Japan: X. Peopling of the Pacific. *American Journal of Physical Anthropology* 51: 619-636.

Ullinger, J.M., Sheridan, S.G., Hawkey, D.E., Turner II, C.G. and Cooley, R. 2005. Bioarchaeological analysis of cultural transition in the southern Levant using dental nonmetric traits. *American Journal of Physical Anthropology* 128: 466-476.

Wood, J.W., Milner, G.R., Harpending, H.C. and Weiss K.M. 1992. The osteological paradox: problems in inferring prehistoric health from skeletal samples. *Current Anthropology* 33: 343-370.

Zakrzewski, S. 2003. Variation in Ancient Egyptian stature and body proportions. *American Journal of Physical Anthropology* 121: 219-229.

# Where Have we Been, Where Are we Now, and What Does the Future Hold? Palaeopathology in the UK over the Last 30 Years, with a Few Bees in my Bonnet

Charlotte Roberts

Department of Archaeology
Durham University
South Road
Durham, DH1 3LE, UK

Email for correspondence: c.a.roberts@durham.ac.uk

**Abstract**

This paper describes the development of palaeopathology in the UK over the last 30 years, documenting how it was dominated by medical doctors, anatomists and dentists in the early years. This has now changed where most scholars derive from archaeology and anthropology backgrounds, and particularly from one year taught masters courses. Key milestones in palaeopathology's development are described, for example the establishment of BABAO, followed by strengths and weaknesses. Strengths include a national organisation (BABAO), many people working generally in bioarchaeology who are knowledge and skills trained, many masters courses that provide that training, and many more cemetery excavations providing skeletal samples for analysis. Weaknesses note that there are too many 'qualified' people working in the discipline, the consequence of the many masters courses that exist in UK universities, too few job/PhD opportunities, too many 'case studies' published compared to elsewhere in the world when compared to population based considerations, too much data on disease in the grey literature, too much concentration of work on specific skeletal samples in particular institutions, and no centralised skeletal database that contains data on all skeletal collections curated in the UK. The future for palaeopathology is considered, and a few 'bees in my bonnet' are noted.

**Keywords:** Disease, Evolutionary Medicine, Biomolecules, Database, Curation

## Introduction

This paper is a general overview of that presented at the Annual Meeting of the British Association of Biological Anthropology and Osteoarchaeology in Cambridge 2010. It covers the development of palaeopathology in the UK, including its history and key people. It documents specific important milestones, and UK contributions (from a global perspective), indicating strengths, weaknesses, opportunities and threats for palaeopathology in the UK, with a few 'pet peeves' or 'bees in my bonnet'. The reader is directed to other publications by the author that document some of the content of this paper in more detail (e.g. Roberts 2006; Roberts and Ingham 2008; Park *et al.* 2009; Roberts 2009; 2010; Roberts and Manchester 2010).

## The Early Years of Paleopathology

Early work in palaeopathology in the UK was primarily undertaken by medical doctors, dentists, anatomists, and nurses, and was very male dominated, unlike today where most people derive from archaeology and/or anthropology and are female. Analyses of evidence of disease took a predominantly clinical approach with little contextualisation of collected data, usually due to personnel not having an archaeological or anthropological background. This led to wonderful stories that were interesting reads, but often the data could not be supported by hard scientific evidence. In relation to the rest of the world, the development of palaeopathology in the UK appears to come rather late compared to other European countries such as the Netherlands, Germany, France, Italy and Portugal (see Roberts and Buikstra in press), but has clear and significant evidence of work from the early 20th century onwards. Some of those early scholars included Alexander Cave, Warren Dawson, Grafton Elliot Smith, Kenneth Oakley and Frederic Wood-Jones, with substantial work being completed by Smith and Wood-Jones on skeletal remains and mummies from Egypt and Sudan (e.g. Elliot Smith and Wood Jones 1910).

It was not until the 1950s that there appeared to be an increase in scholars working with human remains, with two key people developing the study of palaeopathology in significant directions. Those people were Calvin Wells (e.g. 1964) and Don Brothwell (e.g. Brothwell and Sandison 1967), the latter still pushing the discipline forward at the University of York, even though he is officially 'retired'! In more recent times, the late Juliet Rogers (University of Bristol), Simon Hillson and Tony Waldron (Institute of Archaeology, University College (UCL), London), and Keith Manchester (University of Bradford) have also been instrumental in developments in palaeopathology, and specific people have focused on particular areas such as dental pathology (Hillson), joint disease (Rogers, Waldron), and infectious disease (Manchester). However, in the early 1980s when the author first entered the field, there were relatively few scholars practicing palaeopathology in the UK, very little available training, no guidance documents, no national organisation such as the BABAO, no standards for recording, little infrastructure or funding, and importantly (or not!) no email or internet. Since then there have been great advances in all these aspects and loneliness in the profession cannot now be viewed as a challenge to progress!

## Key Milestones in Palaeopathology's Development in the UK

While the UK milestones have been documented elsewhere (Roberts 2006; Roberts in press), it is worth considering their impact on how palaeopathology has developed. In 1990 the first one year taught masters course in the study of human remains was established between the Universities of Bradford and Sheffield, although some training had been available at Sheffield and UCL during the 1980s. This was the first step towards what is now a very different landscape in the UK, one of many trained people and relatively few opportunities for employment in the field. However, this has not deterred (and did not deter) other universities from setting up masters courses focusing on both archaeological and forensic human remains.

At the same time as that first masters course, however, the guidance document PPG 16 (Department of the Environment 1990) came into force whereby all modern building development had to be preceded by developer funded archaeological investigation, including excavation. There rapidly became more opportunities for trained bioarchaeologists, or those people who study human remains, to be involved with excavation and analyses of funerary contexts. It was not until 2004 when standards for data recording were developed and published for the UK (Brickley and McKinley 2004), a full 10 years after those published in the USA (Buikstra and Ubelaker 1994). This followed Roberts and Cox's (2003) express statement that there was a worrying number of skeletal reports in the UK domain whose data were not up to scrutiny, and that standards needed to be established in order for data to be comparable.

In 1998 the BABAO was established which has providing some much needed infrastructure to the overall discipline of bioarchaeology, including an email list, a website (http://www.babao.org.uk), annual conferences, annual reviews of work in the field, and in recent times the development of Codes of Ethics and Practice (http://www.babao.org.uk/index/ethics-and-standards; accessed January 2011). An added development was the establishment of the *International Journal of Osteoarchaeology* in 1991 by Tony Waldron and Ann Stirland which quickly became an alternative outlet for publications on skeletal material from the UK, including palaeopathological evidence.

There are clear differences in how bioarchaeology, and particularly palaeopathology, has developed when compared to the very well established discipline in North America. Their national organisation was formed in 1913 (American Association of Physical Anthropologists - http://www.physanth.org/), and physical anthropology (including bioarchaeology) has been a part of Anthropology departments for many more years than in the UK where 'physical anthropology' remains a part of only a fraction of Anthropology and Archaeology departments in higher education institutions. This means that the subject has had a late introduction into Archaeology and Anthropology undergraduate degrees, and consequently the value of studying human remains has not been appreciated by archaeology as a whole until relatively recently.

However, in spite of the slow development of palaeopathology in the UK, there have been many contributions to the understanding of our past ancestors' experience of disease, including many texts that are widely used around the world (e.g. Brothwell 1981; Waldron 1994; Rogers and

Waldron 1995; Hillson 1996; Cox and Mays 2000; Roberts and Cox 2003; Pinhasi and Mays 2008; Roberts 2009; Roberts and Manchester 2010; Mays 2010a). Whilst most bioarchaeologists in the UK work on inhumed skeletons, there are some who deal with cremated burials, some of whom have contributed considerably to our knowledge of cremated burials, and of course evident pathological changes (e.g. McKinley 2006). Whilst 'Case studies' of specific pathological conditions have been, to date, the most prolific publication generated from the UK, with 'Population studies' a definite 'second', there are signs that those population based studies of health problems in the past are increasing, albeit less so than in North America (see Mays 2010b). In particular, however, the UK has contributed considerably to our understanding of the joint diseases and metabolic disorders in archaeology (e.g. Rogers and Waldron 1995; Brickley and Ives 2008), the infections (e.g. Manchester 2002), the dental diseases (Hillson 1996), and animal diseases (Brothwell 1991; Davies *et al.* 2005), amongst many others. Apart from specific contributions to understanding particular health insults, the UK has also generated for archaeology a plethora of reports on skeletons from funerary contexts (e.g. Wells 1982; White 1988; Miles 1989; Molleson and Cox 1993; Pinter-Bellows 1993; Lilley *et al.* 1994; Powell 1996; Rahtz *et al.* 2000; Fiorato *et al.* 2001; Brickley and Buteux 2006; Mays *et al.* 2007; Waldron 2007; Simmonds *et al.* 2008; Magilton *et al.* 2008; Connell *et al.* in press). There are now much more data available that can be used for comparison; it is also possible to identify gaps in our knowledge about past health in the UK, and also highlight skeletal samples that may be utilised for future research, assuming they remain above ground.

There are also increasingly more integrated holistic approaches to the consideration of illness in the past, and skeletal data for disease that are more useable because of the standardisation of data recording. In addition, because there are more people working in the discipline of bioarchaeology, archaeology as a whole is more aware of our potential contributions. Furthermore, many bioarchaeologists in the UK are called upon to sit on editorial boards of journals, both national and international, review grant applications and publications, and be part of committees for particular organisations. This has also been accompanied by more presentations at conferences, especially internationally, when in the 1980s very few people represented the UK at international meetings. Thus, our discipline is moving forward rapidly and making real contributions to understanding our ancestors' health and how that affected the functioning of their societies.

**Strengths and Weaknesses of Palaeopathology in the UK**

The UK is now in a much stronger contributory position in palaeopathology, from a global perspective. Much of this is due to the huge development in its infrastructure over the last 30 years, already outlined above. We now have:

- A national organisation (BABAO) with around 500 members
- Many people working generally in bioarchaeology who have knowledge and skills training
- Many masters courses that provide that training
- Many more cemetery excavations providing skeletal samples for analysis
- Many more curated skeletal collections
- More finance and facilities for work on human remains
- More studies that integrate different disciplines to access the history of health (e.g. medical history, earth sciences, biomolecular science)

There are also more funding bodies in the UK that are providing financial support for ambitious research projects using cutting edge techniques of analysis (e.g. stable isotope and ancient DNA analyses – Brown and Brown 2011). Alongside this development, a plethora of guidance documents have been published which help archaeologists, bioarchaeologists and museum curators to provide the best 'care and treatment' for our ancestors' remains during excavation, analysis, curation and display (e.g. McKinley and Roberts 1993; Historic Scotland 1997; O'Sullivan and Kilgore 2003; Brickley and McKinley 2004; English Heritage 2004; English Heritage/Church of England 2005; Department for Culture, Media and Sport 2005), including the recent establishment of an Advisory Panel on the Archaeology of Burials in England (APABE - http://www.britarch.ac.uk/apabe/). Finally, the UK has generated, and continues to generate, skeletal samples from a variety of different contexts and dates, ranging from the Late Upper Palaeolithic (*circa* 10,500-8000 BC – Barton 1999) to the post-medieval period (*circa* 1550-1850 AD), and in contexts from prehistoric burial mounds to organised rural and urban churchyard cemeteries and battlefield sites, crypts and hospitals. These sites are located in a variety of environments, including coastal, inland, highland and lowland, and at a range of latitudes, and many museums and other organisations curate remains for further research once the skeletal report has been completed. UK archaeology also provides us with a wealth of archaeological data (artefacts, ecofacts and structures), and often contemporary documentary and illustrative materials, that help us place our biological data for disease into context.

We are now at a point where there is in addition considerable interest in what we as bioarchaeologists do from many 'stake holders', not least the media. The latter has been clearly illustrated in recent television programmes such as 'Meet the Ancestors', 'Time Team', 'Digging Britain', and 'History Cold Case' along with more specialised documentaries often focused on one site, for example 'Headless Romans' (York).

How could there be weaknesses? Inevitably there are areas where bioarchaeology could improve. The following provides an indication of a few weaknesses that need to be worked on, and for some there are real challenges to overcome:

- Too many 'qualified' people working in the discipline in contract archaeology situations, the inevitable consequence of the many masters courses that exist in UK universities
- Too few job/PhD opportunities, or the result of too many masters graduates
- Too many 'case studies' compared to elsewhere in the world, perhaps the legacy of the dominance of the discipline by medical doctors, anatomists, and dentists in the early years (but palaeopathology studies are high overall)
- Too much data on disease in the grey literature
- Too much concentration on specific skeletal samples in particular institutions such that many skeletal samples lie curated in museums but are not used for research
- No centralised skeletal database that contains data on all skeletal collections curated in the UK

We are rather victims of our own success, and this success and interest in bioarchaeology has been exploited by Universities in their enthusiasm to run taught postgraduate courses in bioarchaeology. The consequence? Many masters graduates in bioarchaeology struggle to find employment, although they have many skills that are certainly transferable to other jobs, and there are relatively few funded PhD places to satisfy the demand of those masters graduates who wish to do research. Of course, many of those who come to the UK to do these courses return to their own countries, but the vast majority of students on these courses are UK citizens. With respect to 'case studies', Mays (2010b) has pointed out the contrast between the UK and US, in particular, and our predominant position in numbers published. While more population based studies of health are advocated for the peer reviewed literature (here meaning journals), if 'case studies' are developed for publication, they should provide a statement of their wider significance (period, location, culture, origins, debates), and/or the possibility that they might help future palaeopathological diagnosis (Mays 2010b). This is clearly the aim of the new *International Journal of Palaeopathology* (http://www.elsevier.com/wps/find/journaldescription.cws_home/723943/description#) if 'case studies' are published in this outlet. Finally, much data on disease is not published or widely accessible to all (e.g. see Roberts and Cox 2003 where nearly 40% of reports used for that study were unpublished). This means that they cannot be used for comparative purposes, or to identify gaps in knowledge or future research projects on the remains.

There are a further two (related) concerns. Firstly, much research on UK skeletal collections that has reached publication over the last 20 years concentrates on a limited number of skeletal collections in four geographic locations (comprising 64% of 352 papers in four journals between 1990 and 2009: see Roberts and Mays 2011). There are many possible reasons for this conclusion, including that some collections are well publicised via excellent and informative online databases such as that of the Museum of London (http://www.museumoflondon.org.uk/Collections-Research/LAARC/Centre-for-Human-Bioarchaeology/), or through previous publications, or that some collections may be too remote or take too much time and money to access. Additional factors may also be that work on less 'popular' collections has not been published (e.g. that in masters and PhD theses), that some research has been published in other outlets that were not covered in this study, and finally that some research that has generated many papers and dominated the journals accessed for the study in the last 20 years was research council funded. This latter reason relates to the fact that publication is required as a condition of funding.

In 2003, Roberts and Cox recommended the setting up of a centralised database for skeletal remains in the UK, a database that would be accessible to all and lead to spreading of the handling load on collections around the UK, and provide a more balanced picture of our ancestors' biological profiles, including their disease load. It is well known that excessive handling of skeletal remains can be very damaging to remains that can be very fragile and vulnerable to overuse (Caffell *et al.* 2001). Following unsuccessful, albeit highly rated, bids to the Arts and Humanities Research Council by the author and Andrew Millard, also at Durham University, frequent calls for a database continue. To avoid having a partial view of the health of past people, we need to know the location and nature of skeletal collections in the UK. This would save time for people searching for appropriate samples for research projects, would promote the use of collections nationally and spread the 'handling load', and it might also help museums resist pressure for reburial. Indeed the DCMS (2005: 22) advised: 'Museums should have a policy to compile and make public an inventory of their holdings of human remains'. It should however not be forgotten that there are immense pressures on curators of collections in terms of money, staff, space, demands from more users, and requests for repatriation and/or reburial of human remains.

## The Future for Palaeopathology in the UK

The future is indeed very bright for palaeopathology in the UK, but we should be perhaps more ambitious in what we try to achieve when we analyse human remains from archaeological sites i.e. 'think more outside the box'. There is a tendency by all working in palaeopathology worldwide to do 'more of the same' with different skeletal collections. Generating more searching questions to answer and hypotheses to test using skeletal samples will provide us with more nuanced understandings of past health and disease.

The late Phil Walker recently said that "The only justification for the study of skeletal remains from earlier human populations is that skeletal research yields information that is useful to modern people" (Walker 2008: 13). This is perhaps a statement to which we should pay a bit more heed. There is of course more to palaeopathology than only doing research that is useful to the living. However, it is probably because of the recent development in UK higher education of an emphasis on research that has 'impact' on the wider world and community beyond academia that academics, such as the author, have begun to question their research objectives. Nevertheless, it should be remembered that the U.S. based Paleopathology Association's motto translates into "Let the dead teach the living" (http://www.paleopathology.org/); yes, everything we produce (data and its interpretation) can potentially teach the living about the past, but we could be much more 'inventive' about the information so that it might help the living and contribute to predicting the future. The complimentarity between palaeopathology and the newly emerging discipline of evolutionary (Darwinian) medicine also needs development (Nesse and Williams 1994). This will help us better understand how the last 10,000 years of health changes has set the stage for what we are today (Larsen 2008).

Methods of analysis that can be applied to human remains in the UK have indeed advanced over the last 30 years, with the last 10-15 years seeing an increase in destructive analyses of human remains to measure stable isotopes (diet and mobility) and detect ancient DNA presence (mitochondrial and nuclear). Along with mobility studies primarily using strontium and oxygen isotope data (e.g. Montgomery and Evans 2006), ancient pathogen DNA analyses in the UK have been particularly world leading and have provided us with new information about the origin and evolution of the infectious diseases (e.g. Taylor *et al.* 1999 and see below). Many people in the UK have also been involved with providing data for the Global History of Health Project based at Ohio State University, United States (http://global.sbs.ohio-state.edu/: accessed January 2011). This has been particularly so for the most recent phase focusing on Europe where data on health has been collected in a standard way and collated from 17,000 skeletons across Europe, including the UK. The UK is certainly in a position to continue to contribute to this project as it enters its third phase. It can also through palaeopathology provide a 'long view' of disease focusing on its origin and evolution, in individuals and populations buried in UK funerary contexts, where gene, culture and environment relationships can be explored, using traditional (macroscopic) and non-traditional (e.g. biomolecular) analyses.

However, we should not forget that "Human remains are not just another artefact; they have potency, they are charged with political, evidentiary, and emotional meanings…" (Cassman *et al.* 2007: 1). There are increasing calls for reburial of human remains in the UK, and there is still much work to be done with regard to the laws surrounding burial excavation licenses issued by the Ministry of Justice (although see Pitts 2011; Roberts 2012: 38). Nevertheless, we must not lose sight of the fact that continuous dialogue must be maintained between interested parties for the overall 'good' of the human remains that are under discussion. As Buikstra (2006: 408) has said, 'The need for openness for communication, for mutual respect, and for initiatives that are of interest to all collaborating parties *is* global', and Sayer (2009: 204) has indicated that there is a '...need to continue a constructive contextual dialogue with both the legislators and all religious interest groups within the UK'. It should be remembered that 'Values of the anthropologists who do skeletal research will often differ dramatically from those of the descendants of the people' and that 'This cultural trend toward lack of contact with the dead has greatly increased the cultural gulf between the public that has little familiarity with death and skeletal researchers' (Walker 2008: 5). We are certainly in a position in palaeopathology to educate the general public about the value of human remains study and fill that 'cultural gulf' by bringing death into public and intellectual life (Sayer 2010).

**And Finally.....Some Bees in my Bonnet**

Having worked in palaeopathology for over 25 years, I have developed many 'bees in my bonnet', or 'pet peeves'. There are three major ones that will be briefly highlighted here for readers to ponder.

*1. Activity/Occupation: Can We Recognise It?*

Work is a major part of the life course today and would have been a key part of human behaviour in the past, whether during hunting and gathering, practising agriculture, or working in industries in urban contexts. There is a plethora of papers in the published literature pertaining to this subject. There has always been an interest in reconstructing activity based on skeletal indicators (e.g. Wells 1982), but until recently the scientific basis for doing so has not really been questioned (e.g. see critical evaluations by Waldron 1994; Rogers and Waldron 1995; Jurmain 1999; Jurmain and Roberts 2008; Cardoso and Henderson 2010). The use of skeletal 'markers' such as entheseal changes and osteoarthritis is problematic not least because they can both be caused by many factors, including increasing age. Furthermore, it is not possible to determine exactly what 'activities' a person/population did in any one day, week, month or year, or whether those activities changed through their life course, or seasonally etc. Bioarchaeologists should be much more discerning and careful about attributing 'occupations' to skeletons in the future unless hard scientific data is supportive.

*2. Ancient Pathogen DNA Analysis to Recognise Disease*

As noted above, scholars have used evidence of ancient DNA of pathogens to highlight important facts about infectious disease that were not known prior to this analytical method being applied to human remains. This has included confirmation of macroscopic diagnoses (e.g. Taylor *et al.* 2000), identification of actual frequencies of infections in a 'population' of skeletons that do not necessarily show skeletal signs of the disease (e.g. Gernaey *et al.* 1999), diagnosis of soft tissue diseases such as malaria (Taylor *et al.* 1997), diagnosis of infection from non-specific bone changes (Haas *et al.* 2000), and highlighting the specific organism causing the infection (e.g. Fletcher *et al.* 2003; Zink *et al.* 2004). We now know much more than we ever could about disease because of this development in analysis, but there remain problems about some of the data published and the methods used (see Cooper and Poinar 2000; Roberts and Ingham 2008; Wilbur *et al.* 2009). Some key points that were noted in Roberts and Ingham's 2008 survey of published papers were a lack of adherence to proper authentication procedures, lack of apparent controls for contamination, absence of independent replication of results, and problems with sampling, sample preparation and analytical procedures. There is clearly work to be done to make the data published more scientifically supportable.

*3. Reconstructing Impairment from Skeletal Remains*

Finally, the author would also highlight the care needed when trying to infer impairment and care of the impaired using skeletal remains. This is often done in bioarchaeology, but frequently with no scientific basis to do so (e.g. see Lebel and Trinkaus 2002, and a reply to that study by DeGusta 2003; also see Roberts 2000 for reflections on considering impairment). There have been some developments over the years since Dettwyler's (1991) seminal paper, and some reflective studies of individual skeletons have appeared (e.g. Hawkey 1998; Tilley and Oxenham 2011). Many more of these studies are needed to provide 'role models' for future work in this area. However, studies of the impaired often tend to be of individual skeletons referred to as a 'case'. Therefore, on a related point and from a personal point of view, it would be good to see less use of 'case' and 'specimen' being applied to descriptions of skeletal remains that represent once living people; again, this common practice in palaeopathology probably reflects the heavy influence medical doctors had on the development of palaeopathology in the early years, 'cases' and 'specimens' being commonly used terms used in medicine. Unfortunately, the words 'case' and 'specimen' conjure up glass pots containing human tissue. We should steer clear of using these terms in the future as a mark of respect for those whose remains we study.

Of course, there is still much work to do in palaeopathology in the UK, work that will develop as more skeletal remains from different contexts continue to be excavated. The world of archaeology and museums should, however, heed the conclusions of a now very old but still relevant and important paper (Buikstra and Gordon 1981). This emphasized that continuous curation of skeletal remains enables further information to be generated as new methods develop and more complex questions are generated about the past.

**Literature Cited**


Barton, N. 1999. The Late Glacial or Late Final Upper Palaeolithic colonization of Britain. In: Hunter, J. and Ralston, I. (eds.) *The archaeology of Britain. An introduction from the Upper Palaeolithic to the Industrial Revolution*. Routledge: London. 13-34.

Brickley, M. and Ives, R. (eds.) 2008. *Bioarchaeology of metabolic bone disease*. Academic Press: London.

Brickley, M. and Buteux, S. (eds.) 2008. *St Martin's uncovered: investigations in the churchyard of St Martin's-in-the-Bull Ring, Birmingham, 2001*. Oxbow Books: Oxford.

Brickley, M. and McKinley, J.I. (eds.) 2004. *Recording guidelines for the standards for human remains*. Institute of Field Archaeologists Paper 7. Institute of Field Archaeologists: Reading.

Brothwell, D. 1981. *Digging up bones*. British Museum (Natural History): London.

Brothwell, D. 1991. On zoonoses and relevance to palaeopathology. In: Ortner, D.J. and Aufderheide, A.C. (eds.) *Human paleopathology. Current syntheses and future options*. Smithsonian Institution Press: Washington DC. 18-22.

Brothwell, D. and Sandison, A.T. (eds.) 1967. *Diseases in antiquity*. Charles C. Thomas: Springfield, IL.

Brown, T. and Brown, K. 2011. *Biomolecular archaeology. An introduction*. Wiley-Blackwell: Chichester.

Buikstra, J.E. 2006. Repatriation and bioarchaeology: challenges and opportunities. In: Buikstra, J.E. and Beck, L.A. (eds.) *Bioarchaeology. Contextual analysis of human remains*. Elsevier: London. 389-415.

Buikstra, J.E. and Ubelaker, D. 1994. *Standards for recording human skeletal remains*. Arkansas Archaeological Survey: Fayetteville. Archeological Survey Research Seminar Series 44.

Buikstra, J.E. and Gordon, C.C. 1981. The study and restudy of human skeletal series: the importance of long-term curation. *Annals of the New York Academy of Sciences* 376: 449-465.

Caffell, A.C., Roberts, C.A., Janaway, R.C. and Wilson, A.S. 2001. Pressures on osteological collections: the importance of damage limitation. In: Williams, E. (ed.) *Human remains. Conservation retrieval and analysis. Proceedings of a conference held in Williamsburg, VA, Nov. 7th-11th 1999*. Archaeopress: Oxford. British Archaeological Reports International Series 934. 187-197.

Cardoso, F.A. and Henderson, C.Y. 2010. Enthesopathy formation in the humerus. Data from known age-at-death and known occupation skeletal collections. *American Journal of Physical Anthropology* 141: 550-560.

Cassman, V., Odegaard, N. and Powell, J. (eds.) 2006. *Human remains: a guide for museums and academic institutions*. Altamira Press: Lanham, Maryland.

Connell, B., Gray Jones, A., Redfern, R. and Walker, D. in press. *Spitalfields: a bioarchaeological study of health and disease from a medieval London cemetery. Archaeological excavations at Spitalfields Market 1991-2007*. Volume 3. Museum of London Archaeological Services: London.

Cooper, A. and Poinar, H.N. 2000. Ancient DNA: do it right or not at all. *Science* 289: 1139.

Cox, M. and Mays, S. (eds.) 2000. *Human osteology*

*in archaeology and forensic science*. Greenwich Medical Media: London.

Davies, J., Fabiš, M., Mainland, I., Richards, M. and Thomas, R. (eds.) 2005. *Diet and health in past animal populations: current research and future directions*. Oxbow: Oxford.

DeGusta, D. 2003. Aubesier 11 is not evidence of Neanderthal conspecific care. *Journal of Human Evolution* 45: 821-830.

Department for Culture, Media and Sport. 2005. *Guidance for the care of human remains in museums*. DCMS: London.

Department of the Environment. 1990. *Planning policy guidance note 16*. Her Majesty's Stationery Office: London.

Dettwyler, K. 1991. Can paleopathology provide evidence for 'compassion'? *American Journal of Physical Anthropology* 84: 375-384.

Elliot Smith G. and Wood Jones, F. 1910. *The archaeological survey of Nubia 1907-8. Volume 2. The human remains.* National Printing Department: Cairo.

English Heritage. 2004. *Human bones form archaeological sites. Guidelines for producing assessment documents and analytical reports*. English Heritage in association with the British Association of Biological Anthropology and Osteoarchaeology: Swindon.

English Heritage and Church of England. 2005. *Guidance for best practice of human remains excavated from Christian burial grounds in England*. English Heritage: London.

Fiorato, V., Boylston, A. and Knüsel, C. (eds.) 2001. *Blood red roses. The archaeology of a mass grave from the Battle of Towton AD1461*. Oxbow Books: Oxford.

Fletcher, H.A., Donoghue, H.D., Taylor, G.M., Van der Zanden, A.G.M. and Spigelman, M. 2003. Molecular analysis of *Mycobacterium tuberculosis* DNA from a family of 18th century Hungarians. *Microbiology* 149: 143-151.

Gernaey, A.M., Minnikin, D.E., Copley, M.S., Ahmed, A.M.S., Robertson, D.J., Nolan, J. and Chamberlain, A.T. 1999. Correlation of the occurrence of mycolic acids with tuberculosis in an archaeological populations. In: Pálfi, G., Dutour, O., Deák, J. and Hutás, I. (eds.) *Tuberculosis past and present*. Golden Book Publishers Ltd, Szeged and Tuberculosis Foundation: Budapest, Hungary. 275-282.

Haas, C.J., Zink, A., Molnar, E., Szeimies, U., Resichel, U., Marcsik, A. and Ardagna, Y. 2000. Molecular evidence of different stages of tuberculosis in ancient bone samples from Hungary. *American Journal of Physical Anthropology* 113: 293-304.

Hawkey, D. 1998. Disability, compassion and the skeletal record: using musculoskeletal stress markers (MSM) to construct an osteobiography from early New Mexico. *International Journal of Osteoarchaeology* 8: 326-340.

Hillson, S. 1996. *Dental anthropology*. University Press: Cambridge.

Historic Scotland. 1997. *The treatment of human remains in archaeology*. Historic Scotland Operational Policy Paper 5. Historic Scotland: Edinburgh.

Jurmain, R. 1999. *Stories from the skeleton. Behavioural reconstruction in human osteology*. Gordon and Breach Publishers: Amsterdam.

Jurmain, R. and Roberts, C.A. 2008. Juggling the evidence: the purported 'acrobat' from Tel Brak. *Antiquity* (Project Gallery) 82 (318): http://antiquity.ac.uk/projgall/jurmain/index.html

Larsen, C.S. 2008. *Human origins. Discovering physical anthropology*. WW Norton: London.

Lebel, S. and Trinkaus, E. 2002. Middle Pleistocene remains from the Bau de L'Aubesier. *Journal of Human Evolution* 53: 659-685.

Lilley, J.M., Stroud, G., Brothwell, D. and Williamson, M.H. 1994. *The Jewish burial ground at Jewbury*. Council for British Archaeology: York. The archaeology of York. The medieval cemeteries 12/3.

Magilton, J.R., Lee, F. and Boylston, A. (eds.) 2008. *'Lepers outside the gate'. Excavations at the cemetery of the hospital of St James and St Mary Magdalene, Chichester, 1986-7 and 1993*. Council for British Archaeology: York. Council for British Archaeology Research Report 158 and Chichester Excavations 10.

Manchester, K. 2002. Infective bone changes of leprosy. In: Roberts, C.A., Lewis, M.E. and Manchester, K. (eds.) *The past and present of leprosy. Archaeological, historical, palaeopathological and clinical approaches*. Archaeopress: Oxford. British Archaeological Reports International Series 1054. 69-72.

Mays, S. 2010a. *The archaeology of human bones*. 2nd edition. Routledge: London.

Mays, S. 2010b. Palaeopathology in Britain: a critical analysis of publications with the aim of exploring recent trends (1997-2000). *International Journal of Osteoarchaeology* 20: 497-507.

Mays, S., Harding, C. and Heighway, C. 2007. *Wharram XI: the churchyard*. York University Press: York.

McKinley, J.I. 2006. Cremation…the cheap option? In: Gowland, R. and Knüsel, C. (eds.) *Social archaeology of funerary remains*. Oxbow: Oxford. 81-88.

McKinley, J. and Roberts, C.A. 1993. *Excavation and post-excavation treatment of cremated and inhumed skeletal remains*. Institute of Field Archaeologists: Birmingham. Technical Paper 11.

Miles, A.E.W. 1989. *An early Christian chapel and burial ground on the Isle of Ensay, Outer Hebrides, Scotland with a study of the skeletal remains*. Tempus Reparatum: Oxford. British Archaeological Reports British Series 212.

Molleson, T. and Cox, M. 1993. *The Spitalfields project. Volume 2: the anthropology. The middling sort*. Council for British Archaeology: York. Research Report 86.

Montgomery, J. and Evans, J. 2006. Immigrants on the Isle of Lewis – combining funerary and modern isotope evidence to investigate social differentiation, migration and dietary change in the Outer Hebrides of Scotland. In: Gowland, R. and Knüsel, C. (eds.) *Social archaeology of funerary remains*. Oxbow: Oxford. 122-142.

Nesse, R.M. and Williams, G.C. 1994. *Why we get sick. The new science of Darwinian medicine*. Vintage Books: New York.

O'Sullivan, J. and Killgore, J. 2003. *Human remains in Irish archaeology*. The Heritage Council: Dublin.

Park, V., Roberts, C.A. and Jakob, T. 2009. Palaeopathology in Britain: a critical analysis of publications to explore recent trends. *International Journal of Osteoarchaeology* 19: 1-11.

Pinhasi, R. and Mays, S. (eds.) 2008. *Advances in human palaeopathology*. Wiley: Chichester.

Pinter-Bellows, S. 1993. The human skeletons. In: Crummy, N., Crummy, P. and Crossan, C. (eds.) *Excavations of Roman and later cemeteries, churches and monastic sites in Colchester, 1971-1988*. Archaeological Trust, Colchester. 62-92. Archaeological Report 9.

Pitts, M. 2011. News: human remains to be retained, pending details. *British Archaeology* May/June: 6.

Powell, F. 1996. The human remains. In: Boddington, A. (ed.) *Raunds Furnells. The Anglo-Saxon church and churchyard. Raunds area project*. English Heritage: London. 113-124. Archaeological Report 7.

Rahtz, P.A., Hirst, S. and Wright, S.M. 2000. *Cannington cemetery: excavations 1962-3 of prehistoric, Roman, post-Roman and later features at Cannington Park Quarry, near Bridgwater, Somerset*. Society for the Promotion of Roman Studies: London.

Roberts, C.A. 2000. Did they take sugar? The use of skeletal evidence in the study of disability in past populations. In: Hubert, J. (ed.) *Madness, disability and social exclusion. The archaeology and anthropology of 'difference'*. Routledge: London 46-59.

Roberts, C.A. 2006. A view from afar: bioarchaeology in Britain. In: Buikstra, J.E. and Beck, L.A. (eds.) *Bioarchaeology. Contextual analysis of human remains*. Elsevier: London. 417-439.

Roberts, C.A. 2009. *Human remains in archaeology: a handbook*. Council for British Archaeology: York.

Roberts, C.A. 2010. Adaptation of populations to changing environments: bioarchaeological perspectives on health for the past, present and future. *Bulletins et Mémoires de la Société d'Anthropologie de Paris* 22 (1-2): 38-46.

Roberts, C.A. 2012. *Human remains in archaeology: a handbook*. Revised and reprinted edition. Council for British Archaeology: York.

Roberts, C.A. in press. Development of palaeopathology in the UK. In: Buikstra, J.E. and Roberts, C.A. (eds.) *A global history of paleopathology: pioneers and prospects*. Oxford University Press: New York.

Roberts, C.A. and Buikstra, J.E. in press. Conclusions. In: Buikstra, J.E. and Roberts, C.A. (eds.) *A global history of paleopathology: pioneers and prospects*. Oxford University Press: New York.

Roberts, C.A. and Cox, M. 2003. *Health and disease in Britain: from prehistory to the present day*. Sutton Publishing: Stroud.

Roberts, C.A. and Ingham, S. 2008. Using ancient DNA analysis in palaeopathology: a critical analysis of published papers with recommendations for future work. *International Journal of Osteoarchaeology* 18: 600-613.

Roberts, C.A. and Manchester, K. 2010. *The archaeology of disease*.3rd edition. The History Press: Stroud.

Roberts, C.A. and Mays, S. 2011. Study and restudy of curated skeletal collections in bioarchaeology: a perspective on the UK and its implications for future curation of human remains. *International Journal of Osteoarchaeology* 21: 626-630.

Rogers, J. and Waldron, T. 1995. *Field guide to joint disease in archaeology*. John Wiley and Sons: Chichester.

Sayer, D. 2009. *Ethics and burial archaeology*. Duckworth: London.

Sayer, D. 2010. Archaeology, modernity and the death taboo. *World Archaeology* 42: 481-491.

Simmonds, A., Marquez-Grant, N. and Loe, L. 2008. *Life and death in a Roman city – excavation of a Roman cemetery with a mass grave at 120-122 London Road, Gloucester*. Oxford Archaeology: Oxford. Oxford Archaeology Monograph 6.

Taylor, G.M., Rutland, R. and Molleson, T. 1997. A sensitive polymerase chain reaction method for the detection of plasmodium species DNA in ancient human remains. *Ancient Biomolecules* 1: 193-203.

Taylor, G.M., Goyal, M., Legge, A.J., Shaw, R.J. and Young, D. 1999. Genotypic analysis of *Mycobacterium tuberculosis* from medieval human remains. *Microbiology* 145: 89-904.

Taylor, G.M., Widdison, S., Brown, I.N. and Young, D. 2000. A mediaeval case of lepromatous leprosy from 13th-14th century Orkney, Scotland. *Journal of Archaeological Science* 27: 1133-1138.

Tilley, L. and Oxenham, M.F. 2011. Survival against the odds: modeling the social implication of care provision to seriously disabled individuals. *International Journal of Palaeopathology* 1: 35-42.

Waldron, T. 1994. *Counting the dead. The epidemiology of skeletal populations*. John Wiley and Sons: Chichester.

Waldron, T., with contributions from Rodwell, W. 2007. *St Peter's, Barton-on-Humber, Lincolnshire – a parish church and its community. Volume 2: the human remains*. Oxbow Books: Oxford.

Walker, PL. 2008. Bioarchaeological ethics: a historical perspective on the value of human remains. In: Katzenberg, M.A. and Saunders, S.R. (eds.) *Biological anthropology of the human skeletons*. Wiley-Liss: New York. 3-40.

Wells, C. 1964. *Bones, bodies and disease*. Thames and Hudson: London.

Wells, C. 1982. The human burials. In: McWhirr, A., Viner, L. and Wells, C. (eds.) *Romano-British cemeteries at Cirencester*. Excavations Committee: Cirencester. 135-202.

White, W. 1988. *Skeletal remains from the cemetery of St Nicholas Shambles, City of London*. Museum of London: London.

Wilbur, A.K., Stone, A.C., Roberts, C.A., Pfister, L., Buikstra, J.E. and Brown, T.A. 2009. Deficiencies and challenges in the study of ancient tuberculosis DNA. *Journal of Archaeological Science* 36: 1990-1997.

Zink, A., Sola, C., Reischel, U., Grabner, W., Rastogi, N., Wolf, H. and Nerlich, A. 2004. Molecular identification and characterization of *Mycobacterium tuberculosis* complex in ancient Egyptian mummies. *International Journal of Osteoarchaeology* 14: 404-413.

# The Paleoparasitology of 17th-18th Century Spitalfields in London

Evilena Anastasiou,*[1] Piers D Mitchell[1] and Nigel Jeffries[2]

[1]Department of Archaeology and Anthropology
University of Cambridge
The Henry Wellcome Building
Fitzwilliam Street
Cambridge CB2 1QH, UK

[2]Museum of London Archaeology
Mortimer Wheeler House
46 Eagle Wharf Road
London N1 7ED, UK

*Email for correspondence: ea333@cam.ac.uk

**Abstract**
This presents the paleoparasitological findings from the analysis of five coprolites from 17th and 18th century London. The preserved faeces were analysed using both microscopic and immunological techniques (ELISA). Two parasite species, the whipworm and roundworm were identified, but there was no evidence for dysentery. The results of the present analysis further our knowledge of intestinal health of London's past, and promotes our understanding of the interaction between parasitic disease and the cultural environment. The present study is a part of a major project with Museum of London Archaeology that aims to investigate the introduction and spread of parasitic diseases throughout London's history.

**Keywords:** Paleoparasitology, London, Health, Dysentery, Intestinal Parasites

## Introduction to Parasites and Paleoparasitology

Parasites (παράσιτο; παρά (para)=near + σίτος (sitos)=food) are defined as "any life form, or any organic compound capable of multiplying, that finds its ecological niche in another living form" (Araujo *et al.* 2003: 5-6). Parasites are today one of the major causes of ill health and premature death. Malaria, amoebic dysentery, sleeping sickness, and hookworm infection are but a few examples of commonplace parasitic diseases endemic in many parts of the developing world (Armelagos *et al.* 2005). Inadequate sanitation, lack of clean drinking water and consumption of poorly cooked fish and meat have always been the main causes for the acquisition of the many common intestinal parasites. Parasitic infections have run hand in hand with our evolution (Cox 2002), and thus the parasites found today are either parasites inherited from our ancestors or parasites acquired during our biological and social evolution (Araujo *et al.* 2008). Therefore, even before the appearance of *Homo sapiens* the parasitic diseases have always been important and common health stressors.

The field that studies the parasites that were present in the past is known as paleoparasitology (Ferreira *et al.* 1979) or archaeoparasitology (Reihnard 1990). This allows the extraction and study of parasite markers from archaeological contexts. When found, these parasite markers, which in the majority of cases are the eggs of intestinal species, provide hard evidence for the health status in the past. Paleoparasitology focuses on the intestinal parasites whose eggs survive best in the archaeological record. The intestinal parasites can be categorised into two groups, the protozoa and the helminths (or parasitic worms). The protozoa are single-cell organisms capable of carrying out vital functions such as reproduction, feeding and locomotion with two diagnostic life-cycle stages; the cyst and the adult trophozoite stage (Garcia 2007). The helminths are multicellular organisms with different life-cycles according to their species. They all start their lives as embryonated eggs and they reach adulthood through different stages of larval development, which in some species may occur in intermediate hosts (Bennett 2006).

Although the first paleoparasitological study is thought to date to 1910 (Ruffer 1910), the field started to evolve in its own right after the 1960s, due to methodological and theoretical advancements in both archaeology and parasitology. While the emergence of 'New Archaeology' and the development of interdisciplinary studies in archaeology were the stimuli for increased interest in the parasitic environment of past communities, the work of Callen and Cameron (1960) allowed the extraction of parasites from dehydrated coprolites and disintegrated soil, initiating the methodology currently used in the paleoparasitological studies (Bryant and Dean 2006). Moreover, at the beginning of 1970s, Aidan Cockburn (1971; Cockburn *et al.* 1975) hypothesised the correlation of cultural development with the evolution of infectious diseases, thus further promoting the interest of archaeology in parasitological studies. Today, paleoparasitology has overcome the methodological challenges and scepticism of the past and gained its deserved position as a distinct discipline that gives valuable insights in the health status, hygiene conditions and dietary habits of past communities.

As a field that combines archaeology with parasitology, paleoparasitology is interested both in the antiquity and pathogenicity of the parasitic diseases and in the impact the parasitic diseases had on the cultures of antiquity. Therefore, one of the most important objectives of paleoparasitology is to assess the impact of cultural change on parasitism, as the prevalence of parasites is related to subsistence behaviours, settlement patterns and sanitation, which in turn are influenced by large-scale cultural developments such as agriculture and urbanisation (Calagero *et al.* 2003). Therefore, paleoparasitology tries to explain the connection between the rise of parasitic diseases and the development of complex societies (Reinhard and Araujo 2008). At the same time, it is also interested in the antiquity and pathogenicity of the parasitic diseases, in the antiquity of host-parasite co-evolution and in the prehistoric distribution of parasites (Araujo and Ferreira 1996; Araujo *et al.* 1998; Araujo and Ferreira 2000). This dual interest of the field mirrors the complexity of the parasites' life cycle that both affects and is affected by environmental and cultural factors.

## Materials

For the purposes of the present study, five coprolites in features dated to the 17th and 18th century AD were analysed. The coprolites were retrieved during the excavations conducted by Museum of London Archaeology in the area of Spitalfields, in the East End of London between 1991 and 2004. The five coprolites were found from sieving environmental material of brick-lined cesspools, located in the backyard of residential buildings in Spitalfields (Table 1).

**Table 1:** Information on the coprolites analysed in this study

| Coprolite number* | Found in | Date |
|---|---|---|
| Coprolite [109] <6> | Barrel lined latrine in the backyard of No.23 Duke Street | 1683-1700 |
| Coprolite [2131] <101> | Brick-lined cesspit in the backyard of No. 24 Fort Street | 1730s |
| Coprolite[33363] <764> | Brick-lined cesspit in the backyard of No. 5 Fort Street | 1680-1700 |
| Coprolite[35309] <769> | Brick-lined cesspit in the backyard of No. 8 Steward Street | 1680-1740 |
| Coprolite [35245] <767> | Brick-lined cesspit in the backyard of No. 9 Steward Street | 1680-1740 |

*Number in [ ] refers to the context number, while number in <> refers to the sample number.

The term 'coprolite' (κοπρόλιθος; κόπρος (kopros)= faeces+λίθος (lithos)= stone) was first coined in 1829 by William Buckland (Horne 1985) and has since been used to describe any desiccated or mineralised faecal material. Along with the mummified remains and the soil samples from latrines, cesspools and inhumations, coprolites are one of the most important sources of material for paleoparasitology (Reinhard *et al.* 1986; Bathurst 2005). Besides mummies, coprolites are the only other material that allows for an almost ideal preservation of the parasite eggs and sometimes of the larvae (Araujo and Ferreira 2000). The degree of preservation of the parasite eggs dependent upon the processes involved in transforming the faecal material into coprolites through its desiccation and mineralisation.

The paleoparasitological analysis of coprolites instead of soil samples from latrines and cesspools, presents specific benefits and certain disadvantages, related to the fact that the coprolites, as well as the soil samples from burials, have a limited depositional history as they represent an individual faecal event from an individual defecator (Sobolik 1988; Bathurst 2005). Therefore, when analysing coprolites and/or soil from the pelvic area of burials we can potentially infer the proportion of individuals in a population that suffered from intestinal parasites and the differences in the parasitic load between the different ages, sexes and social classes (Fugassa *et al.* 2006). In contrast to the samples from latrines and cesspools, the analysis of coprolites can only demonstrate which species of intestinal parasite were present in the individuals tested and may not be representative of the wider community from which they came (Mitchell and Tepper 2007). Furthermore, information on how the prevalence of intestinal disease changes throughout time based upon coprolite studies is only as good as the dating of those coprolites.

**Methods**

The five coprolites under study were analysed using microscopic and immunological techniques. For the purposes of the analysis only one gram of each coprolite was analysed. It was thought best to analyse only a part of each coprolite to preserve the rest for the future, as further advances in the field's methodology may enable more complex analysis of the material at a later date.

Prior to the analysis, the samples were submerged for 72 hours in a 0.5% aqueous solution of trisodium phosphate. This process disaggregates the coprolite structure so that the parasite eggs can be viewed as freestanding elements, not obscured by adherent minerals or plant components of the coprolite (Araujo et al., 1998). After their disaggregation, the samples were passed through a series of micro-sieves in order to separate the parasite eggs from the coprolites' components. The eggs of the intestinal parasites have dimensions that range between 30μm to 150μm, depending on the species. Hence, by sieving the samples though increasingly smaller micro-sieves, one can separate the eggs from the larger and smaller contents of the coprolites (Bouchet *et al.* 1999; 2001). For the purposes of the present analysis, the coprolite samples were sieved through three micro-sieves (300μm, 160μm and 20μm). The material with the right dimensions to contain parasite eggs was thus concentrated on the 20μm micro-sieve and was then microscopically examined to identify any parasite eggs. For the present analysis, the use of micro-sieves instead of chemicals such as the hydrochloric and hydrofluoric acid was preferred, since it is safer and more environmentally friendly. The chemicals separate the parasite eggs from the coprolite/soil's components by dissolving any calcium carbonates and any silicates contained in the samples.

With the use of micro-sieves the separation of any helminth eggs from the coprolites' components was rendered possible. However, in contrast with the helminth eggs, the protozoan cysts that cause dysentery cannot usually be identified microscopically, since they are less resistant to taphonomic processes and they rarely survive intact in the archaeological material (Goncalves *et al.* 2004; Le Bailly *et al.* 2008). Therefore, in order to investigate whether any protozoan cysts were also present in the samples, we employed a biomolecular method called ELISA (Enzyme-Linked Immunosorbent Assay). ELISA is able to detect the cyst wall fragments and the proteins secreted uniquely by each of the protozoa that cause dysentery (*Cryptosporidium parvum, Entamoeba histolytica* and *Giardia duodenalis*) via antibodies specific for each microorganism (Goncalves *et al.* 2004; Mitchell *et al.* 2008). In clinical microbiology, ELISA has proven to be more sensitive and specific than microscopy for the detection of the protozoa responsible for dysentery (Addiss *et al.* 1991; Garcia 1999). Additionally, it can also differentiate between the morphologically identical pathological *Entamoeba histolytica* that causes dysentery and the non-pathological *Entamoeba dispar* that causes no symptoms at all (Haque *et al.* 1995; Haque *et al.* 1998; Goncalves *et al.* 2004).

The ELISA kits used for the detection of the protozoan cysts of *Entamoeba histolytica Giardia duodenalis* and *Cryptosporidium parvum* in the coprolites under study, were developed and manufactured by TechLab. The ELISA kits have, according to the manufacturer, a specificity of 100% for all three of the protozoa under study, and a sensitivity of 100% for both *Giardia duodenalis* and *Entamoeba histolytica*. The sensitivity for the *Cryptosporidium parvum* kit is stated to be 97.7%. Each kit has several wells in which few drops of disaggregated samples are placed. A positive sample is demonstrated if the well's colour is turned to deep yellow, quantified by a spectrometer at 450nm. Multiple cysts are required in each well in order to give a positive result, varying from 10-15 cysts for *Giardia duodenalis* to 78-156 for *Cryptosporidium parvum* (TECHLAB® kit booklets).

**Results**

Microscopic examination of the sieved material revealed that two of the five coprolites contained parasite eggs. Coprolite [33363] <764> had eggs of whipworm (*Trichuris trichiura*) and of roundworm (*Ascaris lumbricoides*) (Fig. 1). Coprolite [109] <6> contained multiple eggs of whipworm (*Trichuris trichiura*) (Fig. 2).

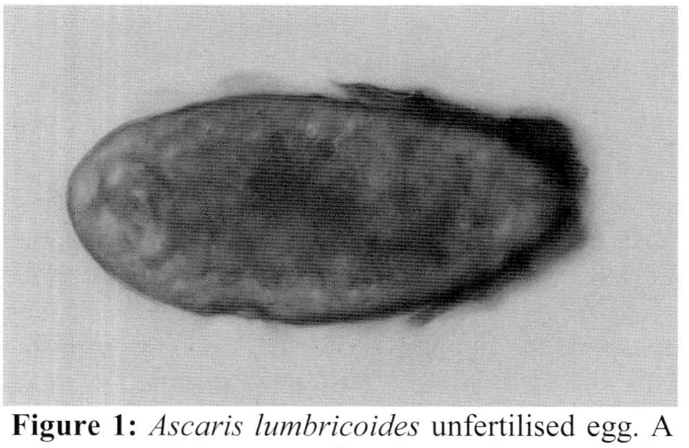

**Figure 1:** *Ascaris lumbricoides* unfertilised egg. A major part of the mammillated coat that covers the outline of the egg has fallen off. The egg is 89.19μm long and 43μm wide.

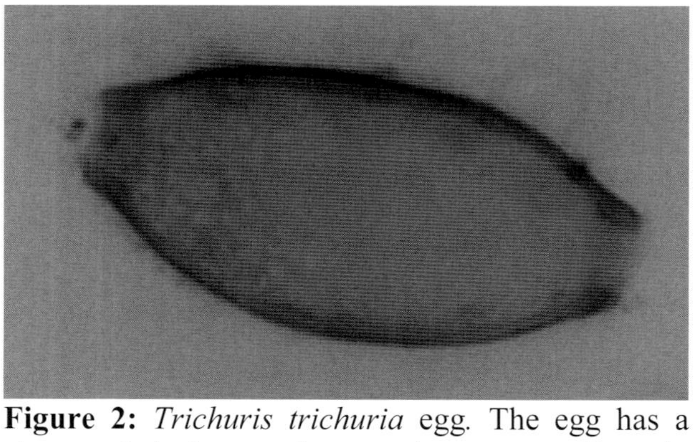

**Figure 2:** *Trichuris trichuria* egg. The egg has a characteristic lemon shape and measures 50μm in length and 23μm in width.

As seen in Figure 1, the roundworm found in coprolite [33363] <764> is unfertilised because it is more elongated than a fertilised egg. The egg has lost the part of the outer mammillated coat, but this is not unusual in archaeological samples. While unfertilised *Ascaris* eggs from non-human species of the genus can appear similar to this, there are several reasons as to why the egg is likely to be *Ascaris lumbricoides*, the human species. The shape and the size of the coprolite is typical for human faeces, the shape and size of the egg matches that of unfertilised *Ascaris lumbricoides* eggs, and the coprolite also contains multiple eggs of the human whipworm (*Trichuris trichiura*). Moreover, the human origin of the coprolite is also supported by the fact that the coprolite came from a cesspool found in the backyard of a house in a residential area of industrialised London, where faeces of farm animals were unlikely to be deposited. Thus, for the above reasons we argue that the roundworm egg found in the coprolite is the human roundworm *Ascaris lumbricoides*.

Roundworms and whipworms are today two of the most common intestinal parasites with a cosmopolitan distribution (Bennet 2006). They both have a faecal-oral transmission, and since they both require moist, warm soils, rich in oxygen to allow for the embryonation of the eggs, they almost always co-occur in the same area and/or even in the same individual (Reinhard and Araujo 2008; Leles *et al.* 2010). This association between roundworms and whipworms has been shown by many paleoparasitological studies both in the Americas and in Europe (Bouchet *et al.* 2003; Goncalves *et al.* 2003).

*Ascaris lumbricoides* is the largest of the intestinal nematodes found in man, with the male being 15-31cm in length and the female 20-49cm. The worms of *Ascaris* are relatively simple structured organisms with a complete digestive tract. Once hatched in the intestines they undergo an incredible migration, with the first stage larvae penetrating intestinal wall and appearing as second stage larvae in the liver within six hours after the infection. In the liver, the larvae develop into their third stage and migrate to the heart and the lungs. Eight to ten days after the infection, the larvae work their way back to the small intestine, where they reach maturity. The mature female then starts to lay about 200,000 eggs per day (Bennet 2006; Garcia 2007). The eggs of the *Ascaris lumbricoides* can be fertilised or unfertilised. The fertile eggs are oval in shape with an irregular bumpy (mammillated) surface, while they normally measure between 45-75μm by 35-50μm. The unfertilised eggs are longer and narrower than the fertile ones, measuring 85-95μm by 35-50μm (Fig.1). Although small burdens with *Ascaris* can be asymptomatic, heavy burdens can cause intestinal blockage and abdominal pain. In children, heavy burdens of roundworms cause nutritional impairment, vitamin deficiencies, anaemia and stunted growth, since children are less able to tolerate parasites that compete with them for energy and nutrients in their food.

*Trichuris trichiura* was the second species identified in the coprolites under study. This parasite is more commonly known as whipworm due to the whip-like form of the adult worm. The female worm reaches 35-50mm in length, while male is smaller with a length of 30-45mm. Whipworms are characterised by an enormously elongated capillary-like oesophagus and by their lemon-shape eggs. The eggs have characteristic bipolar plugs in each end and they measure between 50-54μm by 22-23μm (Fig. 2) (Schmidt and Roberts 2006). Once the embryonated eggs of *Trichuris* are swallowed by the human host, larvae are released into the upper duodenum that either invade the intestinal wall or attach themselves to the villi of the small intestine. After a few days, the larvae migrate towards the caecum, where they attach themselves to the mucosa, their final attachment place. In the caecum, the larvae reach maturity as adult worms three months after the ingestion of the infective eggs. The mature female then starts to lay 2,000-10,000 eggs per day. When passed out with the faeces, the eggs need a period of embryonation in the soil between two weeks to several months before they can re-infect another host (Bennet 2006). Although most infections with whipworms are asymptomatic, a heavy burden may damage the intestinal mucosa due to the adult worm being threaded into the epithelium of the caecum. Moreover, a heavy infection may also cause anaemia, growth retardation and eosinophilia. As was the case for the roundworms, children may exhibit symptoms from a whipworm infection more often than adults (Bennet 2006).

Dysentery was absent in all five of the coprolites under study as tested by ELISA. Dysentery normally causes diarrhoea, which by definition prevents the formation of formed stools and therefore of coprolites. Nevertheless, it was thought important to test the coprolites for dysentery since in the initial steps of infection, before the excystation of the mature cysts into the infective trophozoite stage, diarrhoea is absent. Diarrhoea is also absent in chronic carriers of dysentery organisms, who recover from dysentery to have no further symptoms but still shed the parasites to others in their stool.

**Discussion**

Paleoparasitological studies have been carried out in Britain since 1955, when Taylor (1955) found the eggs of *Trichuris trichiura, Ascaris lumbricoides* and *Dicrocoelium dendriticum* in 12$^{th}$ century AD deposits from Winchester. More paleoparasitological studies followed in Roman and Medieval Winchester (Pike and Biddle 1966; Pike 1967; Pike 1968), Bronze Age Somerset (Jones and Nicholson 1988), Roman and Tudor York (Wilson and Rackham 1976), Medieval Southampton (Pike 1975), Medieval Worcester (Moore 1981), Roman Cambridgeshire (Wells and Dallas 1976), Middle Saxon London (Tibesky and Sidell 2003) and Roman, Saxon and Medieval London (De Rouffignac 1985). The parasitic findings from these sites were eggs of *Trichuris trichiura* (whipworm), *Ascaris lumbricoides* (roundworm), *Taenia* (beef/pork tapeworm), *Dicrocoelium dendriticum* and *Diphyllobothrium latum* (fish tapeworm), *Fasciola hepatica* (liver fluke) and *Echinococcus granulosus* (dog tapeworm).

As far as we are aware, the present study is the first to analyse material from London dated in the early modern times, during the Stuart and Georgian Periods. The five analysed coprolites are dated in the 17$^{th}$ and 18$^{th}$ century, a period during which Spitalfields was renowned for its silk industry, which flourished after the establishment of French Protestant refugees (Hugeunots) in the area. The Hugeunots fled from France after the Revocation of the Edict of Nantes in 1685, and by settling in an area outside the bounds of the City of London, such as Spitalfields, were able to establish their silk industry avoiding the restrictive legislation of the City Guilds (Cox 1996; Thomas 2004). The paleoparasitological analysis of the five coprolites revealed the presence of roundworms and whipworms, species that have already been identified in Britain in the Bronze Age and Roman period contexts respectively (Jones and Nicholson 1988; Wilson and Rackham 1976).

Both roundworms and whipworms are transmitted in the same way, through faecal-oral contamination. Therefore, inadequate sanitation, crowding and contamination of the food and water supplies with faecal waste through its inadequate disposal or through its utilisation as fertiliser, are the main factors that promote infection. It is well known that during the Enlightenment and the Industrial Revolution (17$^{th}$ and 18$^{th}$ centuries) the hygiene conditions that prevailed in London were inadequate to prevent such infections (Molleson and Cox 1993; Roberts and Cox 2003). Almost half of the working class did not have provision for sewage disposal or access to clean water. Although after the mid-18$^{th}$ century the importance of personal hygiene started to be stressed, only a few bathed more often than annually (Roberts and Cox 2003). It is therefore not surprising to find that almost half of the analysed samples were infected with either roundworms or whipworms that are associated with poor sanitation.

Although only five coprolites were analysed for the purposes of this study, the fact that almost half of them were infected with parasites may be suggestive of the proportion of individuals affected by intestinal parasites in 17-18th century Spitalfields. Further paleoparasitological studies in a wider geographical area of London are needed in order to understand better the prevalence of the intestinal diseases and their impact on the health status of the London citizens during the 17th and 18th century.

Additionally, material dated throughout London's history must also be analysed in order to reconstruct the introduction and evolution of the parasitic diseases in the city. Through a wide chronological analysis, the impact of the parasitic diseases on the health status of Londoners, as well as the impact of the hygiene conditions and dietary habits on the transmission of the parasitic diseases will be better understood. Moreover, the impact of human migrations such as the crusades, the discovery of the New World, the African slave trade and British colonialism upon the introduction of new parasitic diseases in London will be better understood. The above underline the importance of the paleoparasitological project organised with the Museum of London Archaeology, of which the present analysis is part.

The present study is the first to use ELISA in an attempt to identify the protozoa that cause dysentery in samples from Britain. This reflects the fact that although ELISA is widely accepted as a highly sensitive, specific and rapid technique in clinical microbiology (Aldeen *et al.* 1998; Garcia *et al.* 2000), until recently its application in archaeoparasitological studies was limited (Goncalves *et al.* 2002; Le Bailly *et al.* 2008; Mitchell *et al.* 2008). Nevertheless, the ability of the immunological techniques to identify parasitic remains in cases where their identification would be impossible with microscopic examination renders them a valuable tool in the advancement of archaeoparasitology (Le Bailly *et al.* 2008). It is our hope that the immunological techniques will start to occupy an ever increasing role in the paleoparasitological studies, so permitting the identification of dysentery from archaeological samples.

As already mentioned, coprolites present some of the best conditions for preservation of parasite eggs. Nonetheless, the loss of the major part of the mammillated coat from the unfertilised *Ascaris* egg, as well as the loss of the bipolar plugs from many *Trichuris* eggs, underlines the need to exercise care when identifying parasite eggs from archaeological contexts. It is always necessary to keep in mind that even species whose eggs have protective structures against the rapid decay, such as the *Ascaridae* and *Trichuridae,* undergo changes after few centuries in the soil. The extent of the changes depends, among other factors, on the parasite species, the acidity of the soil, the time the egg remained in the archaeological record and the method used for the extraction of the egg. It is therefore important to be aware that a parasite egg from an archaeological context will always look different to a certain degree from a modern egg. Therefore, the contextual information of archaeological samples must be kept in mind when interpreting the results of the analysis. In the case of the present study, such an assessment of the contextual information supports the identification of an unfertilised *Ascaris lumbricoides* egg from London.

## Conclusions

Paleoparasitology is a relatively small branch of biological anthropology that provides an innovative approach to analyse and interpret the material from archaeological contexts in order to answer questions of importance for the archaeological discipline. The field has already succeeded in enriching our knowledge regarding the evolution of parasites and their hosts, the migratory paths chosen by prehistoric populations and the consequences of parasitism in past civilisations. The present study identified two parasitic species in two coprolites from 17th and 18th century London, providing an insight into the parasitic environment of the city. As part of a major project that aims to understand the consequences of parasitic disease throughout London's history, the present study is a first step towards the utilisation of the distinct methods that paleoparasitology utilises to understand better the health status, the hygiene conditions and the dietary habits of London's citizens over the centuries.

## Literature Cited

Addiss, D.G., Mathews, H.M., Stewart, J.M., Wahlquist, S.P., Williams, R.M., Finton, R.J., Spencer, H.C. and Juranek, D. 1991. Evaluation of a commercially available enzyme-linked immunosorbent assay for *Giardia lamblia* antigen in stool. *Journal of Clinical Microbiology* 29: 1137-1142.

Aldeen, W.E., Carroll, K., Robison, A., Morrison, M. and Hale, D. 1998. Comparison of nine commercially available enzyme-linked immunosorbent assays for detection of *Giardia lamblia* in fecal specimens. *Journal of Clinical Microbiology* 36: 1338-1340.

Araujo, A. and Ferreira, L.F. 1996. On hookworms and transpacific contact. *Parasitology Today* 12: 454.

Araujo, A., Reinhard, K., Bastos, O.M., Costa, L.C., Pirmez, C., Iniguez, A., Vicente, A.C., Morel, C.M. and Ferreira, L.F. 1998. Paleoparasitology: perspectives with new techniques. *Revista do Instituto de Medicina Tropical de Sao Paulo* 40: 371-376.

Araujo, A. and Ferreira, L.F. 2000. Paleoparasitology and the antiquity of human host-parasite relationships. *Memorias do Instituto Oswaldo Cruz* 95 (Suppl. 1): 89-93.

Araujo, A., Jansen, A.M., Bouchet, F., Reinhard, K., and Ferreira, F.L. 2003. Parasitism, the diversity of life and paleoparasitology. *Memorias do Instituto Oswaldo Cruz* 98 (suppl. 1): 5-11.

Araujo, A., Reinhard, K., Ferreira, F.L. and Gardner, S.L. 2008. Parasites as probes for prehistoric human migrations? *Trends in Parasitology* 24: 112-115.

Armelagos, G.J., Brown, P.J. and Turner, B. 2005. Evolutionary, historical and political economic perspectives on health and disease. *Social Science and Medicine* 61: 755-765.

Bathurst, R.R. 2005. Archaeological evidence of intestinal parasites from coastal shell middens. *Journal of Archaeological Science* 32: 115-123.

Bennett, C. 2006. A-Z guide to parasitology: with diagnosing medical parasites through coprological techniques. Available at:

http://www.soton.ac.uk/~ceb/ (last assessed 10/12/2010).

Bouchet, F., Lefevre, C. and Corbett, W.D. 1999. First paleoparasitological analysis of a midden in the Aleutian Islands (Alaska): results and limits. *The Journal of Parasitology* 85: 369-372.

Bouchet, F., West, D., Lefevre, C. and Corbett, D. 2001. Identification of parasitoses in a child burial from Adak Island (Central Aleutian Islands, Alaska). *Life Sciences* 324: 123-127.

Bouchet, F., Harter, S. and Le Bailly, M. 2003. The state of art of paleoparasitological research in the Old World. *Memorias do Instituto Oswaldo Cruz* 98 (suppl. 1): 95-101.

Bryant, V. M. and Dean, G.W. 2006. Archaeological coprolite science: the legacy of Eric O. Callen (1912-1970). *Palaeogeography, Palaeoclimatology, Palaeoecology* 237: 51-66.

Calagero, S., Reinhard, K., Vinton, S.D. 2003. Inca expansion and parasitism in the Lluta Valley: preliminary data. *Memorias do Instituto Oswaldo Cruz* 98 (suppl. 1): 161-163.

Callen, E.O. and Cameron, T.W M. 1960. A prehistoric diet revealed in coprolites. *New Scientist* 8: 35-40.

Cockburn, A. 1971. Infectious diseases in ancient populations. *Current Anthropology* 12: 45-62.

Cockburn, A., Barraco, R.A., Reyman, T.A. and Peck, W.H. 1975. Autopsy of an Egyptian mummy. *Science* 187: 1155-1160.

Cox, M. 1996. *Life and death in Spitalfields, 1700-1850.* Council for British Archaeology: York.

Cox, F.E.G. 2002. History of human parasitology. *Clinical Microbiology Reviews* 15: 595-612.

De Rouffignac, C. 1985. Parasite egg survival and identification from Hibernia Wharf, Southwark. *London Archaeologist* 5(4) 103: 105.

Ferreira, L.F., Araujo, A. and Confalonieri, U. 1979. Subsidios para a paleoparasitologia do Brasil. I parasitos encotrados em coprolitos no municipio de Unai, Minas Gerais. *Res Congresso Brasiliero de Parasitologia, 1979. Resumos Campinas SP*: 56.

Fugassa, M.H., Araujo, A. and Guichon, R.A. 2006. Quantitative paleoparasitology applied to archaeological sediments. *Memorias do Instituto Oswaldo Cruz* 101 (suppl. 2): 29-33.

Garcia, L.S. 1999. *Practical guide to diagnostic parasitology.* ASM Press: Washington D.C.

Garcia, L.S. 2007. *Diagnostic medical parasitology.* 5th ed. ASM Press: Washington D.C.

Garcia, L.S., Shimizu, R.Y. and Bernand, C.N. 2000. Detection of *Giardia lamblia, Entamoeba histolytica/Entamoeba dispar,* and *Cryptosporidium parvum* antigens in human fecal specimens using the triage parasite panel enzyme immunoassay. *Journal of Clinical Microbiology* 38: 3337-3340.

Goncalves, C.L.M., Araujo, A., Duarte, R., Da Silva, J.P., Reinhard, K., Bouchet, F. and Ferreira, F.L. 2002. Detection of *Giardia duodenalis* antigen in coprolites using a commercially available enzyme-linked immunosorbent assay. *Transactions of the Royal Society of Tropical Medicine and Hygiene* 96: 640-643.

Goncalves, C.L.M., Araujo, A. and Ferreira, F.L. 2003. Human intestinal parasites in the past: new findings and a review. *Memorias do Instituto Oswaldo Cruz* 98 (suppl. 1): 103-118.

Goncalves, C.L.M., Da Silva, L.V., De Andrade, C.M., Reinhard, K., Da Rocha, G.C., Le Bailly, M., Bouchet, F., Ferreira, L.F. and Araujo, A. 2004. Amoebiasis distribution in the past: first steps using an immunoassay technique. *Transactions of the Royal Society of Tropical Medicine and Hygiene* 98: 88-91.

Haque, R., Neville, L.M., Hahn, P. and Petri, W.A. 1995. Rapid diagnosis of *Entamoeba* infection by using *Entamoeba* and *Entamoeba histolytica* stool antigen detection kits. *Journal of Clinical Microbiology* 33: 2558-2561.

Haque, R., Ali, I.K.M., Akther, S. and Petri, W.A. 1998. Comparison of PCR, isoenzyme analysis and antigen detection for diagnosis of *Entamoeba histolytica* infection. *Journal of Clinical Microbiology* 36: 449-452.

Horne, P.D. 1985. A review of the evidence of human endoparasitism in the pre-Columbian New World through the study of coprolites. *Journal of Archaeological Science* 12: 299-310.

Jones, A.K.G. and Nicholson, C. 1988. Recent finds of *Trichuris* and *Ascaris* ova from Britain. *Paleopathology Newsletter* 62: 5-6.

Le Bailly, M., Goncalves, M.L.C., Harter-Lailheugue, S., Prodeo, F., Araujo, A. and Bouchet, F. 2008. New finding of *Giardia intestinali* (eukaryote, metamonad) in Old World archaeological site using immunofluorescence and enzyme-linked immunosorbent assays. *Memorias do Instituto Oswaldo Cruz* 103: 298-300.

Leles, D., Reinhard, K., Fugassa, M., Ferreira, L.F., Iniguez, A.M. and Araujo, A. 2010. A parasitological paradox: why is ascarid infection so rare in the prehistoric Americas? *Journal of Archaeological Science* 37: 1510-1520.

Molleson, T. and Cox, M. 1993. *The Spitalfields project. Volume 2 – the anthropology. The middling sort.* Council for British Archaeology: York. Research Report 86.

Mitchell, P.D. and Tepper, Y. 2007. Intestinal parasitic worm eggs from a crusader period cesspool in the city of Acre (Israel). *Levant* 39: 91-95.

Mitchell, P.D., Stern, E. and Tepper, Y. 2008. Dysentery in the crusader kingdom of Jerusalem: an ELISA analysis of two medieval latrines in the City of Acre (Israel). *Journal of Archaeological Science* 35: 1849-1853.

Moore, D.P. 1981. Life seen from a medieval latrine. *Nature 294*: 644.

Pike, A.W. 1967. The recovery of parasite eggs from ancient cesspit and latrine deposits: an approach to the study of early parasite infections. In: Brothwell, D. and Sandison, A.T. (eds.) *Diseases in antiquity*. CC Thomas: Springfield. 184-188.

Pike, A.W. 1968. Recovery of helminth eggs from archaeological excavations, and their possible usefulness in providing evidence for the purpose of an occupation. *Nature* 219: 303-304.

Pike, A.W. 1975. Parasite eggs. In: Platt, C. and Coleman-Smith, R. (eds.) *Excavations in medieval Southampton*. Leicester University Press: Leicester. 347-348.

Pike, A.W. and Biddle, M. 1966. Parasite eggs in medieval Winchester. *Antiquity* 40: 293-297.

Reinhard, K. 1990. Archaeoparasitology in North America. *American Journal of Physical Anthropology* 82: 145-163.

Reinhard, K.J., Confalonieri, U.E., Herrmanni, B., Ferreira, L.F. and Araujo, A. 1986. Recovery of parasite remains from coprolites and latrines: aspects of paleoparasitological technique. *Homo* 37: 217-239.

Reinhard, K.J. and Araujo, A. 2008. Archaeoparasitology. In: Pearsall, D.M. (ed.) *Encyclopaedia of archaeology*. Elsevier, Academic Press: New York. 494-501.

Roberts, C. and Cox, M. 2003. *Health and disease in Britain: from prehistory to the present day*. Sutton Publishing: Stroud.

Ruffer, M.A. 1910. Note on the presence of '*Bilharzia haematobia*' in Egyptian mummies of the Twentieth Dynasty. *The British Medical Journal* 1: 16.

Schmidt, G.D. and Roberts, L.S. 2006. *Foundations of parasitology*. New York: McGraw-Hill.

Sobolik, K.D. 1988. The importance of pollen concentration values from coprolites: an analysis of Southwest Texas samples. *Palynology* 12: 201-214.

Taylor, E.L. 1955. Parasitic helminths in medieval remains. *Veterinary Record* 67: 218-228.

Thomas, C. 2004. *Life and death in London's East End: 2000 years at Spitalfields*. Museum of London Archaeology Service: London.

Tibesky, K. and Sidell, J. 2003. The parasite remains. In: Malcolm, G., Bowsher, D. and Cowie, R. (eds.) *Middle Saxon London, excavations at the Royal Opera House, 1989-99*. Museum of London Archaeology Service: London. 333-337.

Wells, C. and Dallas, C. 1976. Romano-British pathology. *Antiquity* 50: 53-55.

Wilson, A. and Rackham, D.J. 1976. Parasite eggs. In: Addyman, P.V. and Buckland, P.C. (eds.) *The environmental evidence from the Church Street Roman sewer system*. York Archaeological Trust: York. The Archaeology of York Vol. 14. 32-33.

# Integrated Strategies for the use of Lipid Biomarkers in the Diagnosis of Ancient Mycobacterial Disease

Oona Y-C. Lee[1], Ian D. Bull[2], Erika Molnár[3], Antonia Marcsik[3], György Pálfi[3], Helen D. Donoghue[4], Gurdyal S. Besra[1] and David E. Minnikin*[1]

[1]School of Biosciences
University of Birmingham
Edgbaston, Birmingham B15 2TT, UK

[2]Bristol Biogeochemistry Research Centre
School of Chemistry
University of Bristol, Bristol BS8 1TS, UK

[3]Department of Anthropology
University of Szeged
H-6701 Szeged, Hungary

[4] Research Department of Infection
University College, London W1T 4JF, UK

*Email for correspondence: d.e.minnikin@bham.ac.uk

**Abstract**

The use of ancient DNA and lipid biomarkers has become established for the detection of tuberculosis and leprosy in archaeological material. Long-chain compounds are released by an efficient non-aqueous alkaline extraction and acidic components are converted to stable pentafluorobenzyl (PFB) esters, which can be preserved for immediate or future analysis. These long-chain components are fractionated into non-hydroxylated fatty acid esters and mycolic acid esters. Characteristic profiles of mycolates are recorded by fluorescence high-performance liquid chromatography (HPLC) of pyrenebutyric acid derivatives of PFB esters. Mycocerosate PFB esters are analysed by negative-ion chemical-ionisation gas chromatography-mass spectrometry (NICI-GCMS). In this study, ancient DNA analyses, along with mycolate and mycocerosate profiles, for a representative late 7th century AD skeleton from the Avar period in Hungary, are presented. It will be shown how mycolate and mycocerosate analyses of residual material from an ancient DNA analysis can be used to confirm a mixed leprosy-tuberculosis infection and provide an estimate of the relative amounts of the *M. tuberculosis* and *M. leprae* bacterial load obtained. In the present case, the bone pathology indicated only leprosy, but the biomarker analysis suggested predominance of tuberculosis over leprosy.

**Keywords:** Tuberculosis, Leprosy, Biomarkers, Lipids, Skeletons, Paleopathology

## Introduction

The aim is to develop the use of specific lipid biomarkers, in addition to DNA, in the diagnosis of ancient tuberculosis and leprosy. An integrated approach is used to analyse the established lipid biomarkers, mycolic and mycocerosic acids. The mycolic acids (Fig. 1A) are high molecular weight, 70 to 90 carbon, fatty acids, which are linked into the cell envelope to provide a tough hydrophobic defensive permeability barrier (Minnikin 1982; Minnikin *et al.* 2002). The mycocerosates (Fig. 1B) are multi-methyl branched fatty acids, components of waxes that also contribute to the hydrophobic barrier (Minnikin *et al.* 2002). A brief "Glossary of Technical Terms" is provided later.

In pioneering studies, using fluorescence high performance liquid chromatography (HPLC) of methylanthryl derivatives, mycolic acid profiles complemented the detection of ancient DNA in confirming the presence of tuberculosis in calcified pleura (Donoghue *et al.* 1998) and a medieval skeleton (Gernaey *et al.* 2001). The presence of *Mycobacterium tuberculosis* infection was also found to correlate well with burial records in a skeletal collection from Newcastle Infirmary (Gernaey *et al.* 1998). The fluorescence HPLC protocol was updated to use pyrenebutyric acid (PBA) derivatives of mycolic acid pentafluorobenzyl (PFB) esters (Fig. 1A). Using this method, the oldest proven case of tuberculosis was confirmed in a 9,000 year old female skeleton and an adjacent child (Herschkovitz *et al.* 2008). Similarly, tuberculosis was confirmed in the British Museum Granville Mummy (Donoghue *et al.* 2010) and a case of leprosy was identified from Uzbekistan (Taylor *et al.* 2009). The value of mycocerosate biomarkers for tuberculosis was demonstrated in the Coimbra Skeletal Collection, using negative ion chemical ionisation gas chromatography mass spectrometry (NICI-GCMS) (Redman *et al.* 2009).

This paper illustrates the integrated use of ancient DNA and mycolic and mycocerosic acid analysis in detecting ancient tuberculosis and leprosy, with particular reference to a mixed infection.

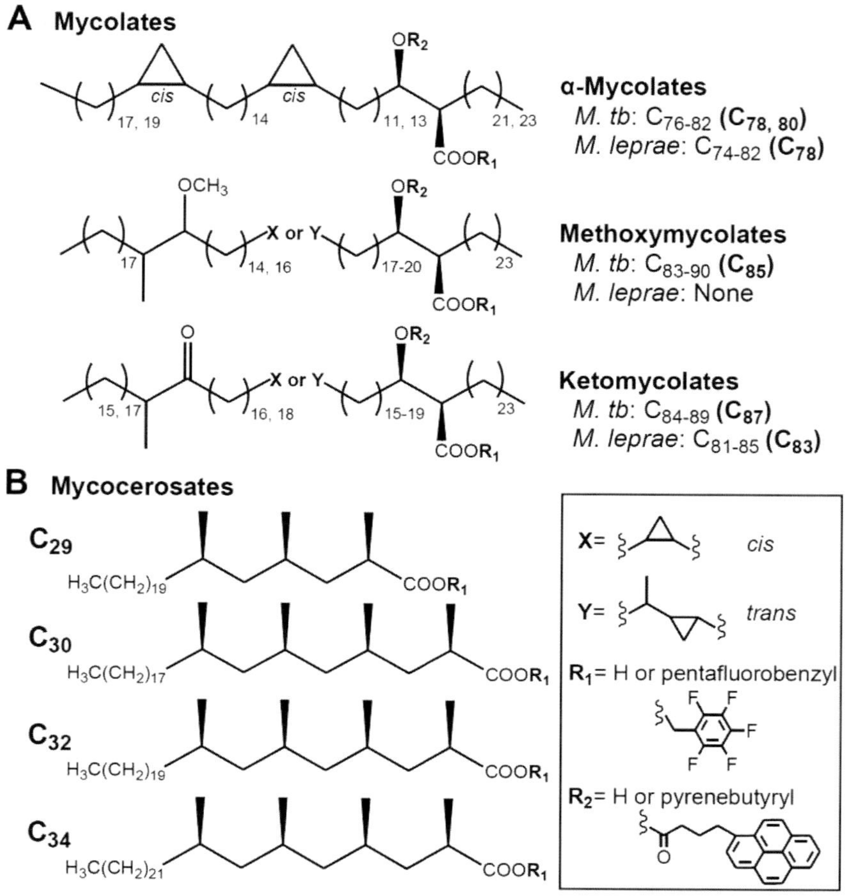


**Figure 1:** Structures of lipid biomarkers. **A:** Mycolic acids ($R_1$ = H, $R_2$ = H) are analysed as pyrenebutyric acid derivatives of pentafluorobenzyl esters ($R_1$ = pentafluorobenzyl, $R_2$ = pyrenebutyryl); major components are shown in **bold** in brackets. **B:** Mycocerosic acids ($R_1$ = H) are analysed as pentafluorobenzyl esters ($R_1$ = pentafluorobenzyl).

## Analytical Methods

The archaeological material studied was a nasal scraping of skeleton KD 517 from the late 7th century site at Kiskundorozsma, Hungary (Molnár *et al.* 2006; Pálfi and Molnár 2009). This was a male, aged 35–40 years, with distinctive paleopathology indicative of leprosy; there was pronounced remodelling of the rhinomaxillary region, including abnormal porosity of the hard palate and slight changes to the tibiae and fibulae. In addition, bilateral porotic criba orbitalia was noted. There was palaeopathology for leprosy and/or tuberculosis in other skeletons from this site, so KD 517 was examined, for both *Mycobacterium leprae* and *M. tuberculosis* complex DNA, using protocols described previously (Donoghue *et al.* 2005).

To analyse lipid biomarkers, the residual extract from the DNA study on KD 517 (Molnár *et al.* 2006) was used along with standard *M. tuberculosis* and *M. leprae* biomass. Alkaline hydrolysis and derivatisation, as described previously (Hershkovitz *et al.* 2008; Redman *et al.* 2009; Taylor *et al.* 2009; Donoghue *et al.* 2010), produced fractions containing pentafluorobenzyl esters of mycocerosic and mycolic acids. The PFB-mycocerosates were analysed by selected ion monitoring negative ion chemical ionisation gas chromatography mass spectrometry (SIM NICI-GCMS) (Redman *et al.* 2009). PFB-mycolates were converted to pyrenebutyric acid (PBA) esters (Fig. 1A), which were analysed by fluorescence HPLC (Hershkovitz *et al.* 2008; Donoghue *et al.* 2010). Profiles were recorded for standard samples of *M. tuberculosis* H37Rv and *M. leprae*, remaining from a previous study (Draper *et al.* 1983).

## Results

In the initial ancient DNA analysis of KD 517, a specific region of the *M. leprae* RLEP region was targeted, as this is present at 32 copies/cell and is therefore very sensitive. A 129-bp amplicon was obtained and confirmed by nested PCR, which yielded a 99-bp product. In addition, primers for the single-copy 18kD antigen gene gave a 136-bp product, confirmed by nested PCR giving a 110-bp amplicon (Donoghue *et al.* 2005). *M. tuberculosis* complex-specific PCR primers for the multi-copy IS*6110* region yielded a 123-bp amplicon that was confirmed by production of a 92-bp nested product.

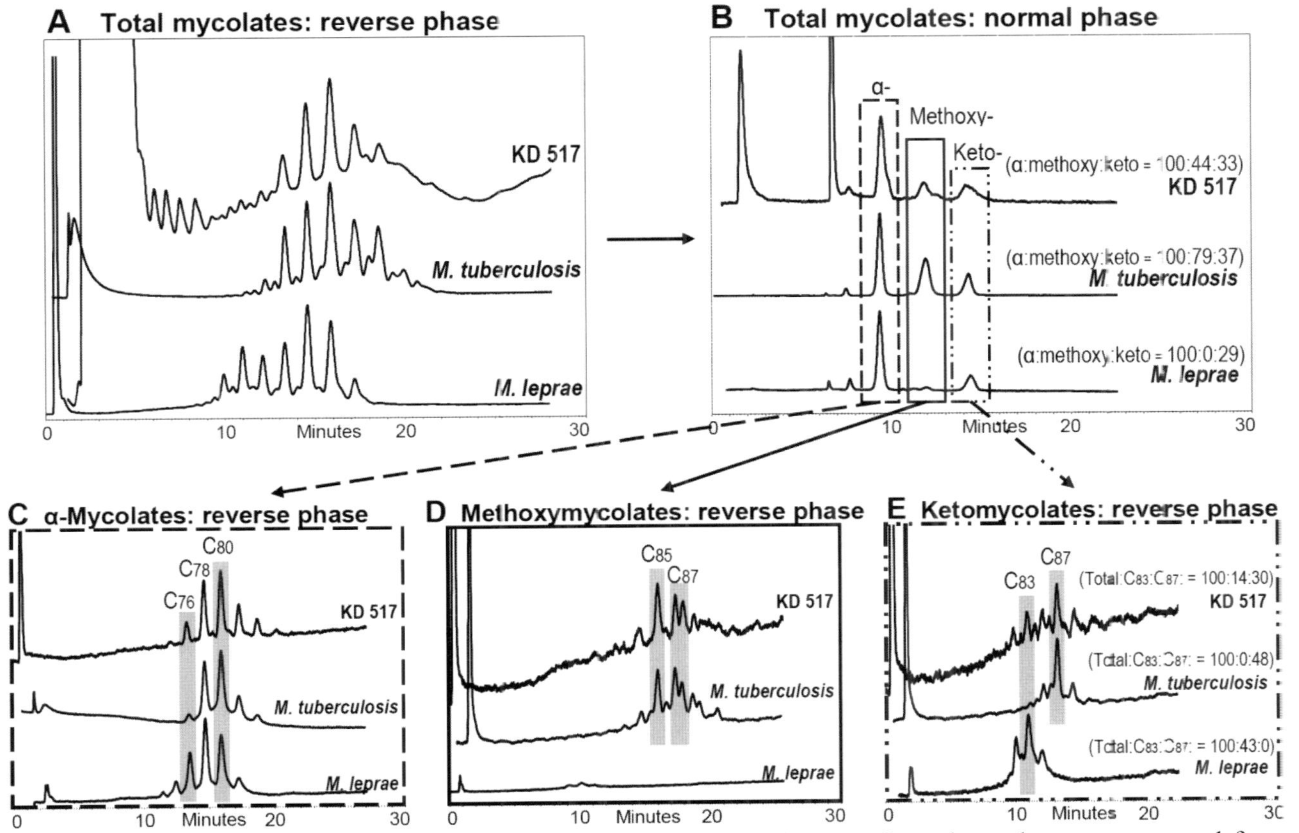


**Figure 2:** HPLC of pyrenebutyric acid derivatives of mycolic acid pentafluorobenzyl esters, prepared from extracts of KD 517 and standard biomass of *M. tuberculosis* and *M. leprae*. **A**: Reverse phase HPLC of total mycolates. **B**: Normal phase HPLC of total mycolates, collected from the reverse phase separation in **A**; the normalised ratios of the α-mycolates, methoxymycolates and ketomycolates, respectively, are in brackets. **C**, **D** and **E**: Reverse phase HPLC of α-mycolate, methoxymycolate and ketomycolates fractions, collected from the normal phase separation in **B**; the normalised ratios of total ketomycolates, $C_{83}$ and $C_{87}$ components, respectively, are shown in brackets in **E**.

The mycolic and mycocerosic acid profiles, obtained from extracts of skeleton KD 517 are shown in Figures 2 and 3, respectively. In the reverse phase HPLC profiles of total mycolates (Fig. 2A), the profile from KD 517 showed a closer superficial resemblance to *M. tuberculosis* than *M. leprae*, suggesting a predominance of the former. The total mycolates (Fig. 2A) were collected and analysed by normal phase HPLC, as shown in Figure 2B. The presence of a probable methoxymycolate component (Fig. 1) in the KD 517 profile was also indicative of *M. tuberculosis*, as methoxymycolates are absent in *M. leprae* (Fig. 2B) (Minnikin *et al.* 1985). The fractions corresponding to α-mycolates were analysed by reverse phase HPLC (Fig. 2C), with a main $C_{80}$ component in KD 517 again suggesting a predominance of *M. tuberculosis*. However, a relatively enhanced proportion of the $C_{76}$ α-mycolate introduced a possibility of leprosy (Fig. 2C). Tuberculosis infection was confirmed by a very clear methoxymycolate reverse phase HPLC profile, corresponding well with that from *M. tuberculosis* (Fig. 2D). The ketomycolate reverse phase HPLC profile from KD 517 showed a main $C_{87}$ component, emphasising the predominance of *M. tuberculosis,* but a significant $C_{83}$ ketomycolate strongly suggested the presence of *M. leprae* (Fig. 2E). The ratio of α-, methoxy- and ketomycolates (100:44:33) in KD 517 (Fig. 2B) was similar to a ratio (100:47:34), calculated for a 3:2 approximate ratio of the *M. tuberculosis* and *M. leprae* standards. Similarly in KD 517, assuming this *M. tuberculosis* to *M. leprae* bacterial loading of 3:2, the total ketomycolates and its component peaks of $C_{83}$ and $C_{87}$ have a ratio of 100:14:30 (Fig. 2E), which corresponds to the calculated value of 100:17:29 for the 3:2 mixture.

The profiles recorded for mycocerosic acids are shown in Figure 3. The mycocerosates of KD 517 displayed four major $C_{29}$, $C_{30}$, $C_{32}$ and $C_{34}$ components (Fig. 3A). This suggests a mixed infection, as the mycocerosates of *M. tuberculosis* lack $C_{34}$ components (Fig. 3B) and those from *M. leprae* have minor amounts of $C_{29}$ mycocerosates (Fig. 3C). The $C_{34}$ component in the profiles from the *M. tuberculosis* standard (Fig. 3B), with a retention time of 27.05 min, is not a mycocerosate, as authentic $C_{34}$ mycocerosates have retention times around 30 min (Fig. 3C). Again, assuming a 3:2 *M. tuberculosis* to *M. leprae* loading, the 27:65:100:81 ratio of the $C_{29}$, $C_{30}$, $C_{32}$ and $C_{34}$ mycocerosates in KD517 (Fig. 3A) corresponded well for the $C_{29}$, $C_{30}$ and $C_{32}$ components in the ratio (28:67:100:42) calculated for the 3:2 mixture, but not so well for the $C_{34}$ mycocerosate.

## Discussion

This communication illustrates how integrated analysis of ancient DNA and the principal lipid biomarkers, mycolic and mycocerosic acids, can provide a clear diagnosis of a mixed infection of ancient tuberculosis and leprosy. Since the DNA protocols use only aqueous extraction media, hydrophobic lipids remain in the residual materials. Strict protocols (Donoghue *et al.* 2005; 2009) were followed in the DNA study to avoid any contamination of the residues, so that they could be examined for lipid biomarkers.

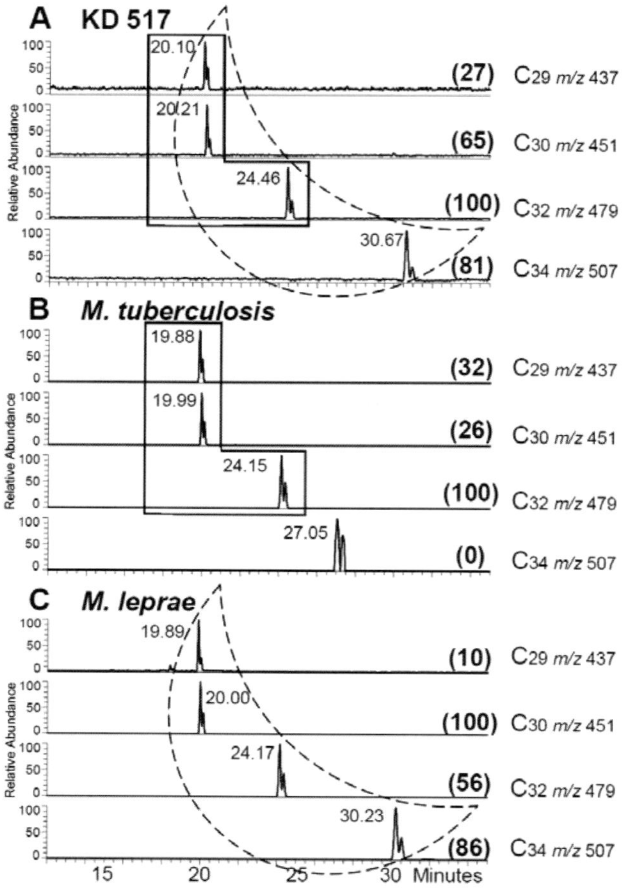


**Figure 3:** Selected ion monitoring NICI GCMS of mycocerosic acid pentafluorobenzyl esters prepared from extracts of KD 517 and standard biomass of *M. tuberculosis* and *M. leprae.* **A:** KD 517. **B:** *M. tuberculosis*. **C:** *M. leprae.* Relative proportions (in brackets) are shown normalised to the main component; values less than **1** are ignored. It was not possible to record the profile for KD 517 on the same day as the standard profiles, so the retention times are not precisely the same; the key factor is the clear recognition of the characteristic pattern.

The ancient DNA results demonstrated the presence of clear amplicons for both leprosy and tuberculosis. There was clearly sufficient well-preserved *M. leprae* DNA to enable amplification of a 136-bp target sequence from the single-copy 18 kD antigen locus. However, only the IS*6110* locus was examined for the *M. tuberculosis* complex. This is multi-copy and the copy number varies between strains. In addition, DNA is inherently less stable than lipid biomarkers and it is likely that its preservation is not consistent, either between different sites on the bacterial genome, or between different microbial species. Therefore, no conclusions can be drawn from the DNA study regarding the relative quantities of microbial DNA from each organism.

The mycolic acid profiles, in Figure 2, show the overall strategy for the recognition of components characteristic of tuberculosis and leprosy. The initial "reverse-phase" mycolate HPLC analysis (Fig. 2A) involves a partition between a "non-polar" hydrophobic surface, with 18-carbon attached long chains, and a relatively "polar" solvent in which the mycolates are only partially soluble. This type of chromatography is essentially a size screen enabling the high molecular weight $C_{70}$ to $C_{90}$ mycolic acids to be distinguished from any mammalian lipids, which all have less than 60 carbons. Total mycolates are collected and subjected to "normal" phase HPLC (Fig. 2B), which separates different mycolate classes dissolved in a relatively "non-polar" solvent on a "polar" surface according to their overall polarity. This polarity is increased in mycolates by adding polar functions to the molecules. The α-mycolates (Fig. 1A) are the least polar but adding a methoxy group increases polarity, as the oxygen atom can bond strongly to the polar silica gel "normal" phase surface. The oxygen atom in the keto group bonds even more strongly to the silica gel so ketomycolates are eluted last (Fig. 2B). The standard normal phase HPLC profiles for *M. tuberculosis* and *M. leprae* are distinguished by the lack of methoxymycolates in the latter (Minnikin *et al.* 1985). The individual mycolate types are collected from the normal phase separation and each is subjected to a second reverse phase analysis to reveal the different homologous components present (Figs 2C-E). For *M. tuberculosis* and *M. leprae,* respectively, the main α-mycolates are $C_{80}$ and $C_{78}$ and the ketomycolates are $C_{87}$ and $C_{83}$, the latter difference being the most discriminatory. The mycolate profiles from KD 517 show features indicating the presence of infection by both *M. tuberculosis* and *M. leprae*. Tuberculosis is confirmed by the presence of methoxymycolates in the normal phase profiles (Fig. 2B) and a highly characteristic methoxymycolate profile, comparing well with that given by the *M. tuberculosis* standard (Fig. 2D).

The ketomycolate profile of KD 517 (Fig. 2E) is particularly informative, showing two distinct clusters of peaks centred on $C_{83}$, for *M. leprae* and $C_{87}$ for *M. tuberculosis*. These two clusters correlate well with the profiles for standard *M. leprae* and *M. tuberculosis* (Fig. 2E). The ratio of the main $C_{87}$ and $C_{83}$ components in the ketomycolate profiles from KD 517 can provide an indication of the relative proportions of tuberculosis and leprosy infections. The profile of the α-mycolate of KD 517 (Fig. 2C) is less informative, with only an enhanced amount of the $C_{76}$ α-mycolate indicating that this may not be a homogeneous tuberculosis infection. Also, the fact that the main α-mycolate in KD 517 is $C_{80}$, rather than $C_{78}$, suggests a predominance of tuberculosis over leprosy. As shown in Results, a 3:2 ratio of tuberculosis to leprosy correlates with the HPLC proportions recorded in Figure 2.

The multimethyl-branched mycocerosic acids (Fig. 1B) are recognisable by their appearance as characteristic double peaks (Fig. 3), resulting from hydrolytic racemisation to give "diastereoisomers" which can be distinguished on gas chromatography (Minnikin *et al.* 1993; Redman *et al.* 2009). Another characteristic recognition feature, for mycocerosates, is the fact that the $C_{29}$ and $C_{30}$ components have almost identical gas chromatographic retention times of around 20 min., in the present study (Fig. 3). Since the $C_{29}$ acid is smaller by one carbon unit (Fig. 1B), it would be expected to be eluted before a $C_{30}$ acid, but mycocerosates with three methyl branches, rather than four, are relatively less volatile, so a characteristic chromatographic coincidence occurs (Fig. 3). The $C_{29}$ and $C_{30}$ mycocerosates are, of course, readily distinguished by their ions at *m/z* 437 and *m/z* 451 (Fig. 3); these ions correspond to negative carboxylate ions (- $COO^-$ ), which are characteristically produced from pentafluorobenzyl esters (Fig. 1B) on NICI mass spectrometry.

The recorded profiles of mycocerosic acids (Fig. 3) gave clear evidence for a tuberculosis-leprosy co-infection. Essentially, in the profile from KD 517 (Fig. 3A), the presence of $C_{34}$ mycocerosate suggests leprosy (Fig. 3C) (Draper *et al.* 1983; Minnikin *et al.* 1993) and enhanced $C_{29}$ is characteristic of tuberculosis (Fig. 3B). As noted above, the $C_{34}$ component, in the profiles from the *M. tuberculosis* standard (Fig. 3B), is not a mycocerosate. The essential patterns for tuberculosis (Fig. 3B) and leprosy (Fig 3D) are highlighted by an "L-shape" and a "crescent shape", respectively. The profile for KD 517 can be considered as a superposition of these two patterns (Fig. 3A). Mass spectrometry is not intrinsically very quantitative, but the assumption that there is a 3:2 predominance of tuberculosis over leprosy is broadly supported by the mycocerosate data.

It must be emphasised that these estimates of disease prevalence have limited accuracy. The mycolate HPLC analysis has the potential to be very accurate, if higher resolution columns are employed; however, under the conditions used, the key peaks in Figure 2 are not all clearly separated. Also, the distribution of tuberculosis and leprosy is unlikely to be uniform throughout skeletons. It is interesting that, in the nasal scraping analysed, there was an apparent predominance of tuberculosis mycolic and mycocerosic acids over those characteristic of leprosy, as the nasal area is a favoured site for leprosy infection. This does not necessarily imply that there were more tubercle than leprosy bacilli in the entire body. Results may also vary over time, according to the relative progression of each individual disease in the infected subject. The proportions of individual mycolates in the *M. tuberculosis* and *M. leprae* standards will also naturally vary somewhat, again diluting the precision of such diagnoses. Overall, although the pathology indicates an early leprosy infection, this is a disease that takes several years to progress to the stage of visible lesions. However, tuberculosis is a more virulent infection that kills the majority of susceptible individuals before any skeletal palaeopathology can develop. Therefore, the finding of a greater proportion of *M. tuberculosis* lipid biomarkers is consistent with the scenario of an individual infected with leprosy succumbing to tuberculosis (Donoghue *et al.* 2005). However, the possibility of death from a totally unrelated cause cannot be discounted.

The present study illustrates the benefit of assembling a wide range of evidence to support, or otherwise, an initial suspicion of mycobacterial disease, based solely on pathology. Detailed pathological investigations (Molnár *et al.* 2006; Pálfi and Molnár 2009) clearly suggested a diagnosis of leprosy in KD 517, with no obvious pathology suggestive of tuberculosis.

It is important when using specific biomarkers, such as DNA and lipids, to follow a strict and well-designed protocol. In recent years, it has been necessary to clearly define important criteria for the use of ancient DNA (Donoghue *et al.* 2009) and mycolic acids (Minnikin *et al.* 2010) in the diagnosis of ancient mycobacterial disease. A significant advantage of lipid biomarkers is that they are detected directly and, due to the great sensitivity of the methods, femtogram quantities can be detected without any amplification. The present study demonstrates the range and rigour of diagnostic data that can be achieved by an integrated, objective approach to biomarker use in the diagnosis of ancient mycobacterial disease. The detection of both DNA and lipid biomarkers in the same sample is a step forward in realising the maximum amount of information from valuable archaeological samples.

## Glossary of Technical Terms

Biomarker: a characteristic discriminatory cellular component.
DNA: deoxyribonucleic acid, a key molecule carrying essential genetic information.
Gas chromatography: a separation process where compounds are carried along in a gaseous "mobile phase" over a discriminatory "stationary phase" in a column.
Lipid: a fatty, waxy cellular material insoluble in water.
Liquid chromatography: a separation process where compounds are carried along in a liquid "mobile phase" over a discriminatory "stationary phase" in a column.
Mass spectrometry: a technique for giving molecules an electric charge (ionisation) and determining their mass by focussing them with magnetic and electrical fields.
PCR: polymerase chain reaction, a means for making multiple copies of DNA fragments.

## Acknowledgements

Support was obtained from The Leverhulme Trust in an Emeritus Fellowship (DEM) and Project Grant F/00 094/BL (GSB, DEM, OY-CL). Provision of access to the UK Natural and Environmental Research Council Mass Spectrometry Unit at the University of Bristol is acknowledged (DEM, IDB).

## Literature Cited

Donoghue, H.D., Spigelman, M., Zias, J., Gernaey-Child, A.M. and Minnikin, D.E. 1998. Demonstration of *Mycobacterium tuberculosis* complex DNA in calcified pleura from remains 1400 years old. *Letters in Applied Microbiology* 27: 265-269.

Donoghue, H.D., Marcsik, A., Matheson, C., Vernon, K., Nuorala, E., Molto, J.E., Greenblatt, C.L. and Spigelman, M. 2005. Co-infection of *Mycobacterium tuberculosis* and *Mycobacterium leprae* in human archaeological samples: a possible explanation for the historical decline of leprosy. *Proceedings of the Royal Society B* 272: 389–394.

Donoghue, H.D., Hershkovitz, I., Minnikin, D.E., Besra, G.S., Lee, O.Y-C., Galili, E., Greenblatt, C.L., Lemma, E., Spigelman, M. and Bar-Gal, G.K. 2009. Biomolecular archaeology of ancient tuberculosis: response to "Deficiencies and challenges in the study of ancient tuberculosis DNA by Wilbur *et al.* (2009)". *Journal of Archaeological Science* 36: 2797-2804.

Donoghue, H.D., Lee, O.Y-C., Minnikin, D.E., Besra, G.S., Taylor, J.H. and Spigelman, M. 2010. Tuberculosis in Dr. Granville's mummy: a molecular re-examination of the earliest known Egyptian mummy to be scientifically examined and given a medical diagnosis. *Proceedings of the Royal Society B* 277: 51-56.

Draper, P., Payne, S.N., Dobson, G. and Minnikin, D.E 1983. Isolation of a characteristic phthiocerol dimycocerosate from *Mycobacterium leprae. Journal of General Microbiology* 129: 859-863.

Gernaey, A.M., Minnikin, D.E., Copley, M.S., Power, J., Ahmed, A.M.S., Dixon, R.A., Roberts, C.A., Robertson, D.J., Nolan, J. and Chamberlain, A. 1998. Detecting ancient tuberculosis. *Internet Archaeology* http://intarch.ac.uk/journal/issue5/gernaey_index.html.

Gernaey, A.M., Minnikin, D.E., Copley, M.S., Dixon, R.A., Middleton, J.C. and Roberts, C.A. 2001. Mycolic acids and ancient DNA confirm an osteological diagnosis of tuberculosis. *Tuberculosis* 81: 259-265.

Hershkovitz, I., Donoghue, H.D., Minnikin, D.E., Besra, G.S., Lee, O.Y-C., Gernaey, A.M., Galili, E., Eshed, V., Greenblatt, C.L., Lemma, E., Bar-Gal, G.K. and Spigelman, M. 2008. Detection and molecular characterization of 9000-year-old *Mycobacterium tuberculosis* from a neolithic settlement in the eastern Mediterranean. *PLoS ONE* 3: e3426.

Minnikin, D.E. 1982. Lipids: complex lipids, their chemistry, biosynthesis and roles. In: Ratledge, C. and Stanford, J.L. (eds.) *The biology of the mycobacteria*. Academic Press: London. 95-184.

Minnikin, D.E., Dobson, G., Goodfellow, M., Draper P. and Magnusson, M. 1985. Quantitative comparison of the mycolic and fatty acid composition of *Mycobacterium leprae* and *Mycobacterium gordonae. Journal of General Microbiology* 131: 2013-2021.

Minnikin, D.E., Besra, G.S., Bolton, R.C., Datta, A.K., Mallet, A.I., Sharif, A., Stanford J.L., Ridell, M. and Magnusson, M. 1993. Identification of the leprosy bacillus and related mycobacteria by analysis of mycocerosate profiles. *Annales de la Société Belge de Médecine Tropicale* 73 (Suppl. 1): 25-34.

Minnikin, D.E., Kremer, L., Dover, L.G. and Besra, G.S. 2002. The methyl-branched fortifications of *Mycobacterium tuberculosis*. *Chemistry and Biology* 9: 545-553.

Minnikin, D.E., Lee, O.Y-C., Pitts, M., Baird, M.S. and Besra, G.S. 2010. Essentials in the use of mycolic acid biomarkers for tuberculosis detection: response to "High-throughput mass spectrometric analysis of 1400-year-old mycolic acids as biomarkers for ancient tuberculosis infection" by Mark *et al.* 2010. *Journal of Archaeological Science* 37: 2407-2412.

Molnár, E., Marcsik, A., Bereczki, Z. and Donoghue, H.D. 2006. Pathological cases from the 7th century in Hungary. 16th European Meeting of the Paleopathology Association, 28 August – 1 September 2006, Fira, Santorini, Greece. *Paleopathology Newsletter Supplement* (ISSN 0148-4737), p33.

Pálfi, G. and Molnár, E. 2009. The paleopathology of specific infectious diseases from Southeastern Hungary: a brief overview. *Acta Biologica Szegediensis* 53: 111-116.

Redman, J.E., Shaw, M.J., Mallet, A.I., Santos, A.L., Roberts, C.A., Gernaey, A.M and Minnikin, D.E. 2009. Mycocerosic acid biomarkers for the diagnosis of tuberculosis in the Coimbra skeletal collection. *Tuberculosis* 89: 267-277.

Taylor, G.M., Blau, S., Mays, S., Monot, M., Lee, O.Y-C., Minnikin, D.E., Besra, G.S., Cole, S.T. and Rutland, P. 2009. *Mycobacterium leprae* genotype amplified from an archaeological case of lepromatous leprosy in Central Asia. *Journal of Archaeological Science* 36: 2408-2414.

# A Comparative Study of Markers of Occupational Stress in Coastal Fishers and Inland Agriculturalists from Northern Chile

Paola V. Ponce

Department of Archaeology
Durham University
South Road
Durham DH1 3LE, UK

Email for correspondence: paolavponce@hotmail.com

**Abstract**
The arrival of agriculture and the study of its impact on health, disease and lifestyle in past populations is one of the goals most often pursued by bioarchaeologists. This study considers the presence of a group of markers of occupational stress (MOS) that are accepted by many in bioarchaeology as representing the impact of physical activity. To examine their presence, two past populations from northern Chile who practised two contrasting subsistence economies, marine hunter-gathering and agricultural farmers, were compared. The skeletal markers analysed were enthesophytes, osteoarthritis, spondylolysis, os acromiale as well as the robusticity of the humerus. The aim of this study was to compare the pattern of these MOS in archaic coastal hunter-gatherers (3rd-2nd millennium BC) with later inland agriculturalists (1st millennium AD). One hundred and seventy-five skeletons of adult males and females curated at the Museo Arqueológico San Miguel de Azapa in Arica, Chile were analysed. It was found that in general both populations were similarly affected by these MOS thus suggesting that the archaic way of life based on marine hunting and gathering and the lifestyle practised by later agricultural and farming populations were fairly equally demanding. In conclusion, this study showed that the arrival of agriculture in northern Chile did not produce a negative impact on the health of the local Native American populations.

**Keywords**: Palaeopathology, Enthesophytes, Osteoarthritis, Spondylolysis, Os Acromiale, Agriculture

## Introduction

The arrival of agriculture in the New World is often perceived under two contrasting paradigms. On the basis of the study of health and disease of the Native American populations, some scholars support the idea that human health declined after the adoption of farming and the rise of civilisation whereas other scholars do not believe this event produced either a negative or positive effect. Two important books, "*Paleopathology at the origins of agriculture*" edited by Cohen and Armelagos (1984) and "*Ancient health, skeletal indicators of agricultural and economic intensification*" edited by Cohen and Crane-Kramer (2007) review a number of studies that cover this topic. The general trend seen in the studies and presented in these books varies according to the skeletal marker considered for analysis, although overall, the evidence of health decline through prehistory is far more common than the evidence of improvement or stability, despite economic and political progress.

In order to test these paradigms, this study compares the presence of a number of markers of occupational stress or MOS in two Amerindian populations from northern Chile that practised two contrasting subsistence economies: marine hunter-gatherers with settled inland agriculturalists. The skeletal markers analysed were enthesophytes, osteoarthritis, spondylolysis, os acromiale as well as the robusticity of the humerus. These markers were chosen because they have been previously used by bioarchaeologists to address a number of social and biosocial aspects of prehistoric lifestyles including how sedentary or physically demanding were the lives of past populations and to explore the impact of a change in subsistence economy from hunting and gathering to farming (see Kennedy 1989; Bridges 1989, Bridges 1991a, Bridges 1991b; Robb 1998; Steen and Lane 1998; Nagy 1998; Larsen 2002; and Havelková *et al.* 2010).

Enthesophytes are bone changes at muscle and ligament insertion sites on bones (Fig. 1). Physical activity and occupation are important aetiological factors for enthesophytes as highlighted by studies carried out in the fields of kinesiology, sports medicine, occupational medicine, biomechanics and applied anatomy (Eller *et al.* 1992; Karlsson *et al.* 1995; Woods *et al.* 2002). However, as with osteoarthritis, enthesophytes are also multifactorial in aetiology. For instance, sex and age as well as trauma and a number of pathological conditions including degenerative (osteoarthritis), inflammatory (ankylosing spondylitis, psoriatic arthritis, Reiter's syndrome), metabolic (acromegaly) and DISH (diffuse idiopathic skeletal hyperostosis) have all been linked to the formation of enthesophytes (Benjamin *et al.* 1992; Ruhoy *et al.* 1998; Resnick 2002; Freemont 2002; Stafford and Youssef 2002). Furthermore, the role of enthesophytes in transmitting forces from tendon and ligament to bone is accompanied by a gradual transition of the forces through four histologically distinctive zones; dense fibrous connective tissue is replaced successively by uncalcified fibrocartilage, calcified fibrocartilage and bone (Benjamin *et al.* 1992; Benjamin and Ralphs 1997). This gradual transition would therefore reflect the difference in loading according to each attachment site and across the sites. As highlighted by Alves Cardoso and Henderson (2010) and Villotte *et al.* (2010) the implications of these mechanical differences are important for the bioarchaeologist because they relate to the normal (non-pathological) appearance of entheses on dry bone.

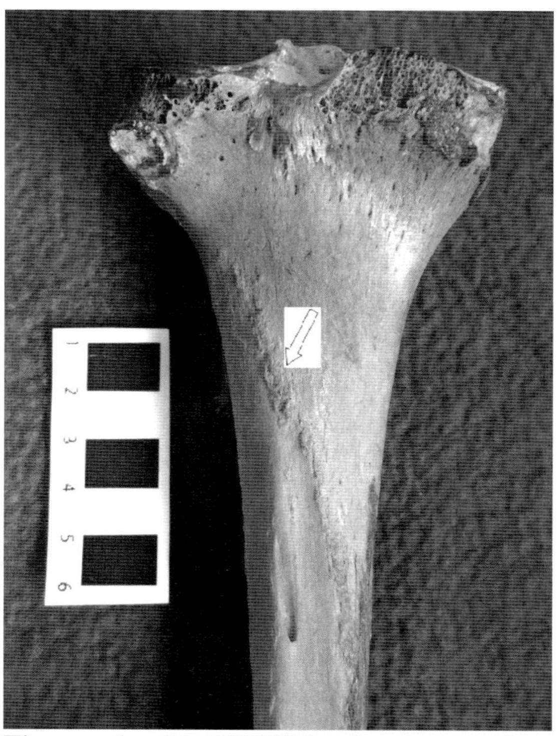

**Figure 1**: Mo1T27C13 showing enthesophyte formation at the *M. soleus* insertion of the left tibia.

Osteoarthritis is a degenerative condition of the diarthrodial joints of the skeleton that produces an alteration of the normal joint anatomy (Coote and Haslam 2004; Bullough 2004a) (Fig. 2). According to modern clinical literature, a combination of intrinsic, as well as extrinsic factors, are involved in its multifactorial aetiology. For instance, age, hormonal changes occurring in women during menopause, developmental deformities, obesity, genetic predisposition, and mechanical factors including joint mal-alignment, joint incongruity, joint overload as well as physical activity and occupation are all risk factors responsible for the condition (Doherty *et al.* 2000; Walker-Bone and Palmer 2002; Jones *et al.* 2002; Bullough 2004b; Christensen *et al.* 2005; Solovieva *et al.* 2005; Andrianakos *et al.* 2006; Grotle *et al.* 2008; Ganz *et al.* 2008).

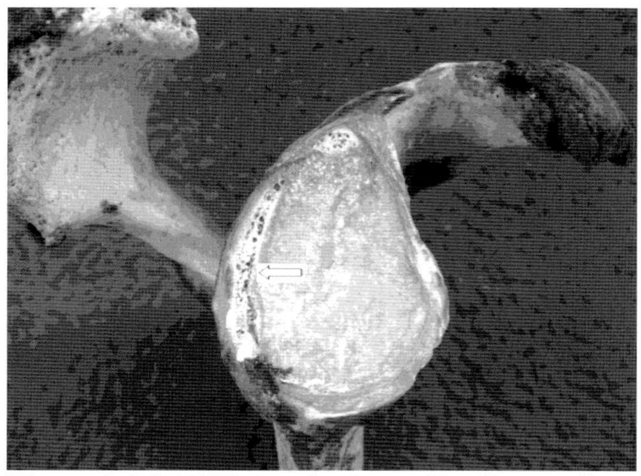

**Figure 2**: Mo1T27 showing loss of hyaline cartilage on the joint margins of the glenoid cavity with underlying porosity of the subchondral bone of the right scapula (glenoid-humeral joint).

Additional MOS considered in this study were spondylolysis and os acromiale. The former condition results from the separation of the neural arches or 'pars interarticularis' of the lumbar vertebrae from their bodies (Fig. 3). Spondylolysis can be found in other sections of the spine, however, this trend diminishes ascending the vertebral column cranially (Resnick and Goergen 2002). Often accepted as a stress fracture (Whiting and Zernicke 2008), spondylolysis has been commonly used as a MOS to indicate vigorous movements of the spine and strenuous physical activity (Merbs 1983, 1996; Arriaza 1997; Fibiger and Knüsel 2005). Os acromiale is a condition that results from the non-fusion of the acromial end of the scapula (Resnick and Goergen 2002) (Fig. 4) and it is believed to result from trauma and repetitive mechanical stress placed on the region of the developing acromion.

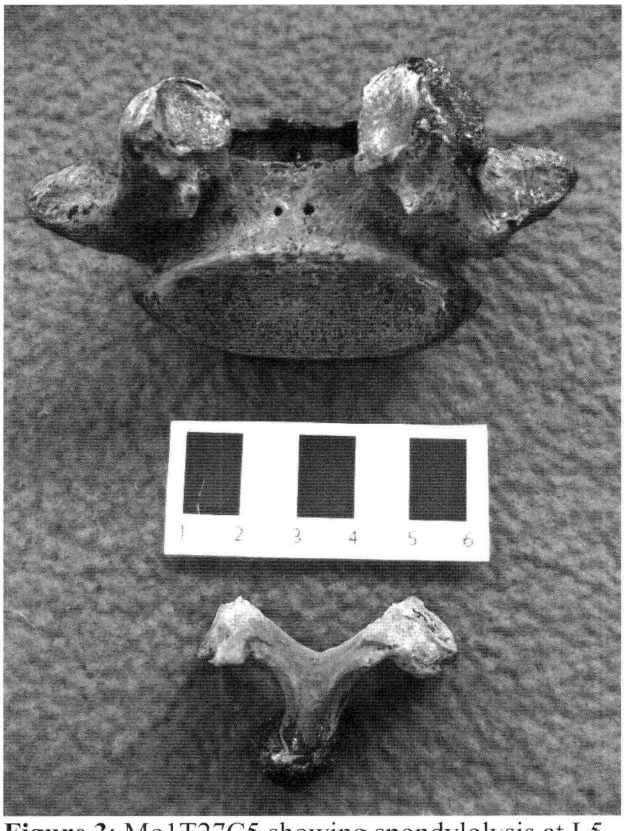

**Figure 3**: Mo1T27C5 showing spondylolysis at L5

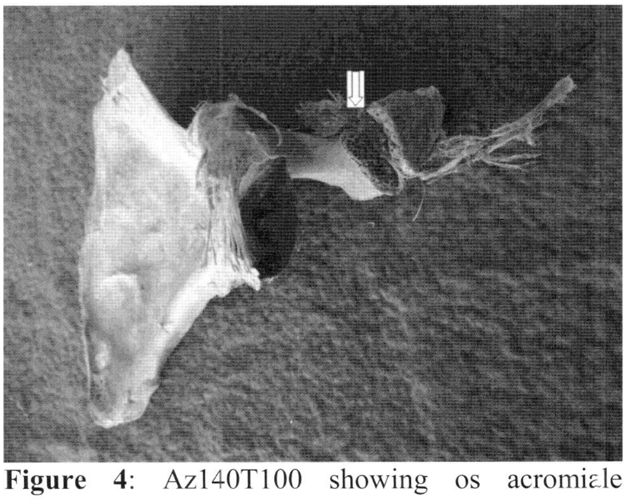

**Figure 4**: Az140T100 showing os acromiale affecting the left acromion.

Finally, according to 'Wolff's Law' and the idea that bones respond to mechanical stimuli by remodelling their internal and external structure in the direction of the functional stress (Pearson and Lieberman 2004; Ruff *et al.* 2006), bioarchaeologists have taken external bone measurements to calculate robusticity indices and thus, to record variation between and within populations through changes in subsistence strategies (e.g., Bridges 1989; Larsen *et al.* 2007). The humeral robusticity index is of particular interest because, according to Knüsel (2007:104), upper limb bones are normally involved in voluntary activities such as manipulation of objects and tools and therefore are more likely to reveal information on activity patterns. On the other hand, age, sex, diet and disease have been found responsible for changing the architecture of bones and for this reason behaviour and physical activity cannot solely explain osteological differences between populations (Jurmain 1999).

## Materials and Methods

The skeletal material analysed for this study is curated at the Museo Arqueológico San Miguel de Azapa, (Archaeological Museum of San Miguel de Azapa), in Arica, Northern Chile. It comprised one hundred and seventy-five skeletons of adult males and females from which 100 belonged to marine hunter-gatherers (3rd-2nd millennium BC) and 75 to inland agriculturalists (1st millennium AD) (Fig. 5). For a detailed demographic profile of the population studied, see Table 1. The former group settled along the Pacific coast, expanding their cultural influence geographically for approximately 1,500km, from Southern Peru to Northern Chile (Arriaza 1994, 1995). This population was characterised by the absence of sophisticated technology; they did not produce pottery, nor did they develop smelting techniques for metals, or use looms for weaving. Their subsistence economy was mainly based on the marine resources such as mackerel, sole, sardines, manta ray, clams, mussels, limpets, and winkles that they fished and gathered along the Pacific coast. As well as fishing, these populations complemented their diet with hunting marine fauna such as sea lions and dolphins in addition to shore birds such as pelicans and cormorants (Focacci and Chacón 1989, Standen 2003). Palaeodietary studies have shown that marine resources constituted about 80% of the diet of these populations whereas terrestrial animals and plants constituted the remainder (Aufderheide *et al.* 1993).

**Table 1:** Sample composition

| Sex | Age | Coastal | Inland |
|---|---|---|---|
| Females | Y-A | 19 | 22 |
| | M-A | 14 | 26 |
| | O-A | 4 | 14 |
| | **Total** | 37 | 62 |
| Males | Y-A | 20 | 14 |
| | M-A | 14 | 21 |
| | O-A | 4 | 3 |
| | **Total** | 38 | 38 |
| **Total** | | 75 | 100 |

Inland agriculturalists on the other hand, were sedentary populations, who settled in large villages where domestic, funerary, administrative and defensive structures were spatially connected. These were located along the lower slopes of the middle course of the Azapa Valley in northern Chile, between 15 and 25 km from the coast and the city of Arica, at 200-250 metres above sea level (Fig. 5).

Inland agriculturalists cultivated different varieties of maize and tubers such as yucca, tapioca, potato and sweet potato. They also grew pumpkins and butternut squashes, chillies, peanuts, quinoa, cotton, coca and different types of beans (Focacci 1981; Muñoz 1983; Alfonso *et al.* 2007). In line with the agricultural way of life in settled villages, a number of other important social and economic events developed during the presence of these populations in the region. These included the development of a sophisticated textile and ceramic industry and the practise of smelting metals.

Sex estimation was carried out by using a combination of dimorphic aspects of the skull and the pelvis according to Bass (2005). Age was assessed whenever possible with a combination of methods observing the degenerative changes of the pubic symphysis, the auricular surface, and the sternal rib ends according to Lovejoy *et al.* (1985), Loth and İşcan (1989) and Brooks and Suchey (1990). The age categories allocated to the skeletons were taken from those proposed by Buikstra and Ubelaker (1994).

The methods used to analyse the presence of enthesophytes and osteoarthritis consisted in observing left and right major upper and lower limb bones of the skeleton. A list of the total 17 chosen muscle and tendon attachment sites is given in Table 2 and the nine joints analysed for the presence of osteoarthritis are listed in Table 3. Osteoarthritis was diagnosed following the criteria of Rogers and Waldron (1995), in other words, when two of the following features (marginal osteophytes and /or new bone on the joint surface; pitting on the joint surface or alteration of the bony contour of the joint) were present. As the joints examined consisted of two articular surfaces, and the changes observed may not always be the same on both surfaces of one joint, it was decided primarily to record them as separate surfaces and treat them as dichotomous variable (present/absent). Thus, following a similar path of analysis as that of enthesophytes, a joint was recorded as positive or 'YES' for osteoarthritis (score of 1) when at least one surface showed the condition. Negative or 'NO' meant that both surfaces did not show changes indicative of osteoarthritis (score of 0).

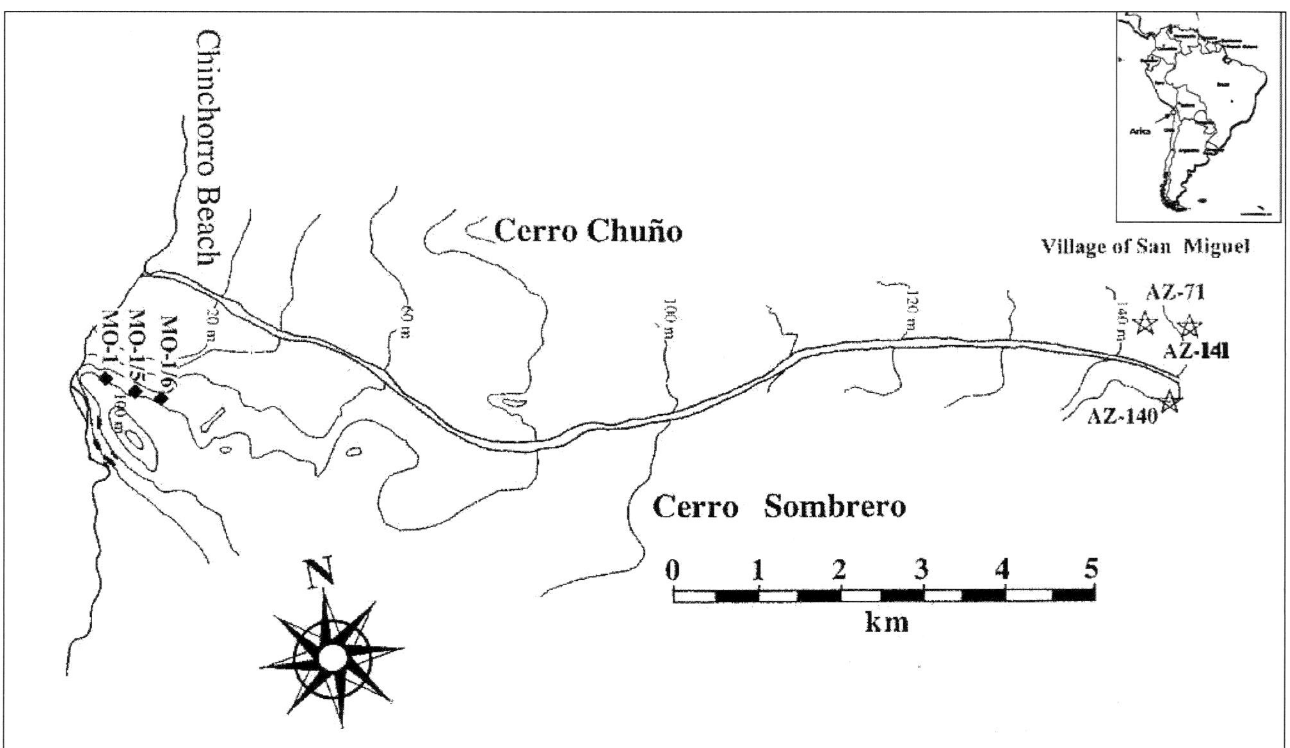


**Figure 5**: Location of the sites studied. Modified from Sutter and Mertz (2004: 133)
Key: ♦ Coastal sites ☆Inland sites

**Table 2:** Grouped entheseal areas chosen for the analysis of enthesophytes.

| Limb | Joint | Bone | Entheses | Muscle/Tendon/Ligament | Type |
|---|---|---|---|---|---|
| Upper | Shoulder | Clavicle | Costal tuberosity | Costo-clavicular ligament | C |
| | | Humerus | Lesser tubercle | *M. subscapularis* | FC |
| | | | Greater tubercle | *M. supraspinatus* | FC |
| | | | | *M. infraspinatus* | FC |
| | | | | *M. teres minor* | FC |
| | | | Deltoid tuberosity | *M. deltoideus* | C |
| | Elbow | Humerus | Medial epicondyle | *M. common flexor origin* | FC |
| | | | | *M. pronator teres* | FC |
| | | | Lateral epicondyle | *M. common ext. origin* | FC |
| | | | | *M. anconeus* | FC |
| | | Radius | Radial tuberosity | *M. biceps brachii* | FC |
| | | Ulna | Olecranon | *M. triceps brachii* | FC |
| | | | Ulnar tuberosity | *M. brachialis* | FC |
| Lower | Hip | Os coxa | Ischial tuberosity | *M. semimembranosus* | FC |
| | | | | *M. semitendinosus* | FC |
| | | | | *M. biceps femoris* | FC |
| | Knee | Femur | Lesser trochanter | *M. iliacus* | FC |
| | | | | *M. psoas major* | FC |
| | | | Greater trochanter | *M. gluteus minimus* | FC |
| | | | | *M. gluteus medius* | FC |
| | | | | *M. piriformis* | FC |
| | | | | *M. obturator internus* | FC |
| | | | | *M. obturator externus* | FC |
| | | | Linea aspera | *M. adductor brevis* | FC |
| | | | | *M. adductor magnus* | C |
| | | | | *M. gluteus maximus* | FC |
| | | | | *M. vastus medialis* | C |
| | | | | *M. vastus lateralis* | C |
| | | Tibia | Tibial tuberosity | *M. quadriceps femoris* | FC |
| | | | Soleal line | *M. soleus* | C |
| | Ankle | Calcaneus | Calcaneal tuberosity | Achilles tendon | C |

Note: (FC) is fibrocartilaginous entheses and (C) is cartilaginous entheses.

Spondylolysis and os acromiale were similarly analysed as dichotomous variables. Spondylolytic defects were scored as present (score of 1) when at least one pars interarticularis showed signs of separation and os acromiale was scored as present when a fragment resulted from the non-fusion of the acromion of the scapula.

Entheseal areas along with joints, vertebrae and acromia 'Unavailable' for study were scored as such if at least one or both surfaces were unavailable for observation due to the presence of soft tissues still attached near to the entheseal/articular area, as well as when a bone or bones were absent, missing or broken. Osteoarthritis secondary to trauma was also not considered in the final score.

**Table 3**: Joints analysed for the presence of OA

| Limb | Region | Joint |
|---|---|---|
| Upper | Shoulder | Acromial-clavicular |
| | | Glenoid-humeral |
| | Elbow | Humeral-ulnar |
| | | Humeral-radial |
| | | Radial-ulnar |
| Lower | Hip | Coxal-femoral |
| | Knee | Femoral-tibial |
| | | Femoral-patellar |
| | Ankle | Tibial-talar |

With regards to the humeral robusticity index, two measurements were taken on the humerus using an osteometric board and an electronic calliper following the descriptions provided by Bass (2005) (Table 4). The formula used to calculate the index was: [least circumference of shaft x 100]/ maximum length of humerus.

Dichotomous scores were counted and two types of prevalence rate calculations were computed for the five MOS analysed in this study. Following Waldron (2007), true prevalence rates were calculated by determining the ratio of n/N, 'n' being the numerator resulting from the total number of osseous elements affected with the condition and 'N' the denominator, resulting from the total number of osseous elements present for the particular sex category considered. Crude prevalence rates were calculated by determining the ratio of n/N, 'n' being the numerator resulting from the total number of individuals affected with the condition, and 'N' the denominator, resulting from the total number of individuals sampled, regardless of preservation of specific bone elements. These two types of prevalence rates were calculated because the lack of consensus and standard methods in studying these MOS prompted the necessity for reporting true and crude prevalence rates in order to provide more opportunities for comparisons with other published data.

**Table 4**: External measurements of humerus (from Bass 2005: Fig. 3-40)

| Bone | Measurement | Definition | | Marks |
|---|---|---|---|---|
| Humerus | Maximum length | Distance from the most superior point on the head of the humerus to the most inferior on the trochlear | (A-B) | 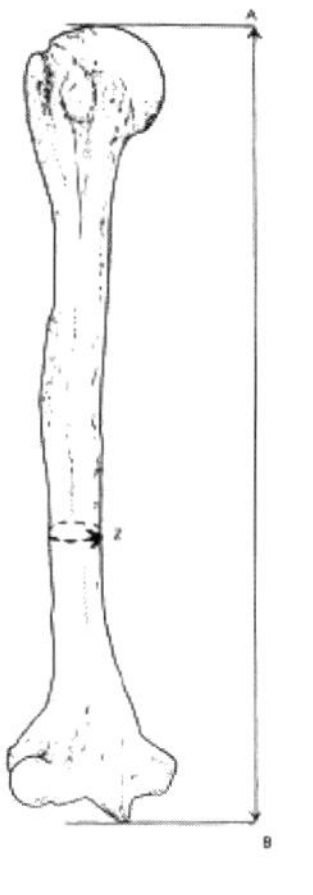 |
| | Circumference | Least circumference of the shaft taken at about the second one-third distal to the deltoid tuberosity | (Z) | |

Statistical analysis common to all MOS consisted of a series of Pearson Chi-square tests. These were calculated on true prevalence rate calculations. Mays (2010) suggested that inferential statistical tests such as Chi-square should not be used on data quantified by individual anatomical elements (bones, teeth) but only on individuals. On the other hand, as crude prevalence rates represent a gross under-estimate of the real prevalence of a pathological condition (Roberts and Cox 2003:401), all statistical tests performed in this study were based on true prevalence rate results.

On the basis that physical activities practised by males and females are often different, comparisons of these MOS were performed between same sex individuals belonging to different groups rather than grouping both sexes together. Intra-group comparisons were outside the scope of this study as these have been addressed elsewhere, see Ponce (2010a).

The analysis of MOS according to age was not possible due to the nature of the sample composition (Table 1). In other words, the small number of individuals in each age category and the uneven composition between coastal and inland groups did not allow for a reliable comparative statistical analysis.

Furthermore, a series of t-tests were calculated for the measurements taken on the humerus with the objective of comparing the differences between sample means. When the independent t-test was impossible to calculate due to a non-normal distribution of data, the Mann-Whitney U test was used instead. The level of statistical significance was always set at $p<0.05$. In cases where the assumption of expected values greater than five (>5) was not met, a Fisher's exact test was used instead. Finally, a two-tailed significance test was considered for all statistical tests used because there were no expectations about the direction of the difference between the samples.

## Results

The results for enthesophytes, osteoarthritis, spondylolysis, os acromiale and the humeral robusticity index are shown in Tables 5-9. Inter-group sex comparison of enthesophytes (Table 5) suggested that coastal and inland females showed more variation in the patterning and distribution compared to the males. Chi-square analysis based on total true prevalence rates revealed that female agriculturalists were significantly more affected by enthesophytes than coastal females $X^2$=5.092 (df =1) $p<0.05$. Males of both groups on the other hand, showed a highly significant difference only at the knee and non-significant differences at the remaining entheseal areas. Chi-square analysis based on total true prevalence rates of entheses analysed also revealed no significant differences between both groups $X^2$=0.709 (df =1) $p>0.05$.

**Table 5**: Chi-square test results of the association between enthesophytes and sex

| Sites | | Females | | | | Males | | | |
|---|---|---|---|---|---|---|---|---|---|
| | | True n/N | % | $x^2$ (df=1) | p | True n/N | % | $x^2$ (df=1) | p |
| Shoulder | Coastal | 45/107 | 42.1 | 4.478 | 0.037 | 68/121 | 56.2 | 0.950 | >0.05 |
| | Valley | 197/367 | 53.7 | | | 111/219 | 50.7 | | |
| Elbow | Coastal | 58/132 | 43.9 | 0.282 | >0.05 | 88/148 | 59.5 | 2.724 | >0.05 |
| | Valley | 216/464 | 46.6 | | | 131/257 | 51.0 | | |
| Hip | Coastal | 35/39 | 89.7 | 5.190 | 0.038 | 28/41 | 68.3 | 3.643 | >0.05 |
| | Valley | 62/87 | 71.3 | | | 49/58 | 84.5 | | |
| Knee | Coastal | 129/216 | 59.7 | 8.860 | 0.003 | 131/207 | 63.3 | 14.852 | <0.001 |
| | Valley | 365/514 | 71.0 | | | 235/298 | 78.9 | | |
| Ankle | Coastal | 1/2 | 50.0 | Fisher | >0.05 | 5/5 | 100.0 | Fisher | >0.05 |
| | Valley | 51/58 | 87.9 | | | 20/27 | 74.1 | | |
| Total | Coastal | 268/496 | 54.0 | 5.092 | 0.027 | 320/522 | 61.3 | 0.709 | >0.05 |
| | Valley | 891/1490 | 59.8 | | | 546/859 | 63.6 | | |

Note: both right and left hand sides as well as all age categories were pooled. True prevalence: (n) is the number of entheses affected and (N) is the number of entheses available for study. Crude prevalence: (n) is the number of individuals affected and (N) the number of individuals with entheses available for study. Chi-square analysis was performed on true prevalence values.

**Table 6**: Chi-square test results of the association between osteoarthritis and sex

| Sites | | Females | | | | Males | | | |
|---|---|---|---|---|---|---|---|---|---|
| | | True n/N | % | $\chi^2$ (df=1) | p | True n/N | % | $\chi^2$ (df=1) | p |
| Shoulder | Coastal | 28/76 | 36.8 | 3.492 | >0.05 | 23/81 | 28.4 | 0.696 | >0.05 |
| | Valley | 55/215 | 25.6 | | | 30/129 | 23.3 | | |
| Elbow | Coastal | 54/147 | 36.7 | 4.087 | >0.05 | 69/169 | 40.8 | 3.490 | >0.05 |
| | Valley | 94/341 | 27.6 | | | 68/215 | 31.6 | | |
| Hip | Coastal | 20/66 | 30.3 | 1.771 | >0.05 | 26/58 | 44.8 | 5.137 | 0.026 |
| | Valley | 47/117 | 40.2 | | | 18/70 | 25.7 | | |
| Knee | Coastal | 28/113 | 24.8 | 0.805 | >0.05 | 27/100 | 27.0 | 1.225 | >0.05 |
| | Valley | 55/186 | 29.6 | | | 23/112 | 20.5 | | |
| Ankle | Coastal | 6/61 | 9.8 | 0.618 | >0.05 | 1/45 | 2.2 | Fisher | >0.05 |
| | Valley | 7/108 | 6.5 | | | 3/54 | 5.6 | | |
| Total | Coastal | 136/463 | 29.4 | 0.876 | >0.05 | 146/453 | 32.2 | 7.591 | >0.05 |
| | Valley | 258/967 | 26.7 | | | 142/580 | 24.5 | | |

Note: As for Table 5, above.

The results obtained for the association between osteoarthritis and sex (Table 6) showed that with the only exception of the hip joint where coastal males were more affected than inland males, the remainder inter-group sex comparisons did not reveal statistical differences ($X^2$=0.876, df=1, p>0.05 and $X^2$=7.591, df=1, p>0.05 based on total true prevalences between females and males respectively).

The analysis of spondylolysis according to sex was not possible to be carried out between coastal and inland females (Table 7a) as expected counts were smaller than five for the Chi-square test. The alternative Fisher's exact test revealed no significant differences between both groups (Fisher's exact= 1.000 (df=1) p>0.05). On the other hand, coastal males (Table 7b) were significantly more affected by spondylolysis than inland agriculturalists ($X^2$=7.659 (df=1) 0.005 p<0.05).

**Table 7a**: Prevalence rates of spondylolysis according to sex (Females)

| Vertebra | Females | | | | | | | | $X^2$ (df=1) | p |
|---|---|---|---|---|---|---|---|---|---|---|
| | Coastal | | | | Inland | | | | | |
| | True n/N | % | Crude n/N | % | True n/N | % | Crude n/N | % | | |
| L1 | 0/28 | 0.0 | 0/28 | 0.0 | 0/48 | 0.0 | 0/48 | 0.0 | - | - |
| L2 | 0/29 | 0.0 | 0/29 | 0.0 | 0/49 | 0.0 | 0/49 | 0.0 | - | - |
| L3 | 0/27 | 0.0 | 0/27 | 0.0 | 0/49 | 0.0 | 0/49 | 0.0 | - | - |
| L4 | 0/26 | 0.0 | 0/26 | 0.0 | 0/50 | 0.0 | 0/50 | 0.0 | - | - |
| L5 | 1/27 | 3.7 | 1/27 | 3.7 | 3/50 | 6.0 | 3/50 | 6.0 | - | - |
| L6 | 0/2 | 0.0 | 0/2 | 0.0 | 0/0 | 0.0 | 0/0 | 0.0 | - | - |
| Total | 1/139 | 0.7 | 1/30 | 3.3 | 3/246 | 1.2 | 3/52 | 5.8 | Fisher | >0.05 |

Note: all age categories were pooled. True prevalence: (n) is the number of vertebrae affected and (N) is the number of vertebrae available for study. Crude prevalence: (n) is the number of individuals affected and (N) is the number of individuals available with at least one lumbar vertebra present for study.

**Table 7b**: Prevalence rates of spondylolysis according to sex (Males)

| Vertebra | Males | | | | | | | | $X^2$ (df=1) | p |
|---|---|---|---|---|---|---|---|---|---|---|
| | Coastal | | | | Inland | | | | | |
| | True n/N | % | Crude n/N | % | True n/N | % | Crude n/N | % | | |
| L1 | 0/28 | 0.0 | 0/28 | 0.0 | 0/34 | 0.0 | 0/34 | 0.0 | - | - |
| L2 | 0/29 | 0.0 | 0/29 | 0.0 | 0/33 | 0.0 | 0/33 | 0.0 | - | - |
| L3 | 0/26 | 0.0 | 0/26 | 0.0 | 0/34 | 0.0 | 0/34 | 0.0 | - | - |
| L4 | 1/21 | 4.8 | 1/21 | 4.8 | 0/31 | 0.0 | 0/31 | 0.0 | - | - |
| L5 | 9/27 | 33.3 | 9/27 | 33.3 | 2/32 | 6.2 | 2/32 | 6.2 | - | - |
| L6 | 0/1 | 0.0 | 0/1 | 0.0 | 0/1 | 0.0 | 0/1 | 0.0 | - | - |
| Total | 10/132 | 7.6 | 9/31 | 29 | 2/165 | 1.2 | 2/34 | 5.9 | 7.659 | 0.007 |

Note: all age categories were pooled. True prevalence: (n) is the number of vertebrae affected and (N) is the number of vertebrae available for study. Crude prevalence: (n) is the number of individuals affected and (N) the number of individuals available with at least one lumbar vertebra present for study.

Inter-group sex comparisons on the basis of os acromiale were not possible to be carried out between coastal and inland females as the former group did not exhibit any evidence of the condition (Table 8a). Comparisons between males (Table 8b) were not possible to be calculated with Chi-square test because of low expected counts, but the alternative Fisher's exact test revealed no significant differences between these groups (Fisher's exact= 0.277 (df=1) p>0.05).

Finally, the results obtained for the humeral robusticity index between coastal and inland males and females (Tables 9a-b) were not statistically significant (Mann-Whitney=1938.000, p>0.05 for females and T-test=1.082 (df=95), p>0.05 for males).

**Table 8a**: Prevalence rates of os acromiale according to sex (Females)

| Acromia | Females | | | | | | | | $x^2$ (df=1) | p |
|---|---|---|---|---|---|---|---|---|---|---|
| | Coastal | | | | Inland | | | | | |
| | True n/N | % | Crude n/N | % | True n/N | % | Crude n/N | % | | |
| Right | 0/22 | 0.0 | 0/26 | 0.0 | 2/53 | 3.8 | 3/56 | 5.4 | - | - |
| Left | 0/21 | 0.0 | | | 2/53 | 3.8 | | | - | - |
| Total | 0/43 | 0.0 | 0/26 | 0.0 | 4/106 | 3.8 | 3/56 | 5.4 | - | - |

Note: all age categories were pooled. True prevalence: (n) is the number of acromia affected and (N) is the number of acromia available for study. Crude prevalence: (n) is the number of individuals affected and (N) is the number of individuals available with at least one acromion present for study.

**Table 8b**: Prevalence rates of os acromiale according to sex (Males)

| Acromia | Males | | | | | | | | $x^2$ (df=1) | p |
|---|---|---|---|---|---|---|---|---|---|---|
| | Coastal | | | | Inland | | | | | |
| | True n/N | % | Crude n/N | % | True n/N | % | Crude n/N | % | | |
| Right | 4/21 | 19.0 | 4/26 | 15.4 | 2/30 | 6.7 | 2/34 | 5.9 | - | - |
| Left | 1/22 | 4.5 | | | 1/29 | 3.4 | | | - | - |
| Total | 5/43 | 11.6 | 4/26 | 15.4 | 3/59 | 5.1 | 2/34 | 5.9 | Fisher | >0.05 |

Note: all age categories were pooled. True prevalence: (n) is the number of acromia affected and (N) is the number of acromia available for study. Crude prevalence: (n) is the number of individuals affected and (N) is the number of individuals available with at least one acromion present for study.

**Table 9a**: Independent means t-test comparing humeral robusticity (Females)

| Index | | Coastal fishers | | | | | Inland agriculturalists | | | | | T-test | df | p |
|---|---|---|---|---|---|---|---|---|---|---|---|---|---|---|
| | | Females | | | | | Females | | | | | | | |
| | | n | Min | Max | Mean | Sd | n | Min | Max | Mean | Sd | | | |
| Humeral Robusticity | R | 21 | 17.6 | 22.1 | 20.0 | 1.2 | 54 | 17.7 | 24.2 | 19.9 | 1.3 | Mann-Whitney 493.000 | | >0.05 |
| | L | 16 | 17.8 | 22.5 | 19.7 | 1.3 | 54 | 17.8 | 23.4 | 19.9 | 1.2 | Mann-Whitney 383.000 | | >0.05 |
| | R+L | 37 | 17.6 | 22.5 | 19.9 | 1.2 | 108 | 17.7 | 24.2 | 19.9 | 1.3 | Mann-Whitney 1938.000 | | >0.05 |

Note: (n) is the number of cases; (Min) is the minimum value; (Max) is the maximum value; (Sd) is the standard deviation; (df) is the degrees of freedom. All ages were pooled. Mann Whitney statistical test calculated when the independent t-test was not possible to be calculated due to a non-normal distribution.

**Table 9b**: Independent means t-test comparing humeral robusticity (Males)

| Index | | Coastal fishers | | | | | Inland agriculturalists | | | | | T-test | df | p |
|---|---|---|---|---|---|---|---|---|---|---|---|---|---|---|
| | | Males | | | | | Males | | | | | | | |
| | | n | Min | Max | Mean | Sd | n | Min | Max | Mean | Sd | | | |
| Humeral Robusticity | R | 21 | 18.9 | 23.4 | 21.0 | 1.4 | 27 | 17.1 | 22.4 | 20.3 | 1.1 | -1.775 | 46 | >0.05 |
| | L | 19 | 18.2 | 23.3 | 20.1 | 1.4 | 30 | 18.1 | 22.9 | 20.2 | 1.2 | Mann-Whitney 282.000 | | >0.05 |
| | R+L | 40 | 18.2 | 23.4 | 20.5 | 1.4 | 57 | 17.1 | 22.9 | 20.2 | 1.2 | 1.082 | 95 | >0.05 |

Note: (n) is the number of cases; (Min) is the minimum value; (Max) is the maximum value; (Sd) is the standard deviation; (df) is the degrees of freedom. All ages were pooled. Mann Whitney statistical test calculated when the independent t-test was not possible to be calculated due to a non-normal distribution.

## Discussion

On the assumption that the MOS analysed in this study are related to workload and physical activity, the mechanical stress involved in hunting and gathering marine fauna during the 3rd-2nd millennium BC as well as practising agriculture during the 1st millennium AD of northern Chile appears to be similar for males and females. The only exception was represented by enthesophytes where inland females were more affected than coastal females and also by spondylolysis where coastal males were more affected than inland males. On the other hand, a variety of other mechanisms that are not necessarily activity-related and sex-based such as hormonal changes and normal variation of bone responding to stress could have also played a role. The presence of enthesophytes is also positively correlated with age and these groups were not the exception. As found by Ponce (2010b) the Kendall's tau-b correlation between enthesophytes and age confirms this idea.

Coastal and inland males and females were similarly affected by osteoarthritis regardless the physical activity and the subsistence economy practised. The only exception was the hip joint, which was significantly more affected in coastal males compared to inland males. The analysis of individual joints also showed no significant differences in involvement among these populations. With particular attention to this joint, Waldron (1995, 1997) and Baetsen *et al.* (1997) suggested that the pattern of hip OA has changed over time, indicating a steady decrease in prevalence rate from the early pre-medieval period to the modern period in European populations. This temporal trend in the prevalence of OA has led a number of scholars working with skeletons from Native American populations to propose that, with the shift from a subsistence economy based on hunting and gathering to agriculture, there was a decrease in the condition (Walker and Hollimon, 1989; Larsen *et al.* 2007; Danforth *et al.* 2007). On the other hand, Hutchinson *et al.* (2007) and Marquez Morfín and Storey (2007) observed a temporal increase in OA.

The present study showed that regardless of sex and the time period, both coastal and inland males and females were equally affected by osteoarthritis, thus confirming the idea that this is the most common degenerative condition affecting humans worldwide (Bullough, 2004a). Furthermore, as found by Ponce (2010b) in a study conducted with these populations, OA was positively correlated with age therefore posing a question on its reliability as a MOS.

The data on spondylolysis showed that coastal males were more affected than inland males. Clinical studies have suggested that there are two basic movements regarded as potentially predisposing to lysis of the pars interarticularis, repetitive spinal flexion and extension. The physical activities, sports and occupations that have been mentioned as requiring these movements are throwing sports, weight lifting, artistic gymnastics, rowing, wrestling, football, cricket and diving among others (Rossi and Dragoni, 1990; Soler and Calderón, 2000; Bono, 2004). Although weight lifting, throwing activities and rowing might have been performed by coastal males as daily activities, it would be difficult to confirm if the aetiology of spondylolysis in their cases was triggered by any of these. On the other hand, as indicated by a number of family and twin studies (Albanese and Pizzutillo, 1982; Young and Koning, 2003) the underlying hereditary potential and congenital malformation of the laminae cannot be disregarded as contributory aetiological factor.

Inland agriculturalists on the other hand, appeared, according to these findings, not to have suffered such a negative effect on the spine. The absence of reports of spondylolysis in other Amerindians who practised a similar subsistence economy raises a question regarding the implication for these activities in the aetiology of the condition.

With regards to os acromiale it was not possible to determine Chi-square analysis between coastal and inland females because the former group did not present any example of the condition. Assuming that os acromiale results from physical activity, it could be suggested that there was a marked sexual division of labour among coastal males and females although future studies involving a larger number of acromia might give a more definite answer. On the other hand, sex bias in the presence of os acromiale will tend to favour the trauma theory, according to Case *et al.* (2006), following the assumption that a sexual division of labour and sport preference exists between sexes.

Modern clinical studies have suggested that os acromiale is commonly linked to sports and athletes engaged in 'overhead' activities, or physical activity where repetitive overhead arm motions are combined with abduction and external rotation of the arm such as in volleyball, handball, tennis, badminton and swimming (Pećina and Bojanić, 1993; Pagnani *et al.* 2006; Demetracopoulos *et al.* 2006). In line with this idea, bioarchaeological studies have suggested a connection between os acromiale and archery and the use of projectiles in general (Stirland, 1987, 2000; Knüsel, 2007). The use of arrows, bows, atlatls and harpoons is consistent with 'overhead' activities and with the archaeological record of coastal hunter-gatherers (Arriaza, 1995). However, it cannot be confirmed if these activities were directly responsible for the aetiology of this condition as os acromiale can occur in response to a genetic predisposition to non-fusion of the acromion.

Finally, the metric analysis also showed that males and females were equally robust and hypertrophic in their upper limbs. Assuming that bones respond to mechanical stimuli by remodelling their structure in the direction of the functional stress, as explained by 'Wolff's Law', it could be suggested that the trends found with the robusticity index could be interpreted as resulting from equal mechanical demands and workload. However, the well known bone morphology influencing variables including diet and hormonal changes with age, as well as nutritional and inheritance influences, should not be ruled out as influential aetiological factors.

To summarise, on the basis of the MOS analysed in this study, the arrival of agriculture in northern Chile cannot be regarded as a negative event in the health of the local populations. Fairly equal distributions of the conditions analysed in this study along with the results for the robusticity index, have suggested that both sexes were subjected to a similar degree of physical stress despite the contrasting subsistence economies practised by these populations. On the other hand, the multifactorial aetiology of these MOS should not be dismissed because, as reviewed earlier, all the conditions analysed in this study including the external bone measurements can respond to multiple factors other than solely to physical activity.

Besides the multifactorial origin of these MOS, a number of other issues not always considered by bioarchaeologists are worthy of mention. Firstly, although bone changes can result from subjecting the skeleton to repetitive tasks over a long period of time, Jurmain (1999) has emphasised that the many varied activities that human beings put their bodies through during their lives should similarly be considered. On the contrary, Merbs (1983) has argued that despite the variety of activities to which humans expose their bodies, even during one entire day, there are certain activities that are performed repetitively over and over again if they are necessary for survival. In this context Arriaza (1995) emphasised that, because food is essential to survival, the pursuit of dietary needs can became a primary determinant of behaviour.

Secondly, apart from the type, duration and range of activities performed by human beings during their lives, there are other factors such as ethnicity, sex, age, diet and genetics that may affect or influence the way people practise a specific activity, along with how the activity affects the body (Jurmain 1999). Being able to evaluate the role played by these individual variables in human skeletal remains can prove challenging. In this context, it is hoped that the analysis of other skeletal markers other than those analysed in this study will contribute to better understanding the effect that the arrival of agriculture had on the health of the Native American populations.

## Conclusion

On the basis of the MOS analysed in this study, it is suggested that the lifestyle of coastal populations during the 3rd millennium BC could be regarded to be as physically demanding as that practised by inland populations settled in the Azapa valley of northern Chile during the 1st millennium AD. Whether these similarities correlate to similarities in levels of specific/general activity is highly debatable because of the many aetiological factors that can cause these MOS. However, the results found in this study followed those obtained by a number of scholars involved in the study of physical activity, health and the arrival of agriculture among prehistoric Amerindian populations. These studies support the idea that human health did not necessarily decline after the adoption of farming and the rise of civilisation. Hence, the gradual transition towards a sedentary way of life and the reliance on food production in northern Chile did not represent a negative impact to the health of these prehistoric populations.

## Acknowledgements

The author would like to thank her supervisors, Prof Charlotte Roberts and Dr Andrew Millard for their help and guidance throughout the course of her PhD and also the support of Durham University, the Durham Doctoral Fellowship Award and the Rosemary Cramp Fund.

## Literature Cited

Albanese, M. and Pizzutillo, P. 1982. Family study of spondylolysis and spondylolisthesis. *Journal of Pediatric Orthopedics* 2: 496-499.

Alfonso, M., Standen, V. and Castro, V. 2007. The adoption of agriculture among Northern Chile populations in Azapa Valley, 9000-1000 BP. In: Cohen, M. and Crane-Kramer, G. (eds.) *Ancient health. Skeletal indicators of agricultural and economic intensification*. University Press of Florida: Gainesville Fl. 114-129.

Alves Cardoso, F. and Henderson, C. 2010. Enthesopathy formation in the humerus: data from known age-at-death and known occupation skeletal collections. *American Journal of Physical Anthropology* 141: 550-560.

Andrianakos, A., Kontelis, L., Karamitsos, D., Aslanidis, S., Georountzos, A., Kaziolas, G., Pantelidou, K., Vafiadou, E. and Dantis, P. 2006. Prevalence of symptomatic knee, hand, and hip osteoarthritis in Greece. The ESORDIG study. *The Journal of Rheumatology* 33: 2507-2513.

Arriaza, B. 1994. Tipología de las momias Chinchorro y evolución de las practicas de momificación. *Chungará* 26: 11-24.

Arriaza, B. 1995. *Beyond death. The Chinchorro mummies of Ancient Chile*. Smithsonian Institution: Washington DC.

Arriaza, B. 1997. Spondylolysis in prehistoric human remains from Guam and its possible etiology. *American Journal of Physical Anthropology* 104: 393-397.

Aufderheide, A., Muñoz, I. and Arriaza, B. 1993. Seven Chinchorro mummies and the prehistory of northern Chile. *American Journal of Physical Anthropology* 91: 189-201.

Baetsen, S., Bitter, P. and Bruintjes, T. 1997. Hip and knee osteoarthritis in an eighteenth century urban population. *International Journal of Osteoarchaeology* 7: 628-630.

Bass, W. 2005. *Human osteology. A laboratory and field manual*. Archaeological Society: Missouri.

Benjamin, M. and Ralphs J. 1997. Tendons and ligaments – an overview. *Histology and Histopathology* 12: 1135-1144.

Benjamin, M., Newell, R., Evans, E., Ralphs, J. and Pemberton, D 1992. The structure of the insertions of the tendons of biceps brachii, triceps and brachialis in elderly dissecting room cadavers. *Journal of Anatomy* 180: 327-332.

Bono, C. 2004. Low-back pain in athletes. *Journal of Bone and Joint Surgery* 86-A: 382-396.

Bridges, P. 1989. Changes in activities with the shift to agriculture in the Southeastern United States. *Current Anthropology* 30: 385-394.

Bridges, P. 1991a. Degenerative joint disease in hunter-gatherers and agriculturalists from the Southeastern United States. *American Journal of Physical Anthropology* 85: 379-391.

Bridges, P. 1991b. Skeletal evidence of changes in subsistence activities between the Archaic and Mississippian time periods in Northwestern Alabama. In: Powell, M., Bridges, P. and Mires, A.

(eds.) *What mean these bones? Studies in southeastern bioarchaeology*. University of Alabama Press: Tuscaloosa, Al. 89-101.

Brooks, S. and Suchey, J. 1990. Skeletal age determination based on the os pubis: a comparison of the Acsádi-Nemeskéri and Suchey-Brooks methods. *Human Evolution* 5: 227-238.

Buikstra, J. and Ubelaker, D. 1994. *Standards for data collection from human skeletal remains*. Research Series 44. Arkansas Archeological Survey: Fayetteville, Ar.

Bullough, P. 2004a. *Orthopaedic pathology*. Mosby: Edinburgh.

Bullough, P. 2004b. The role of joint architecture in the etiology of arthritis. *Osteoarthritis and Cartilage* 12: 2-9.

Case, D., Burnett, S. and Nielsen, T. 2006. Os acromiale: population differences and their etiological significance. *Homo* 57: 1-18.

Christensen, R., Astrup, A. and Bliddal, H. 2005. Weight loss: the treatment of choice for knee osteoarthritis? A randomized trial. *Osteoarthritis and Cartilage* 13: 20-27.

Cohen, M. and Armelagos, G. (eds.) 1984. *Paleopathology at the origins of agriculture*. Academic Press: New York.

Cohen, M. and Crane-Kramer, G. (eds.) 2007. *Ancient health. Skeletal indicators of agricultural and economic intensification*. University Press of Florida: Gainesville, Fl.

Coote, A. and Haslam, P. 2004. *Rheumatology and orthopaedics*. Mosby: Edinburgh.

Danforth, M., Jacobi, K., Wrobel, G. and Glassman, S. 2007. Health and the transition to horticulture in the South-Central United States. In: Cohen, M. and Crane-Kramer, G. (eds.) *Ancient health. Skeletal indicators of agricultural and economic intensification*. University Press of Florida, Gainesville, Fl. 65-79.

Demetracopoulos, C., Kapadia, N., Herickhoff, P., Cosgarea, A. and McFarland, E. 2006. Surgical stabilization of os acromiale in a fast-pitch softball pitcher. *American Journal of Sports Medicine* 34: 1855-1859.

Doherty, M., Spector, T. and Serni, U. 2000. Session 1: epidemiology and genetics of hands osteoarthritis. *Osteoarthritis and Cartilage* 8 (Suppl A): 14-15.

Eller, N., Skylv, B., Ostri, B., Dahlin, E., Suadicani, P. and Gyntelberg, F. 1992. Health and lifestyle characteristics of professional singers and instrumentalists. *Occupational Medicine* 42: 89-92.

Fibiger, L. and Knüsel, C. 2005. Prevalence rates of spondylolysis in British skeletal populations. *International Journal of Osteoarchaeology* 15: 164-174.

Focacci, G. 1981. Nuevos fechados para la época del Tiahuanaco en la arqueología del norte de chile. *Chungará* 8: 63-77.

Focacci, G. and Chacón, S 1989. Excavaciones arqueológicas en los faldeos del Morro de Arica sitios Morro 1/6 y 2/2. *Chungará* 22: 15-62.

Freemont, A. 2002. Enthesopathies. *Current Diagnostic Pathology* 8: 1-10.

Ganz, R., Leunig, M., Leunig-Ganz, K. and Harris, W. 2008. The etiology of osteoarthritis of the hip. *Clinical Orthopaedics and Related Research* 466: 264-272.

Grotle, M., Hagen, K., Natvig, B., Dahl, F. and Kvien, T. 2008. Obesity and osteoarthritis in knee, hip/or hand: an epidemiological study in the general population with 10 years follow-up. *Musculoskeletal Disorders* 9: 132-136.

Havelková, P., Villotte, S., Velemínský, L., Poláček, L. and Dobisíková, M. 2011. Enthesopathies and activity patterns in the early medieval great Moravian population: evidence of division of labour. *International Journal of Osteoarchaeology* 21(4): 487-504.

Hutchinson, D., Norr, L. and Teaford, M. 2007. Outer coast foragers and inner coast farmers in late prehistoric North Carolina. In: Cohen, M. and Crane-Kramer, G. (eds.) *Ancient health. Skeletal indicators of agricultural and economic intensification*. University Press of Florida, Gainesville, Fl. 52-64.

Jones, G., Cooley, H. and Stankovish, J. 2002. A cross sectional study of the association between sex, smoking, and other lifestyle factors and osteoarthris of the hand. *The Journal of Rheumatology* 29: 1719-1724.

Jurmain, R. 1999. *Stories from the skeleton. Behavioral reconstruction in human osteology*. Gordon and Breach Sciences Publishers: New York.

Karlsson, M., Vergnaud, P., Delmas, P. and Obrant, K. 1995. Indicators of bone formation in weight lifters. *Calcified Tissue International* 56: 177-180.

Kennedy, K. 1989. Skeletal markers of occupational stress. In: İşcan, M. and Kennedy, K. (eds.) *Reconstruction of life from the skeleton*. Wiley-Liss: New York. 129-160.

Knüsel, C. 2007. Activity-related skeletal change. In: Fiorato, V., Boylston, A. and Knüsel, C. (eds.). *Blood red roses. The archaeology of a mass grave from the battle of Towton AD 1461*. Oxbow Books: Oxford. 103-118.

Larsen, C. 2002. Bioarchaeology: the lives and lifestyles of past people. *Journal of Archaeological Research* 10: 119-166.

Larsen, C., Hutchinson, D., Stojanowski, C., Williamson, M., Griffin, M., Simpson, S., Ruff, C., Schoeninger, M., Norr, L., Teaford, M., Driscoll, E., Schmidt, C. and Tung, T. 2007. Health and lifestyle in Georgia and Florida. Agricultural origins and intensification in regional perspectives. In: Cohen, M. and Crane-Kramer, G. (eds.) *Ancient health. Skeletal indicators of agricultural and economic intensification*. University Press of Florida, Gainesville, Fl. 20-34.

Loth, S. and İşcan, M. 1989. Morphological assessment of age in the adult: the thoracic region. In: İşcan, M. (ed). *Age markers in the human skeleton*. Charles C. Thomas: Springfield, Il. 105-136.

Lovejoy, C., Meindl, R., Pryzbeck, T. and Mensforth, R. 1985. Chronological metamorphosis of the auricular surface of the ilium: a new method for the determination of age at death. *American Journal of Physical Anthropology* 68: 15-28.

Marquez Morfín , L. and Storey, R. 2007. From early village to regional center in Mesoamerica: an investigation of lifestyles and health. In: Cohen, M. and Crane-Kramer, G. (eds.) *Ancient health. Skeletal indicators of agricultural and economic intensification*. University Press of Florida: Gainesville Fl. 80-91.

Mays, S. 2010. *The archaeology of human bones*. London: Routledge.

Merbs, C. 1983. *Patterns of activity-induced pathology in a Canadian Inuit population*. Mercury Series 119. National Museum of Man: Ottawa, Canada.

Merbs, C. 1996. Spondylolysis and spondylolisthesis: a cost of being an erect biped or a clever adaptation? *Yearbook of Physical Anthropology* 101(S23): 201-228.

Muñoz, I. 1983. El poblamiento aldeano en el valle de Azapa y su vinculación con Tiwanaku (Arica-Chile). Asentamientos Aldeanos en los Valles Costeros de Arica. *Documento de Trabajo* 3: 43-94.

Nagy, B. 1998. Age, activity, and musculoskeletal stress markers. *American Journal of Physical Anthropology* 26: 168-169 [abstract].

Pagnani, M., Mathis, C. and Solman, C. 2006. Painful os acromiale (or unfused acromial apophysis) in athletes. *Journal of Shoulder and Elbow Surgery* 15: 432-435.

Pearson, O. and Lieberman, D. 2004. The aging of Wolff's "Law": ontogeny and responses to mechanical loading in cortical bone. *Yearbook of Physical Anthropology* 47: 63-99.

Pećina, M. and Bojanić, I. 1993. *Overuse injuries of the musculoskeletal system*. CRC Press: London.

Ponce P. 2010a. Biosocial aspects of sexual division of labour among prehistoric Chinchorro people. *Society, Biology & Human Affairs* 75: 41-65.

Ponce, P. 2010b. *A comparative study of activity-related skeletal changes in 3rd-2nd millennium BC coastal fishers and 1st millennium AD inland agriculturists in Chile, South America*. Unpublished PhD thesis. Durham University.

Resnick, D. 2002. Diffuse idiopathic skeletal hyperostosis (DISH): ankylosing hyperostosis of Forestier and Rotes-Querol. In: Resnick, D. (ed.) *Diagnosis of bone and joint disorders*. W. B. Saunders: Philadelphia, Pa. 1477-1503.

Resnick, D., Goergen, T. 2002. Physical injury: concepts and terminology. In: Resnick, D. (ed.) *Diagnosis of bone and joint disorders*. W.B. Saunders: Philadelphia, Pa. 2627-2782.

Robb, J. 1998. The interpretation of skeletal muscle sites: a statistical approach. *International Journal of Osteoarchaeology* 8: 363-377.

Roberts, C., Cox, M. 2003. *Health and disease in Britain: from prehistory to the present day*. Sutton Publishing: Stroud.

Rogers, J. and Waldron, T. 1995. *A field guide to joint disease in archaeology*. John Wiley & Sons: Chichester.

Rossi, F. and Dragoni, S. 1990. Lumbar spondylolysis: occurrence in competitive athletes. Updated achievements in a series of 390 cases. *Journal of Sports Medicine and Physical Fitness* 30: 450-452.

Ruhoy, M., Schweitzer, M. and Resnick, D. 1998. Enthesopathy. In: Klippel, J. and Dieppe, P. (eds.) *Rheumatology*. Mosby: London. 1-6.

Ruff, C., Holt, B. and Trinkaus, E. 2006. Who's afraid of the big bad Wolff?: "Wolff's Law" and bone functional adaptation. *American Journal of Physical Anthropology* 129: 484-498.

Soler, T. and Calderón, C. 2000. The prevalence of spondylolysis in the Spanish elite athlete. *American Journal of Sports Medicine* 28: 57-62.

Solovieva, S., Vehmas, T., Riihimäki, H., Luoma, K. and Leino-Arjas, P. 2005. Hand use and patterns of joint involvement in osteoarthritis. A comparison of female dentists and teachers. *Rheumatology* 44: 521-528.

Stafford, L. and Youssef, P. 2002. Spondyloarthropathies: an overview. *Internal Medicine Journal* 32: 40-46.

Standen, V. 2003. Bienes funerarios del cementerio Chinchorro Morro1: descripción, análisis e interpretación. *Chungará* 35: 175-207.

Steen, S. and Lane, R. 1998. Evaluation of habitual activities among two Alaskan Eskimo populations based on musculoskeletal stress markers. *International Journal of Osteoarchaeology* 8: 341-353.

Stirland, A. 1987. A possible correlation between os acromiale and occupation in the burials from the Mary Rose. *Proceedings of the Fifth European Meeting of the Paleopathology Association*. Paleopathology Association: Siena, Italy.

Stirland, A. 2000. *Raising the dead. The skeleton crew of King Henry VIII's great ship, the Mary Rose*. John Wiley & Sons: Chichester.

Sutter, R. and Mertz, L. 2004. Nonmetric cranial trait variation and prehistoric biocultural change in the Azapa Valley, Chile. *American Journal of Physical Anthropology* 123: 130-145.

Villotte, S., Castex, D., Couallier, V., Dutour, O., Knüsel, C. and Henry-Gambier, D. 2010 Enthesopathies as occupational stress markers: evidence from the upper limb. *American Journal of Physical Anthropology* 142: 224-234.

Waldron, T. 1995. Changes in the distribution of osteoarthritis over historical time. *International Journal of Osteoarchaeology* 5: 385-389.

Waldron, T. 1997. Osteoarthritis of the hip in past populations. *International Journal of Osteoarchaeology* 7: 186-189.

Waldron, T. 2007. *Palaeoepidemiology. The measure of disease in the human past*. Left Coast Press: Walnut Creek Ca.

Walker, P. and Hollimon, S. 1989. Changes in osteoarthritis associated with the development of a maritime economy among southern California Indians. *International Journal of Anthropology* 4: 171-183.

Walker-Bone, K. and Palmer, K. 2002. Musculoskeletal disorders in farmers and farm workers. *Occupational Medicine* 52: 441-450.

Whiting, W. and Zernicke, R. 2008. *Biomechanics of musculoskeletal injury*. Human Kinetics: Champaign, Il.

Woods, C., Hawkins, R. and Hodson, A. 2002. The football association medical research programme: an audit of injuries in professional football-analysis of preseason injuries. *British Journal of Sports Medicine* 36: 436-441.

Young, K. and Koning, W. 2003. Spondylolysis of L2 in identical twins. *Journal of Manipulative and Physiological Therapeutics* 26: 196-201.

# The Human Remains from the Medieval Islamic Cemetery of Can Fonoll, Ibiza, Spain: Preliminary Results

Xenia-Paula Kyriakou[1], *Nicholas Márquez-Grant[2,3], Helen Langstaff[1], Cara Samuels[1], Carrie Springs Pacelli[1], Jonathan Castro[4], Joan Roig[4] and Elena F. Kranioti[1]

[1]Forensic Anthropology
School of History, Classics and Archaeology
The University of Edinburgh
Edinburgh UK

[2] Cellmark Forensic Services, Abingdon, UK

[3] Institute of Human Sciences
School of Anthropology and Museum Ethnography
University of Oxford, Oxford, UK

[4] Freelance Archaeologist, Ibiza, Spain

*Email for correspondence: nmarquez-grant@cellmark.co.uk

**Abstract**
Skeletal remains constitute the most direct evidence of past populations. Osteological data, integrated with historical and archaeological information, are necessary for a thorough analysis of ancient populations. Here we present the study of a medieval Islamic cemetery excavated in Ibiza, Spain. The cemetery contained 167 single inhumations with the skeletons lying on their right side and facing Mecca following the traditional Muslim burial ritual. This paper focuses on the biological and demographic profile of the population with reference to metric data, skeletal and dental pathology.

Interestingly, there is a lack of infant burials and of individuals over 45 years of age while the majority of the individuals were estimated to be young adults. Although only a small sample was well preserved to provide adequate measurements, stature estimates indicate that both male and females were shorter compared to other, earlier, later and contemporary populations from the Iberian Peninsula and the Balearic Islands. Preliminary observations revealed some pathological conditions including cribra orbitalia and osteoarthritis. The results of this work provide an invaluable insight into Ibiza's Moorish period, as well as that of the Balearic Islands, whereas the findings of this study will contribute to the osteological and palaeopathological record of European anthropology and medieval archaeology.

**Keywords**: Ibiza, Islamic, Palaeopathology

## Introduction

Ibiza, part of the Balearic Islands, is located in the western Mediterranean Sea, near the eastern coast of the Iberian Peninsula. Due to its location, the island has been settled and ruled by many different populations including, but not limited to the following: Phoenicians, Carthaginians, Romans, Byzantines and Moors (McMillan and Boone 1999). The Moors are believed to have brought significant changes to the island including transformations regarding language, social structure and technology. Evidence from stable isotope analysis of 21 individuals from Es Soto in Ibiza show a unique dietary pattern compared to earlier populations (Fuller *et al.* 2010). Although there are few Islamic sites already excavated and studied in Ibiza (e.g. Gómez-Bellard 1989; Márquez-Grant 1999; 2000) at present the total number of individuals available for comparison are less than one hundred and data is quite limited and still unpublished. Consequently very little is known so far for the biological characteristics of the *Ibicenco Muslims*. The present study aims to contribute to fill that gap by providing information on the population of Can Fonoll, the largest Islamic cemetery excavated so far in Ibiza and probably in the Balearic Islands. Can Fonoll was a rural cemetery on the SW of the island and has provided information regarding the lifestyle of the inhabitants of Ibiza between the 10th and 13th centuries AD (Fig. 1).

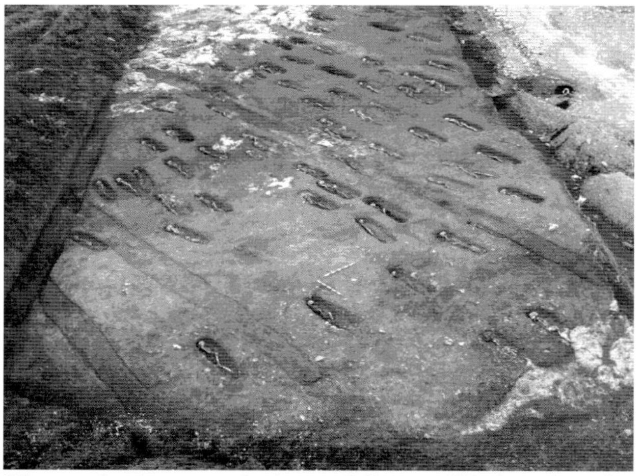

**Figure 1:** A general view of Sector IV showing the positions of the graves.

The present work is a summary of a much larger monograph publication (in preparation) which aims to reconstruct the demographic profile and investigate physical characteristics of the population, assess the health status, assess the level of inter/intra-personal violence, reconstruct living conditions and if possible throw light on the social status of the people of Can Fonoll. It is hoped that the skeletal analysis will contribute to further our understanding of the Islamic period in the island and also to contribute to the osteological and palaeopathological record for this region and for Spain in general. In order to address these aims, the minimum number of individuals was calculated, their age-at-death and sex were estimated where possible, in addition to obtaining information on physical characteristics such as cranial shape and stature. The range and extent of pathological conditions were also explored.

## Material and Methods

The excavation took place between 2006 and 2008 which recorded a total of 167 burials dating between the 10th and 13th centuries AD (Castro Orellana 2009). From these 167 graves, a total of 154 skeletons were preserved and lifted from the ground, thus submitted for osteological analysis contributing towards the demography and palaeopathology of the Can Fonoll population. Examination of the remains was undertaken in May 2010 by the present authors from the University of Edinburgh under the supervision of Dr E. Kranioti and with the assistance of Dr N. Márquez-Grant. The majority of the assemblage comprised articulated skeletons representing various age groups and both sexes. These skeletons were buried in single inhumation burials, lying on their right side and facing SE towards Mecca (Fig. 2).

After the bones had been cleaned, the skeletal material was primarily examined macroscopically in accordance with recognized international guidelines (e.g. Ferembach *et al.* 1980; Buikstra and Ubelaker 1994; Brickley and McKinley 2004).

The minimum number of individuals (MNI) present in each burial was calculated based on the number of the most frequently repeated element(s), combined with age-at-death and sex considerations.

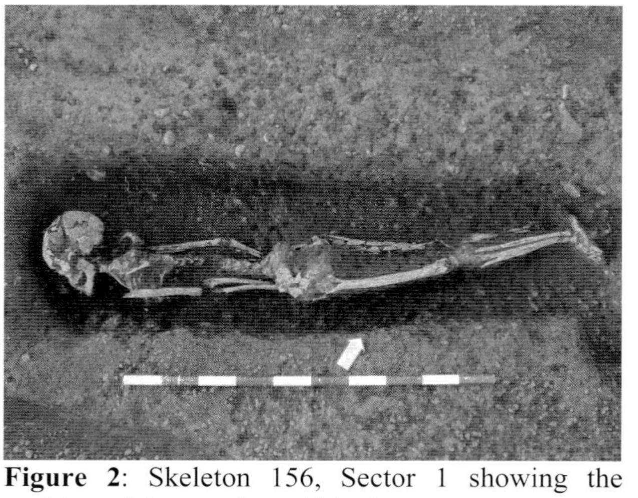

**Figure 2**: Skeleton 156, Sector 1 showing the position of the remains within the grave.

Subadult age-at-death estimation was based primarily on the observation of the stage of dental development (Smith 1991; Ubelaker 1999), followed by the stage of epiphyseal fusion and by diaphyseal long bone length (see Scheuer and Black 2000). Wherever possible, a combination of methods was used to estimate age-at-death in adults (>18 years) (Bedford *et al.* 1993). This took into account late fusing epiphyses (e.g. clavicle, sacrum), the characteristics of the auricular surface (Lovejoy *et al.* 1985; Buckberry and Chamberlain 2002) and the pubic symphysis (Katz and Suchey 1986; Brooks and Suchey 1990), and dental attrition (Miles 1963; Brothwell 1981).

Sexually dimorphic features of the pelvis were employed to estimate skeletal sex in adults (Buikstra and Ubelaker 1994). Cranial traits were found to be ambiguous and were not considered in the present study (Langstaff 2010). A number of standard measurements taken on the femur, the humerus and the mandibular ramus were employed for sex determination, since univariate and multivariate functions extrapolated from a previous analysis on this population were proven successful (Langstaff 2010).

A standard set of cranial and post-cranial measurements (after Martin and Saller 1957; Krogman and İşcan 1986; Buikstra and Ubelaker 1994) was taken on the adult skeletons. Stature was estimated based on sex-specific formulae for the femur (Pearson 1898; Trotter 1970; Robins and Shute 1986). Femora with obvious pathological lesions and trauma were not considered as this would have affected the measurements.

Cranial, dental and post-cranial non-metric analysis was undertaken by following the guidelines primarily set out by Hauser and De Stefano (1989) and Buikstra and Ubelaker (1994) (see Pacelli 2010 for a list of dental traits identified in the population of Can Fonoll).

Dental health was assessed by examining the frequency of conditions such as dental caries, dental calculus, ante-mortem tooth loss, periodontitis and periapical cavities. In addition, enamel hypoplasia was recorded since it may provide an insight into physiological stress during childhood. Enamel hypoplasias (linear type) were scored following the guidelines of the *Fédération Dentaire Internationale* (1982); dental caries scoring followed the recommendations by Hillson (2001); dental calculus the classification of Brothwell (1981); and periapical lesions the nomenclature by Dias and colleagues (Dias and Tayles 1997; Dias *et al.* 2007).

All skeletons were examined for pathological conditions based on the recommendations by Roberts and Connell (2004). When present, lesions were diagnosed with reference to standard texts (e.g. Ortner and Putschar 1981; Aufderheide and Rodríguez-Martín 1998). Since many studies make inferences about the health status of the population by examining growth (including stature), sexual dimorphism, possible indicators of anaemia (e.g. cribra orbitalia), periostitis, trauma and osteoarthritis (e.g. Bush and Zvelebil 1991; Steckel *et al.* 2002), these conditions will be the focus of the Can Fonoll palaeopathological analysis. Only bones or articular surfaces with cortical bone in sufficient condition (falling within the surface preservation IFA grades 0-3, McKinley 2004) were considered for calculating the prevalence of osteoarthritis. Further information on recording of specific palaeopathological conditions is included in the following section.

## Results

### *Skeletal Preservation*

Approximately 69% of the sample comprised skeletons that were less than 25% complete, followed by the second largest group of skeletons (18.8%) which were between 25% and 50% complete. Only 2.5% (4 skeletons) were over 75% complete. In addition to the bulk of skeletons being incomplete, regrettably most of them were also in very poor condition with regard to surface erosion and fragmentation. This limited the age-at-death and sex estimations as well as palaeopathological diagnosis. Table 1 includes the percentage of skeletons classified into the different grades of bone surface preservation following the classification of McKinley (2004). Since six skeletons were only represented by teeth, the total number of skeletons considered for Table 1 is 148.

**Table 1:** Condition of the skeletons in the Can Fonoll assemblage. Note: '0' represents an excellent condition and '5' or '5+' extensive penetrating erosion affecting the bone profile.

| Bone condition (McKinley 2004) | Number of skeletons | % of sample |
|---|---|---|
| 0 | 0 | 0 |
| 1 | 0 | 0 |
| 2 | 0 | 0 |
| 3 | 2 | 1.2 |
| 4 | 20 | 12.9 |
| 5 | 44 | 28.5 |
| 5+ | 82 | 53.2 |
| Total skeletons | 148 | - |

Most skeletons displayed a significant degree (grades 4-5+) of surface erosion. This degree of preservation affected the assessment of palaeopathological conditions (e.g. periostitis). In addition, in excess of 90% of the skeletons were highly fragmented, meaning multiple post-mortem breaks usually resulting in small (<5 cm) fragments or splinters and involving over 75% of the bones in the skeleton. This was a considerable limitation particularly for metrical analysis.

*Demographic Information*

The medieval assemblage from Can Fonoll comprised 21 subadults, 112 adults and 21 skeletons of unknown age-at-death. Table 2 provides the summary data for the population and the percentages of deaths in each category. Unfortunately, due to poor preservation of pelvic bones, at least 95 adults could only be aged based on dental attrition, which is a problem to bear in mind although dental attrition has proved to be relatively reliable for some archaeological populations from Ibiza (Márquez-Grant 2006).

Among the adults, 23 were females or possibly females, 35 were males or possibly males and the sex assessment of the remaining individuals was not possible. The results shown in Figure 3 do not illustrate an expected U-shaped mortality curve (Waldron 1994). The profile obtained reveals an absence of perinates, neonates and infants (<1 year of age), a surprisingly high number of deaths in the young adult age category and an absence of over 45-year-olds (Fig. 3). Previous spatial analysis of burials according to age-at-death and sex has revealed no specific clusters or patterns (Langstaff 2010).

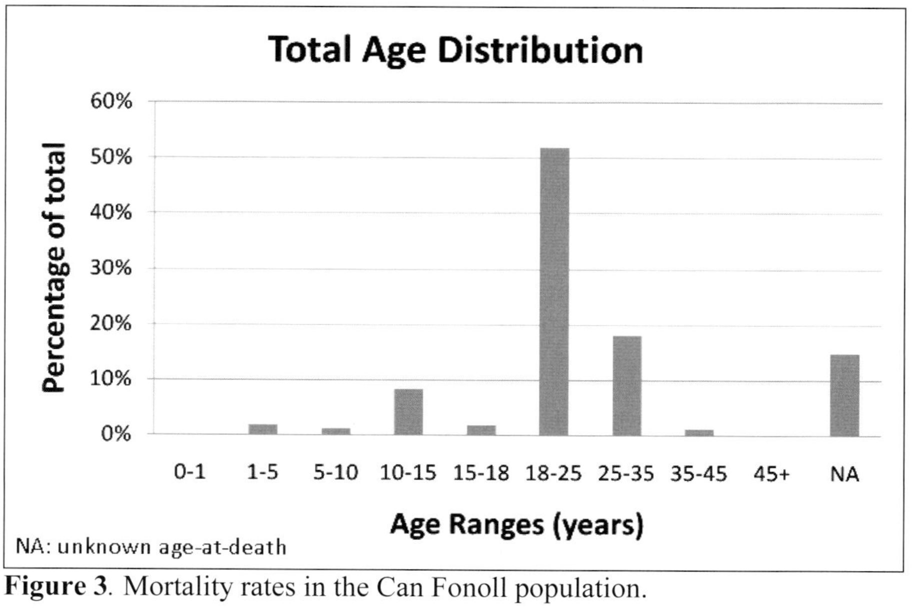


**Figure 3**. Mortality rates in the Can Fonoll population.

**Table 2:** Age and sex distribution of the Can Fonoll assemblage (number of individuals)

| Age category | F | F? | M? | M | ? | TOTAL | % |
|---|---|---|---|---|---|---|---|
| Perinate | - | - | - | - | 0 | 0 | 0 |
| Neonate | - | - | - | - | 0 | 0 | 0 |
| <1 year | - | - | - | - | 0 | 0 | 0 |
| 1-5 years | - | - | - | - | 3 | 3 | 1.9 |
| 5-10 years | - | - | - | - | 2 | 2 | 1.3 |
| 10-15 years | - | - | - | - | 13 | 13 | 8.4 |
| 15-18 years | - | - | - | - | 3 | 3 | 1.9 |
| Subadult (age unknown) | - | - | - | - | 0 | 0 | 0 |
| 18-25 years | 14 | 3 | 4 | 19 | 40 | 80 | 51.9 |
| 25-35 years | 5 | 0 | 0 | 9 | 14 | 28 | 18.1 |
| 35-45 years | 0 | 0 | 0 | 2 | 0 | 2 | 1.3 |
| >45 years | 0 | 0 | 0 | 0 | 0 | 0 | 0 |
| Adult (age unknown) | 1 | 0 | 0 | 1 | 0 | 2 | 1.3 |
| Unknown age | 0 | 0 | 0 | 0 | 21 | 21 | 13.6 |
| TOTAL | 20 | 3 | 4 | 31 | 96 | 154 | 100 |

*Physical Characteristics*

From the 36 measurements (Martin and Saller 1957; Krogman and İşcan 1986; Buikstra and Ubelaker 1994) which were considered for the best preserved adult skulls (N=90), only a limited amount of information was obtained. Table 3 presents the descriptive statistics for the available measurements on the adult crania and mandibles from Can Fonoll. This data may serve for comparative studies employing Principal Component Analysis.

Sex was available for 58 individuals and sexual dimorphism was explored by means of ANOVA for six measurements only due to small sample size. Chin height and minimum ramus breadth were the only two variables found to differ significantly ($p<0.05$) between males and females. However, the sample was too small to properly explore sexual dimorphism.

A t-test analysis between this Islamic sample and a modern Spanish one (Río Muñoz 2000) indicates that out of 10 measurements considered, only four were found to differ significantly ($p<0.05$) between the groups (Table 4). In all these cases, the Islamic individuals showed greater values. We have assumed a canonical distribution in both groups in order to make the comparisons and we used similar size samples to minimize biases. However a larger sample is needed in order to depict accurately the differences between the two groups. This is a common limitation when analyzing archaeological samples with poor preservation.

Descriptive statistics for humeral and femoral measurements exploring sexual dimorphism are available from the authors upon request, and the discriminant functions derived from these may serve other anthropologists analyzing material from other sites in Ibiza. For the purpose of the present paper, only long bone measurements from the femur are presented for stature calculation (Table 5).

At a first glance the formulae of Pearson and of Robins and Shute give very similar estimates for males but it seems that the latter equations underestimate females. A paired student t-test was performed between the estimates according to Pearson and according to Robins and Shute and there was a significant difference ($p<0.05$) between the means for females which indicates that one of the equations introduces a large error. Trotter and Gleser formulae for White Females provided values closer to those given by applying Pearson's method. It must be stressed however that the limited sample size may have introduced bias in the results and therefore a larger sample is necessary in order to properly test the validity of the equations. This is a common problem in archaeological samples where the number of intact long bones is very limited and therefore any effort to reconstruct stature results problematic.

Female femora were on average 16 cm shorter than males. Taking Pearson's method, the average male height was 159.4 cm, with a range from 154.6 cm to 168 cm. The average female stature was 150.5 cm (range 139-161 cm).

*Non-Metrical Variation*

All adult skeletons were examined for presence or absence of non-metric traits. Data was obtained on 22 cranial and 19 post-cranial traits. In addition, the presence of 21 dental morphological traits was also assessed (Pacelli 2010). The data was extremely limited due to the fragmented nature of the assemblage and when results were obtained these did not provide any information regarding activity or habitual posture, or genetic relations. Further information on frequencies for each trait can be obtained from the authors.

*Dental Health Status*

Dental information was recovered from 135 skeletons (88.31% of the sample). Table 6 provides a brief summary of frequencies of oral pathology in the sample. Data for dental caries and ante-mortem tooth loss are first presented according to anterior (incisors, canines) and posterior (premolars, molars) teeth as recommended in the literature (e.g. Hillson 2001). No caries correction factors were applied to this population.

Low frequencies were observed for dental caries, dental calculus, ante-mortem tooth loss and periapical lesions. No frequencies of enamel hypoplasia could be obtained due to the poor state of preservation of the teeth although it can be said that these lesions were found on at least six permanent teeth from two different individuals. Periodontitis could not be assessed due to the high degree of fragmentation and post-mortem erosion on the mandibles and maxillae.

**Table 3**: Descriptive statistics of cranial and mandibular measurements (both sexes pooled).

| | N | Minimum | Maximum | Mean | SD |
|---|---|---|---|---|---|
| Cranial Length | 17 | 123.00 | 215.00 | 173.35 | 26.38 |
| Nasion-Bregma | 13 | 97.15 | 117.80 | 108.16 | 6.56 |
| Bregma-Lambda | 15 | 112.36 | 190.06 | 124.03 | 19.05 |
| Lambda-Opisthion | 8 | 73.16 | 135.00 | 98.97 | 19.34 |
| Lambda-Inion | 8 | 12.71 | 108.53 | 61.37 | 25.93 |
| Inion-Opisthion | 4 | 43.00 | 99.21 | 59.63 | 26.51 |
| Frontal Arc | 5 | 104.00 | 152.00 | 129.40 | 17.50 |
| Parietal Arc | 6 | 100.00 | 150.00 | 125.83 | 16.09 |
| Occipital Arc | 3 | 112.00 | 163.00 | 131.67 | 27.43 |
| Biasterion breadth | 3 | 111.78 | 115.87 | 113.71 | 2.05 |
| Cranial Breadth | 9 | 125.90 | 145.00 | 137.21 | 5.38 |
| Max Frontal Breadth | 3 | 113.94 | 135.00 | 126.31 | 11.00 |
| Min Frontal Breadth | 6 | 90.39 | 103.58 | 96.16 | 5.86 |
| Mastoid Height R | 29 | 19.17 | 34.50 | 25.5 | 4.38 |
| Mastoid Height L | 14 | 19.05 | 33.67 | 24.89 | 4.20 |
| Chin Height | 18 | 23.67 | 36.85 | 29.68 | 3.79 |
| Bicondylar Breadth | 15 | 95.60 | 132.00 | 114.62 | 8.7 |
| Bigonial Breadth | 14 | 86.00 | 119.00 | 101.18 | 8.59 |
| Bimental Breadth | 8 | 41.90 | 51.00 | 45.82 | 2.68 |
| Min Ramus Breadth | 37 | 26.28 | 39.38 | 32.52 | 3.04 |

**Table 4:** T-differences for cranial and mandibular dimensions between the Can Fonoll population and a Modern Spanish sample (both sexes pooled). *p<0.05

| | Medieval Islamic | | | Modern Spanish | | | T-differences |
|---|---|---|---|---|---|---|---|
| **Measurements** | **N** | **Mean** | **SD** | **N** | **Mean** | **SD** | **between the samples** |
| Cranial Length | 17 | 173.35 | 26.38 | 30 | 178.67 | 8.47 | -0.807 |
| Nasion-Bregma | 13 | 108.16 | 6.56 | 30 | 110.33 | 5.35 | -1.142 |
| Lambda-Opisthion | 8 | 98.97 | 19.34 | 30 | 94.33 | 4.54 | 0.673 |
| Cranial Breadth | 9 | 137.21 | 5.38 | 30 | 135.53 | 4.76 | 0.9 |
| Mastoid Height R | 28 | 25.73 | 4.28 | 30 | 11.03 | 2.16 | *16.329 |
| Mastoid Height L | 15 | 25.03 | 4.08 | 30 | 10.93 | 2.27 | *12.450 |
| Chin Height | 18 | 29.68 | 3.79 | 30 | 31.73 | 4.17 | -1.709 |
| Bicondylar Breadth | 14 | 114.62 | 8.7 | 30 | 113.7 | 5.38 | 0.433 |
| Bigonial Breadth | 14 | 101.18 | 8.59 | 30 | 96.0 | 6.29 | *2.260 |
| Min Ramus Breadth | 37 | 32.52 | 7.32 | 30 | 29.73 | 2.33 | *4.139 |

**Table 5:** Stature (in cm) computed from the adult skeletons from Can Fonoll

| Skeleton | Sex | Bone | Side | Max length (mm) | Pearson (1898) | Robins and Shute (1986) | Trotter and Gleser 'Blacks' (Trotter 1970) | Trotter and Gleser 'Whites' (Trotter 1970) |
|---|---|---|---|---|---|---|---|---|
| 62 | M | Femur | L | 410 | 158.4 | 158.3 | 156.86+/-3.94 | 159.2 +/-3.27 |
| 51 | M | Femur | L | 400 | 156.5 | 156.2 | 154.75+/-3.94 | 156.8+/-3.27 |
| 54 | M | Femur | L | 390 | 154.6 | 154.1 | 152.64+/-3.94 | 154.4+/-3.27 |
| 17 | M | Femur | R | 461 | 168.0 | 169.0 | 167.621+/-3.94 | 171.3+/-3.27 |
| **Average male** | | **Femur** | | **415.25** | **159.4** | **159.4** | **158.0+/-3.94** | **160.4+/-3.27** |
| 43 | F | Femur | L | 395 | 149.7 | 142.5 | 151.3+/3.41 | 151.7+/-3.72 |
| 63 | F | Femur | R | 390 | 148.7 | 141.5 | 150.1+/3.41 | 150.4+/-3.72 |
| 49 | F | Femur | R | 340 | 139.0 | 130.8 | 138.5+/3.41 | 138.1 +/-3.72 |
| 98 | F | Femur | R | 410 | 152.6 | 145.7 | 154.8+/3.41 | 155.4+/-3.72 |
| 114 | F | Femur | R | 405 | 151.6 | 144.7 | 153.6+/3.41 | 154.1+/-3.72 |
| 132 | F | Femur | R | 455 | 161.3 | 155.4 | 165.2+/3.41 | 166.5+/-3.72 |
| **Average female** | | **Femur** | | **399.16** | **150.5** | **143.4** | **152.3+/3.41** | **152.7+/-3.72** |

**Table 6:** Summary of oral pathology in the population

| Condition | Deciduous | Permanent (Subadult ages) | Permanent (Adult ages) | Total |
|---|---|---|---|---|
| Total teeth present | 127 | 396 | 2476 | 2999 |
| Dental caries | 3/78 (3.8) | Ant = 1/150 (0.6)<br>Post = 17/243 (6.9)<br>Tot = 18/393 (4.5) | Ant = 32/916 (3.4)<br>Post = 223/1487 (14.9)<br>Tot = 255/2403 (10.6) | Dec: 3.8%<br>Per: 9.7% |
| Calculus | 0/77 (0) | 0/413 (0) | 63/2347 (2.6) | Dec: 0%<br>Per: 2.2% |
| Ante-mortem tooth loss | - | - | Ant = 4/959 (0.4)<br>Post = 62/1588 (3.9)<br>Tot=66/2547 (2.5) | 2.5% |
| Periapical lesions (alveoli observed) | 1/486 (0.2%) | | 0/2398 (0) | 0.0% |

Codes: Ant = anterior teeth (incisors and canines); Post = posterior teeth (premolars and molars); Tot = total; Dec = Deciduous teeth; Per = Permanent teeth

*Skeletal Pathology*

The poor preservation of the sample impeded an assessment of pathological conditions on most skeletons. Nevertheless, there was evidence for metabolic conditions, osteoarthritis and trauma. Although periostitis is routinely assessed (e.g. see Steckel *et al.* 2002) and would have provided information regarding living conditions and health status, unfortunately due to significant weathering (erosion) of the bone surface it was not possible to score presence or absence of these lesions. Where a lesion was observed, it was described in detail including the stage of healing, location, severity and extent.

*Cribra Orbitalia*

Cribra orbitalia was identified when the surface of the orbital roofs presented pits of varying size and density and which differed (e.g. smooth edges) from post-mortem damage. In this medieval population, abnormal pitting was observed on five adult skeletons and one subadult skeleton. The prevalence in the population was 8.82% (6/68 crania).

*Osteoarthritis and Degenerative Joint Disease (DJD)*

Every joint surface was scored for presence or absence of osteoarthritis (OA) in adults. Presence of OA was characterised by eburnation or at least the presence of two of the following modifications on the joint surface: sub-chondral pitting, bone growth (osteophytes) and ante-mortem contour change (Rogers and Waldron 1995). Every surface had to be at least 75% preserved for observation, including both the joint surface and the joint margins. Figure 4 summarizes the crude prevalence (from the total of adult individuals in the assemblage) of osteoarthritis. Due to the problems of limited preservation of the sample, the data available have to be taken as a *minimum* when obtaining frequencies and therefore may not reflect the actual percentage of cases in the population. A total of eight skeletons showed evidence of joint degeneration including the areas of the temporo-mandibular joint, the neck, the shoulder and the hands.

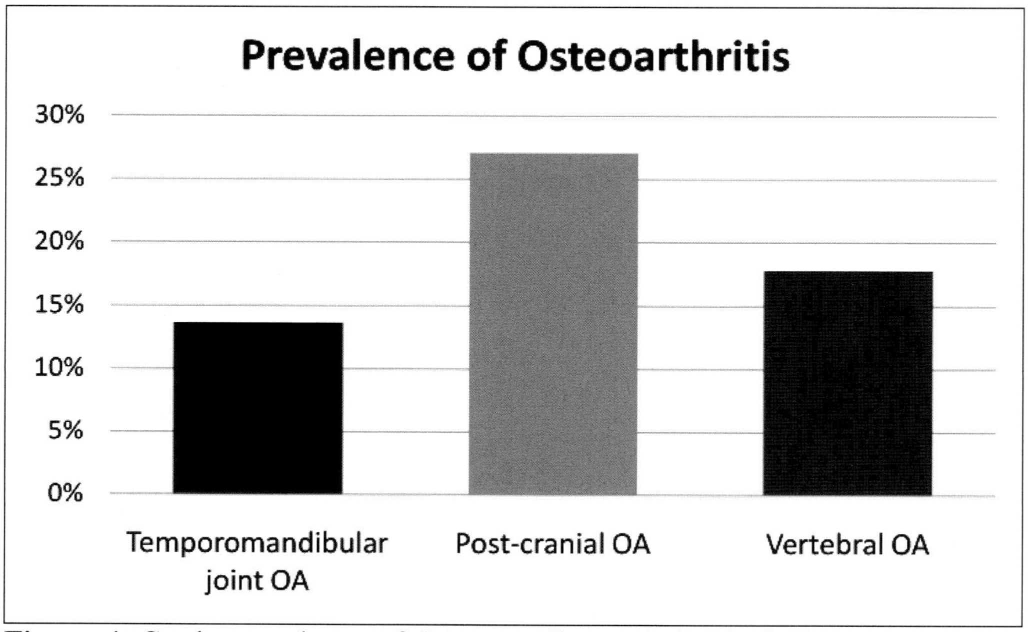


**Figure 4**. Crude prevalence of OA according to individuals (N = 112 adults); temporomandibular joint OA = 13.6%, post-cranial OA =27.1% and vertebral OA = 17.8%.

*Trauma*

Out of 90 well preserved crania, two (2.2%) showed evidence of trauma. The first case involved a healed depressed fracture on the right parietal. The second case presented a healed fracture on the left temporal bone affecting the region of the auditory meatus and the mastoid process. This caused resorption of the external auditory meatus and altered the normal morphology of the bone. A radiograph and a CT scan were obtained and infection was ruled out as a probable cause.

In the postcranial skeleton, only a left clavicle had a healed fracture on its midshaft. Most of the skeletons in the assemblage were incomplete and the crude prevalence for post-cranial trauma is low with a frequency of 0.6% individuals affected (1/148).

No peri-mortem trauma was identified in the sample. However, excavation records provide evidence of an arrowhead in contact with the vertebral column of one individual, but poor preservation of the bone could not verify any skeletal injury.

*Other Conditions*

There are a number of other conditions that were not the focus of this paper but contribute to the osteological and palaeopathological record of medieval Ibiza. Adult skeleton (skeleton 469, burial 136) presented early stages of fusion of the sacro-iliac joint. The most likely diagnosis for this is an inflammatory arthropathy such as ankylosing spondylitis (AS), although it can occur in infection and other conditions. The exact aetiology of AS is somewhat unknown but genetic factors are considered to play a significant role, with most sufferers having a specific gene called HLA-B27, which has been found in around 80% of Mediterranean cases, over 90% of Northern European cases, and around 50% of African-Americans. By contrast, this gene is only present in 8% of Caucasoids and around 2-3% of African-Americans who do not have AS (Khan 2002: 2). Ankylosing Spondylitis may also appear secondary to Familial Mediterranean Fever (FMF), a hereditary auto-inflammatory disorder mainly found within individuals of Mediterranean origin or ancestry. Arthritis is one of the manifestations of this disorder, and in some cases it develops into ankylosing spondylitis (Knockaert *et al.* 1989; Cosan *et al.* 2010).

Two adult skeletons (skeletons 189 and 213, from burials 43 and 51 respectively) presented abnormal bowing of the humeri. Computed Tomography (CT) was utilized to examine these bones radiographically in order to exclude previous trauma as the main causal factor. A potential diagnosis for these is healed rickets or osteomalacia, but neither of the two skeletons had any other bony lesions to further support this hypothesis.

A probable case of Eagle's Syndrome may have been present on an adult skull (skeleton 54, burial 16). Although fragmentary, a rather elongated styloid process measuring a minimum of 33.39 mm was present on the skeleton (Eagle 1937; 1948; 1949; Moffat *et al.* 1977). Finally, a potential lytic lesion appeared to be present on the incomplete orbital roof of skeleton 475 (burial 138). A diagnosis cannot be made given the fragmentary nature of the skeleton.

**Discussion**

In spite of some of the caveats mentioned above such as sample representativity and preservation affecting primarily age-at-death estimation and palaeopathological analysis, the information obtained provides some insight into the lifestyle and living conditions of a rural Muslim community in medieval Ibiza. It also raises questions for further research

*Demography*

Both juvenile and adult individuals, females and males, were represented in the assemblage and no clustering according to these parameters is obvious in the cemetery (Langstaff 2010). In spite of the problems inherent in palaeodemography including sample representativity, accuracy of age and sex estimation, excavation sampling process and that the mortality rates obtained only represent a mean of the entire use of the cemetery among other problems (e.g. Bocquet-Appel and Masset 1982; Boddington 1987; Waldron 1994; Chamberlain 2000a; 2000b); the demographic data obtained revealed an unexpected lack of infants buried in the cemetery, an apparent absence of individuals over the age of 45 years, and an unexpected bulk of young adult deaths. The lack of infants among the skeletons buried in the cemetery often indicates their burial elsewhere. However, it is not typical of contemporary examples from Ibiza (Márquez-Grant *pers. obs.*) or from Islamic cemeteries in mainland Spain (e.g. Guijo *et al.* no date).

If different funerary practices or problems with preservation do not account for this lack of infants and children younger than five years of age, a much higher mortality rate would have been expected (Hewlett 1991; Chamberlain 2000b). Deaths occurring in the first few years of life would tend to be associated, if not by cultural practices such as infanticide, with factors that affect mortality rates today including diarrhea, malaria, measles and respiratory infections, especially affecting individuals who are malnourished (Rousham and Humphrey 2002). A high percentage of deaths in the young adult category would be typical of a 'catastrophic assemblage' (Margerison and Knüsel 2002) but the absence of mass graves, the relatively long time span of the cemetery and the low - if any - evidence of interpersonal violence do not account for this. One possible factor for this 'anomaly' is the age-at-death estimation based on dental wear which raises concerns of reliability, although it has proven to have some success in other archaeological populations from Ibiza (Márquez-Grant 2006).

*Physique and Appearance*

Fragmentation and condition of the bone provided little opportunity to investigate the physical characteristics of the population. Data on cranial shape was obtained and can be employed for future biodistance analysis. When some of these measurements are compared with a modern Spanish sample, the medieval crania from Can Fonoll were found to be larger for both males and females.

Difficulties are always encountered when deciding what formulae to use in the computation of stature. The formulae by Pearson (1898) is commonly used in Spain and often used in southern European populations (Formicola 1993: 352). This method alongside others including Trotter and Gleser's 1952 and 1958 methods for 'Blacks' (Trotter 1970) has proven to be more reliable than Trotter and Gleser's method for 'Whites', for Spanish and a number of Mediterranean populations (Lalueza-Fox 1998). Since North African immigration may be expected due to the location and history of Ibiza, formulae modified from Trotter and Gleser's equations for 'Blacks' were also employed (Robins and Shute 1986). We decided to accept the stature estimates according to Pearson so that we could be consistent when comparing with other Spanish populations. Although the sample size is small and warrants caution, these means at present are lower compared to other medieval Islamic and Christian populations from Spain (e.g. Guijo *et al.* no date; Du Souich 1979; López Martínez 2002) and compared to earlier populations from Ibiza (Márquez-Grant 2006). Changes in stature over time can be explained by environmental factors such as nutrition, health, climate, altitude, social and economic status, culture, and migrations (Ulijaszek 1998), and this may be explored in the future.

### *Health Status and Living Conditions*

A number of palaeopathological lesions or conditions were employed to attempt to understand the health status and living conditions of the population. Since the analysis of dentitions recovered from archaeological sites can offer an insight into the type of diet and the level of oral hygiene of the population, an assessment of dental health was undertaken. Among the factors contributing to the presence of dental defects are malnutrition, infectious disease, diabetes, trauma, neonatal disturbances, psychological stress, genetic background but largely poor living conditions overall (eg. see Pindborg 1982; Dobney and Goodman 1991). The presence of some hypoplasias would be the result of physiological stress (e.g. caused by illness and malnutrition) in some individuals.

Low prevalence of cribra orbitalia have also been reported in this assemblage and are much lower than any preceding Punic and Roman populations from the island (Márquez-Grant 2006). Pathogen load could play a major role in its prevalence (Stuart-Macadam 1992). In particular, attention has been given to the possible role of iron deficiency anaemia on these lesions (El-Najjar *et al.* 1976; Stuart-Macadam 1998), although other contributing factors must be considered too (e.g. see Polo Cerda *et al.* 1999; Wapler *et al.* 2004; Walker *et al.* 2009). The presence of these lesions reflects some chronic health problem which generally results from a complex combination of factors associated with diet, population aggregation, contaminated water, plagues, zoonoses, population movement and inefficient waste disposal (Kent 1986; Holland and O'Brien 1997). Whether one or more of these explanations could be applied to the population of Can Fonoll in Ibiza, would depend on data obtained during future archaeological, historical and palaeo-environmental research.

Osteoarthritis is of multifactorial aetiology (Weiss and Jurmain 2007). Whether it is a valid marker of occupational stress is a matter of debate. However, even though a condition that goes hand-in-hand with growing old, when appeared in specific patterns or it more severely affects less biomechanically active joints such as those other than the hip, followed by the shoulder, then osteoarthritis might have some occupational significance. Osteoarthritis was evident on the skull (temporo-mandibular joint), neck, shoulders, and hands. Modifications at the temporo-mandibular joint may be related to dental functions such as attrition (Hodges 1991), although there was a larger number of young adults showing slight attrition. In young adults, osteoarthritis developed at the shoulder and hand could have been influenced by repetitive mechanical strain (Weiss and Jurmain 2007). The results show a minimum frequency of affected individuals since many articular surfaces were incomplete due to poor preservation and the results given were crude according to individuals affected.

### *Trauma and Level of Violence*

The level of trauma was low in the population and in those skeletons where trauma was present, some treatment or care for the patient must have facilitated the healing process, reflected by the well-healed fractures (slight overlapping, slight shortening, slight angulation).

Low trauma rates may suggest a low level of conflict even though the extent of soft tissue trauma is unknown. No fractures were observed on the hand bones, ulnae or any other bones apart from one clavicle; and no obvious peri-mortem trauma was observed. These low frequencies may be suggestive of times of social and political stability (Lessa and Mendonça de Souza 2004: 385) yet the poor preservation of the assemblage may be impeding additional discoveries of this type. However, such a conclusion may not be unlikely and probably is applicable for the Can Fonoll population. Yet, historical as well as archaeological sources should be combined to verify this interpretation; further study is required with regard to the context in which an arrowhead was found within a burial.

*Diet and Oral Hygiene*

The rate of dental caries falls within the range for the medieval period in the Iberian Peninsula (see Lalueza-Fox and González Martín 1999). Stable isotope analysis on an urban Islamic population in Ibiza, shows an increase in marine consumption at this time as well as an increase in carbohydrates and a decrease in meat consumption in comparison with other periods (Fuller *et al.* 2010).

Apart from dental caries, oral pathology is low in the population. Low percentages of dental diseases may also reveal good levels of oral hygiene, although it is necessary to bear in mind that young adults comprise the majority of the population.

**Concluding Remarks**

This study has presented data obtained from the anthropological study of the largest medieval Islamic skeletal assemblage to date in Ibiza, Spain. Despite the poor preservation, a number of aims have been addressed and a number of questions raised. Of interest is the absence of infants buried in the cemetery and this renders the question of why might this be. Further comparative work and research on funerary practices may help to address the issue. The majority of deaths in the young adult categories is suspicious and questions arise with regard to the reliability of the methods employed and the need to undertake further tests with skeletons of known age from skeletal development or pelvic indicators and perhaps the omission of the third molar which due to its variation in eruption may be lowering the average age estimation. If these frequencies and the lack of over 45-year-olds appear to be real, however, explanations may be sought taking into account a wider biocultural approach.

With regard to cranial shape, differences have been observed between the Islamic and Modern collections and this motivates a research interest into cranial shape over time in the island and with comparisons with other regions, in order to potentially examine microevolution and understand potential immigration.

Cribra orbitalia, linear enamel hypoplasia and stature may be reflective of poor living conditions in this rural population. However, these frequencies are much lower than those obtained from more ancient populations (see Márquez-Grant 2006). Future statistical analysis comparing Can Fonoll with other Ibizan populations and also future analyses on more Islamic assemblages will be able to confirm or reject this interpretation. Indeed, there are problems such as preservation, the age factor and small sample size, in addition to the complexity of interpreting palaeopathological data, however it may also be that there is a real trend reflecting lower physiological stress or better adaptiveness of the population to the environment in medieval Ibiza. The exception to this may be stature which may reveal some stunting compared to other contemporary populations but only increased sample sizes from different periods will be able to confirm or refute such a hypothesis.

Osteoarthritis was prevalent in the sample and surprisingly so in a population comprised largely of young adults, assuming age-at-death estimation is correct. The rates provided are crude at present but nevertheless provide a minimum percentage of individuals affected. There have been ethnographic studies observing local farmers using Islamic agricultural techniques and it may be of interest to see if any research questions can be addressed linking both data together.

Trauma is low in this population. Although evidence for warfare is lacking, two cases possibly reflect interpersonal violence. Once more data is obtained in the future from other medieval Islamic assemblages, it would be important to interpret and discuss these palaeopathological results with historians and archaeologists who specialize in medieval Ibiza.

Oral pathology also improves here with time and the caries indicates a higher level of increased reliance on carbohydrates compared to other earlier populations. The low frequencies of oral pathology in a largely young sample, nevertheless may suggest good levels of oral hygiene.

**Acknowledgments**

The Ibiza 2010 Edinburgh Field School would like to thank all the local archaeologists for their hospitality and their help regarding the archaeological survey. The authors would like to thank Dara Fleming-Farrel, Sara Harris and

Francesca Migliaccio for their contribution in data collection. Special thanks to the Department of Radiology of the Can Misses Hospital in Eivissa (Ibiza) for allowing the use of Radiography and Computed Tomography for the complete examination of the collection. The accommodation and traveling expenses were sponsored by the Abercromby Fund and the University of Edinburgh training assistance grants. EFK like to thank Jim Crow for his invaluable support during our effort to prepare the team for the 2010 Ibiza anthropological survey, and for encouraging us to continue to provide training and research opportunities to the MSc students in Archaeology.

**Literature Cited**

Aufderheide, A.C. and Rodríguez-Martín, C. 1998. *The Cambridge encyclopedia of human paleopathology.* Cambridge University Press: Cambridge.

Bedford, M.E., Russell, K.F., Lovejoy, C.O., Meindl, R.S., Simpson, S.W. and Stuart-Macadam, P. 1993. Test of the multifactorial aging method using skeletons with known ages-at-death from the Grant Collection. *American Journal of Physical Anthropology* 91: 287-297.

Bocquet-Appel, J.P. and Masset, C. 1982. Farewell to paleodemography. *Journal of Human Evolution* 11: 321-333.

Boddington, A, 1987. From bones to population: the problem of numbers In: Boddington, A., Garland, A.N. and Janaway, R.C. (eds.) *Death, decay and reconstruction. Approaches to archaeology and forensic science.* Manchester University Press: Manchester. 180-197.

Brickley, M. And McKinley, J.I. (eds.) 2004. *Guidelines to the standards for recording human remains.* Institute of Field Archaelogists Paper Number 7. British Association for Biological Anthropology and Osteoarchaeology and Institute of Field Archaeologists: Southampton and Reading.

Brooks, S.T. and Suchey, J.M. 1990. Skeletal age determination based on the os pubis: a comparison of the Acsadi-Nemeskéri and Suchey-Brooks methods. *Human Evolution* 5: 227–238.

Brothwell, D.R. 1981. *Digging up bones.* Oxford University Press/British Museum: Oxford.

Buckberry, J.L. and Chamberlain, A.T. 2002. Age estimation from the auricular surface of the ilium: a revised method. *American Journal of Physical Anthropology* 119: 231-239.

Buikstra, J.E. and Ubelaker, D.H. (eds.) 1994. *Standards for data collection from human skeletal remains.* Arkansas Archeological Survey: Fayetteville, Arkansas. Research Series No. 44.

Bush, H. and Zvelebil, M. 1991. Pathology and health in past societies: an introduction. In Bush, H. and Zvelebil, M. (eds.) *Health in past societies. Biocultural interpretations of human skeletal remains in archaeological contexts.* Tempus Reparatum: Oxford. 3-9. BAR International Series 567.

Castro Orellana, J. 2009. La intervenció arqueològica al sector IV de la necròpolis medieval islàmica de Can Fonoll, durant el seguiment arqueològic del nou accés a l'aeroport d'Eivissa. *Quaderns d'Arqueologia Ebusitana* I: 112-119.

Chamberlain, A. 2000a. Problems and prospects in palaeodemography. In: Cox, M. and Mays, S. (eds.) *Human osteology in archaeology and forensic science.* Greenwich Medical Media Ltd: London. 101-115.

Chamberlain, A. 2000b. Minor concerns: a demographic perspective on children in past societies. In: Sofaer Derevenski, J. (ed.) *Children and material culture.* Routledge: London. 206-212.

Cosan, F.C., Üstek, D., Oku, B., Duymaz-Tozkir, J., Cakiris, A., Abaci, A., Ocal, L., Aral, O. and Gül, A. 2010. Association of familial Mediterranean fever–related MEFV variations with ankylosing spondylitis. *Arthritis & Rheumatism* 62: 3232–3236.

Dias, G. and Tayles, N. 1997. 'Abscess cavity' – a misnomer. *International Journal of Osteoarchaeology* 7: 548-554.

Dias, G., Prasad, K. and Santos, A.L. 2007. Pathogenesis of apical periodontal cysts: guidelines for diagnosis in paleopathology. *International Journal of Osteoarchaeology* 17: 619-626.

Dobney, K. and Goodman, A. 1991. Epidemiological studies of dental enamel hypoplasias in Mexico and Bradford: their relevance to archaeological skeletal studies. In: Bush, H. and Zvelebil, M. (eds.) *Health in past societies. Biocultural interpretations of human skeletal remains in archaeological contexts.* Tempus Reparatum: Oxford. 81-100. BAR International Series 567.

Du Souich, P. 1979. Estudio antropológico de la necrópolis medieval de la Torrecilla (Arenas del Rey, Granada). *Antropología y Paleoecología Humana* 1: 27-40.

Eagle, W.W. 1937. Elongated styloid process: report of two cases. *Archives of Otolaryngology* 25: 584-586.

Eagle, W.W. 1948. Elongated styloid process: further observations and a new syndrome. *Archives of Otolaryngology* 47: 630-640.

Eagle, W.W. 1949. Symptomatic elongated styloid process: report of two cases of styloid process-Carotid artery syndrome with operation. *Archives of Otolaryngology* 49: 490-503.

El-Najjar, M.Y., Ryan, D.J., Turner II, C.G. and Lozoff, B. 1976. The etiology of porotic hyperostosis among the prehistoric and historic Anasazi Indians in southwestern United States. *American Journal of Physical Anthropology* 44: 477-488.

Fédération Dentaire International. 1982. An epidemiological index of developmental defects of dental enamel (DDE Index). *International Dental Journal* 32: 159-167.

Ferembach, D., Schwidetzky, I. and Stloukal, M. 1980. Recommendations for age and sex diagnoses of skeletons. *Journal of Human Evolution* 9: 517-549.

Formicola, V. 1993. Stature reconstruction from long bones in ancient population samples: an approach to the problem of its reliability. *American Journal of Physical Anthropology* 90: 351-358.

Fuller, B., Márquez-Grant, N. and Richards, M.P. 2010. Investigation of diachronic dietary patterns on the islands of Ibiza and Formentera, Spain: evidence from carbon and nitrogen stable isotope ratio analysis. *American Journal of Physical Anthropology* 143: 512-522.

Guijo, J.M., Pecero, J.C. and Lacalle, R. n.d. Estudio antropológico. In: Romo, A. (ed). *Intervención arqueológica en la Plaza de España. Écija. Memoria Final. Volumen 1, Memoria 1.* 247 - 291

Gómez-Bellard, F. 1989. *Antropología Médica en Ibiza.* Colección Tesis Doctorales núm. 104/89. Editorial de la Universidad Complutense de Madrid. Facsímil de la Tesis Doctoral presentada en 1987: Madrid.

Hauser, G. and De Stefano, G.F. 1989. *Epigenetic variants of the human skull.* Schweizerbart, Stuttgart.

Hewlett, B.S. 1991. Demography and childcare in preindustrial societies. *Journal of Anthropological Research* 47(1): 1-37.

Hillson, S. 2001. Recording dental caries in archaeological human remains. *International Journal of Osteoarchaeology* 11: 249-289.

Hodges, D.C. 1991. Temporomandibular joint osteoarthritis in a British skeletal population. *American Journal of Physical Anthropology* 85: 367-377.

Holland, T.D. and O'Brien, M.J. 1997. Parasites, porotic hyperostosis, and the implications of changing perspectives. *American Antiquity* 62: 183-193.

Katz, D. and Suchey, J.M. 1986. Age determination of the os pubis. *American Journal of Physical Anthropology* 69: 427-435.

Kent, S. 1986. The influences of sedentism and aggregation on porotic hyperostosis and anaemia: a case study. *Man* 21: 605-636.

Khan, M.A. 2002. Ankylosing spondylitis: introductory comments on its diagnosis and treatment. *Annals* of the Rheumatic Diseases 61: *iii3-iii7*

Knockaert, D.C. Malysse, I.G. and Peetermans, W.E. 1989. Ankylosing spondylitis. An unusual manifestation of familial Mediterranean fever. Report of a case complicated by amyloidosis and polyneuropathy. *Clinical Rheumatology* 8(3): 408-412

Krogman, W.M. and İşcan, M.Y. 1986. *The human skeleton in forensic medicine.* 2nd ed. Charles C. Thomas: Springfield, Illinois.

Lalueza-Fox, C. 1998. Stature and sexual dimorphism in ancient Iberian populations. *Homo,* 49: 260-272.

Lalueza-Fox, C. and González Martín, A. 1999. Oral pathology on the Iberian Peninsula and Balearic Islands from the Mesolithic to present times. *Homo* 50: 54-65.

Langstaff, H. 2010. *Demographic data of the Can Fonoll Islamic population from Ibiza, Spain.* Unpublished MSc thesis, University of Edinburgh.

Lessa, A. and Mendonça De Souza, S. 2004. Violence in the Atacama Desert during the Tiwanaku period: social tension? *International Journal of Osteoarchaeology* 14: 374-388.

López Martínez, B. 2002 *Los pobladores del antiguo reino de León: antropometría, paleodemografía, paleopatología.* Universidad de Leon: Leon.

Lovejoy, C.O., Meindl, R.S., Pryzbeck, T.R. and Mensforth, R.P. 1985. Chronological metamorphosis of the auricular surface of the ilium: a new method for the determination of adult skeletal age at death. *American Journal of Physical Anthropology* 68: 15-28.

Margerison, B.J. and Knüsel, C.J. 2002. Paleodemographic comparison of a catastrophic and an attritional death assemblage. *American Journal of Physical Anthropology* 119: 134-143.

Márquez-Grant, N. 1999. A palaeopathological comparison between two Mediterranean populations from the island of Ibiza, Spain. Unpublished MSc dissertation, University of Sheffield.

Márquez-Grant, N. 2000. Estudio antropológico de la necrópolis islámica de Es Soto (Ibiza). Unpublished report for the Consell Insular d'Eivissa i Formentera, Ibiza.

Márquez-Grant, N. 2006. *A bioanthropological perspective of the Punic period as evidenced by the analysis of human skeletal remains* Unpublished DPhil Thesis, University of Oxford.

Martin, R. and Saller, K. 1957 *Lehrbuch der Anthropologie.* Fischer: Stuttgart.

McKinley, J.I. 2004. Compiling a skeletal inventory: disarticulated and co-mingled remains. In: Brickley, M. and McKinley, J.I. (eds.) *Guidelines to the standards for recording human remains.* British Association for Biological Anthropology and Osteoarchaeology and Institute of Field Archaeologists: Southampton and Reading. Institute of Field Archaeologists Paper Number 7. 14-17.

McMillann, P.G., and Boone L.J. 1999. Population history and the Islamization of the Iberian Peninsula: skeletal evidence from the Lower Alentejo of Portugal. *Current Anthropology* 40: 719-726

Miles, A.E.W. 1963. The dentition in the assessment of individual age in skeletal material. In: Brothwell, D.R. (ed.) *Dental anthropology.* Pergamon: Oxford. 191-209.

Moffat, D.A, Ramsden, R.T. and Shaw, H.J. 1977. The styloid process syndrome: aetiological factors and surgical treatment. *The Journal of Laryngology and Otology* 91: 279-294

Ortner, D.J. and Putschar, W.G.J. 1981. *Identification of pathological conditions in human skeletal remains.* Smithsonian: Washington D.C. Smithsonian Contributions to Anthropology 28.

Pacelli, C.S. 2010. *Evaluation of morphological dental variants expressed on human dental remains from a necropolis in Ibiza, Spain.* Unpublished MSc thesis, University of Edinburgh.

Pearson, K. 1898. Mathematical contributions to the theory of evolution. On the reconstruction of the stature of prehistoric races. Royal Society of London: London. *Philosophical Transactions of the Royal Society of London*, Series A, 192. 169-244

Pindborg, J.J. 1982. Aetiology of developmental enamel defects not related to fluorosis. *International Dental Journal* 32: 123-134.

Polo Cerdà, M., Miquel Freucht, M.J. and Villalaín Blanco, J.D. 1999. Un modelo experimental de cribra orbitalia: estudio preliminar. In: Sánchez Sánchez, J.A. (ed.) *Actas del V Congreso Nacional de Paleopatología (Alcalá la Real, 1999).* 201-212.

Río Muñoz, P.A. del 2000. Estudio antropológico-forense, antropométrico y morfológico, de la colección de la Escuela de Medicina Legal de Madrid. Unpublished DPhil thesis, Universidad Complutense de Madrid.

Roberts, C. and Connell, B. 2004. Guidance on recording palaeopathology. In: Brickley, M. and

McKinley, J.I. (eds.), *Guidelines to the standards for recording human remains.* British Association for Biological Anthropology and Osteoarchaeology and Institute of Field Archaeologists: Southampton and Reading. Institute of Field Archaeologists Paper Number 7. 34-39.

Robins, G. and Shute, C.C.D. 1986. Predynastic Egyptian stature and physical proportions. *Human Evolution* 1: 313-324.

Rogers, J. and Waldron, T. 1995. *A field guide to joint disease in archaeology*. John Wiley and Sons: Chichester.

Rousham, E.K. and Humphrey, L.T. 2002. The dynamics of child survival. In: Macbeth, H. and Collinson, P. (eds.) *Human population dynamics: cross-disciplinary perspectives* 14. Cambridge University Press: Cambridge. Biological Society Symposium Series. 124-140.

Scheuer, L. and Black, S. 2000. *Developmental juvenile osteology*. Academic Press: London.

Smith, B.H. 1991. Standards of human tooth formation and dental age assessment. In: Kelley, M.A. and Larsen, C.S. (eds.) *Advances in dental anthropology*. Wiley-Liss: New York. 143-168.

Steckel, R.H., Rose, J.C., Larsen, C.S. and Walker, P.L. 2002. Skeletal health in the Western Hemisphere from 4000 B.C. to the present. *Evolutionary Anthropology* 11: 142-155.

Stuart-Macadam, P. 1992. Porotic hyperostosis: a new perspective. *American Journal of Physical Anthropology* 87: 39-47.

Stuart-Macadam, P. 1998. Iron deficiency anemia: exploring the difference. In: Grauer, A. and Stuart-Macadam, P. (eds.) *Sex and gender in paleopathological perspective.* Cambridge University Press: Cambridge. 45-63.

Trotter, M. 1970. Estimation of stature from intact long limb bones. In Stewart, T.D. (ed.) *Personal identification in mass disasters.* [*Report of a seminar held in Washington, D.C., 9-11 December 1968, by arrangement between the support services of the Department of the Army and the Smithsonian Institution*]. National Museum of Natural History, Smithsonian Institution: Washington D.C. 71-83.

Ubelaker, D.H. 1999. *Human skeletal remains. Excavation, analysis, interpretation.* 3rd ed. Taraxacum: Washington D.C.

Ulijaszek, S.J. 1998. The secular trend. In: Ulijaszek, S.J., Johnston, F.E. and Preece, M.A. (eds.) *Cambridge encyclopedia of human growth and development.* Cambridge University Press: Cambridge. 395-398.

Waldron, T. 1994. *Counting the dead. The epidemiology of skeletal populations.* John Wiley & Sons: Chichester.

Walker, P.L., Bathurst, R.R., Richman, R., Gjerdrum, T. and Andrushko, V.A. 2009. The causes of porotic hyperostosis and cribra orbitalia: a reappraisal of the iron-deficiency-anemia hypothesis. *American Journal of Physical Anthropology* 139: 109-125.

Wapler, U., Crubézy, E. and Schultz, M. 2004. Is cribra orbitalia synonymous with anemia? Analysis and interpretation of cranial pathology in Sudan. *American Journal of Physical Anthropology* 123: 333-339.

Weiss, E. and Jurmain, R. 2007. Osteoarthritis revisited: a contemporary review of aetiology. *International Journal of Osteoarchaeology* 17: 437-450.

# A New Known Age and Sex Collection at the Natural History Museum, London

Gabrielle Delbarre, Margaret Clegg*, Robert Kruszynski** and Heather Bonney

Department of Palaeontology
Natural History Museum
Cromwell Road
London SW7 5BD, UK.

*Email for correspondence: m.clegg@nhm.ac.uk
** Email for access to remains: r.kruszynski@nhm.ac.uk

**Abstract**

Skeletal remains of known age and sex are particularly important in research to act as comparators to validate and test methods which can then be applied to fossil, archaeological and modern human remains. Few such collections exist and those that are available are used widely in research in many different disciplines. Within the modern human remains collection at the Natural History Museum (NHM) there are individuals which evidence suggested might be of known age and sex, however the information had never been checked or collected together.

During 2009-2010 a project was undertaken to identify and verify the provenance of these remains. The aim was to establish an additional fully documented collection of known age and sex individuals drawn from a much wider geographical area than the widely known Christ Church Spitalfields crypt sample also held at the NHM. Evidence from the registers and index cards at the NHM were used to identify the potential known age and sex individuals. The potential sources of evidence for this information were located and then checked. The initial survey produced 610 records for potential known age and sex individuals. The study identified 109 individuals with verifiable age and sex and a further 98 individuals for whom sex could be accurately documented. There are at least an additional 104 individuals who require more investigation to verify these details. This collection will now be made available for research access.

**Keywords:** Human Remains, Known Age and Sex, Museum Records, Provenance

The research importance of human remains of known age and sex within the disciplines of medicine, physical anthropology and archaeology, in research as diverse as forensic science, growth studies and palaeodemography is well-known (Cox and Mays 2000; Roberts 2009). Such collections provide researchers with comparators that can be used to validate research in relation to fossil, archaeological, and modern human remains which are of unknown age and sex. Known age and sex collections make possible the testing of models that have been developed to infer the age and sex of individuals (in both ancient and modern populations) for which this information is lacking or incomplete (Hoppa and Fitzgerald 1999; White and Folkens 2005). For example, the blind study carried out on a sample of 363 teeth from known age and sex individuals by Wittwer-Backofen *et al.* (2004) to test tooth-cementum annulation as a method to estimate the age of adults showed a high correlation between the estimated and chronological ages (Wittwer-Backofen *et al.* 2004). Known age and sex collections are also heavily used in forensic anthropological research which often seeks to describe new methods for defining living biological characteristics from an individual's remains. They additionally form an essential part of the competency testing process which may eventually become part of the regulatory requirement in the UK. Sexual dimorphism is a continuous variable and reported observer error rates vary widely – most papers on sexing from morphological features of the pelvis report accuracy as being between 84% and 96% (Rogers and Saunders 1994; Volk & Ubelaker 2002).

Few such collections exist in the UK or elsewhere and those that are available are used widely in research in many different disciplines (Roberts 2009; Roberts and Mays 2010). The most notable examples in the UK are the remains from the crypts of Christ Church Spitalfields and St. Brides Fleet

Street. Both collections are of European origin and date to the late 18th and early 19th century. Other European collections include two Portuguese collections at Lisbon and Coimbra both late 19th and early 20th century and a similar collection in Athens. There are also several collections in the US, including the Terry Collection, mostly from dissection rooms or unclaimed cadavers and these are either of European or African American origin. The majority of collections are therefore European or African American in origin. Few collections exist from other parts of the world with the major exception of South Africa which holds both European and African remains.

During 2009-2010 a project was undertaken at the NHM to identify and verify the provenance of modern individuals for whom initial evidence suggested they might be of known age and sex[1]. The aim was to establish a fully documented collection of known age and sex individuals with a far wider geographic spread than is currently available to researchers.

## Methodology

The methodology is based on best practice for the provenance of human remains. It is drawn from the methods used by many other institutions, including the Smithsonian Institution in Washington DC (Hanchant 2004; Ousley *et al.* 2005). The techniques used were originally developed as part of the provenancing process for remains claimed for return to their country of origin.

Initial data was taken from departmental registers (Fig. 1), index cards (Fig. 2) and catalogues of remains at the NHM and used to identify as exhaustively as possible a list of potentially known age and sex individuals in the NHM collection. The personal details (age, sex, name) of each potential individual were entered into a database together with the names of their collectors, donors, previous holding institutions, dates of collection, donation and transfer of the remains between donors and/or institutions.

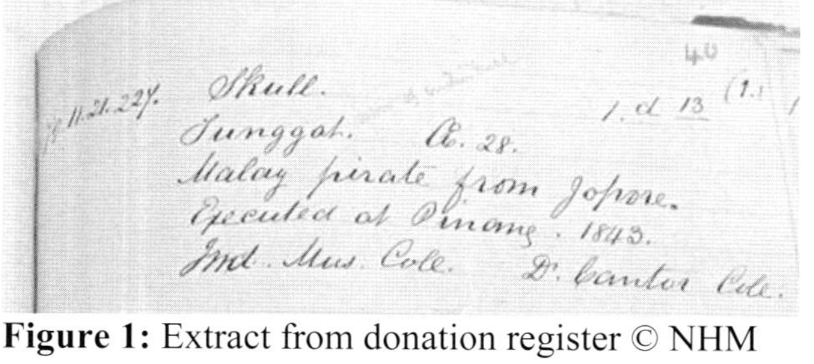
Skull.
Junggah. Æ. 28.
Malay pirate from Johore.
Executed at Penang. 1843.
Ind. Mus. Coll. Dr. Cantor Coll.

**Figure 1:** Extract from donation register © NHM

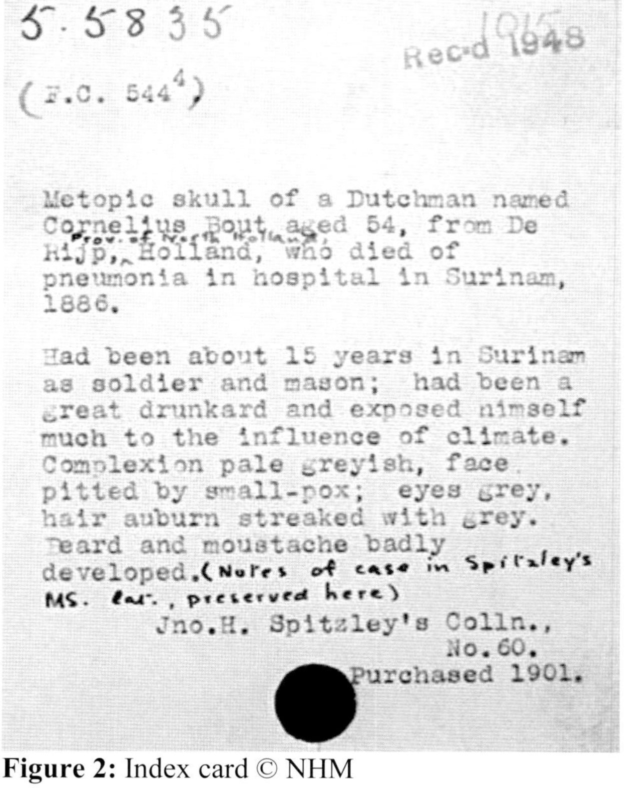
5.5835
Rec'd 1948
(F.C. 544$^4$)

Metopic skull of a Dutchman named Cornelius Bout, aged 54, from De Rijp, Prov. of North Holland, Holland, who died of pneumonia in hospital in Surinam, 1886.

Had been about 15 years in Surinam as soldier and mason; had been a great drunkard and exposed himself much to the influence of climate. Complexion pale greyish, face pitted by small-pox; eyes grey, hair auburn streaked with grey. Beard and moustache badly developed. (Notes of case in Spitzley's MS. Cat., preserved here)

Jno.H. Spitzley's Colln., No. 60. Purchased 1901.

**Figure 2:** Index card © NHM

The initial process enabled the original holding institution to be identified, thus aiding in the location of any relevant documentation, both in the UK and abroad. Online searches were made to either find or when possible access historic sources. The relevant institutions, including, museums and university archives, public record offices and libraries were visited if feasible. Whenever a visit was not possible, for example if the institution was overseas, then the institutions archivists, museum curators, librarians and academics were contacted to obtain copies of original documents.

The NHM archives and those of other named institutions were searched for donation and transfer letters and a wide range of other documents including minutes of Trustees meetings; accession books, catalogues of donation, purchase ledgers and museum staff correspondence, reports and diaries. As it was not uncommon in the past for human remains to be transferred without their full documentation (Clegg 2009), this allowed for the initial records to be checked against original sources and ensured that all information about the individuals has been transferred with them.

Historical documents were checked to provide evidence of actual age and sex for the individuals. They included birth and death registers, hospital records, medical and necrological registers as well as and reports on preparations of specimens. Additionally, the diaries, letters and notebooks of donors and collectors were examined for any extra detail that might improve provenance. In the case of remains donated by scientists (e.g. medical practitioners, naturalists) a literature search was carried out to search for articles and publications that have been written about the remains.

The assessment of age and sex is based solely on *historical sources*, that is, not on direct observation of the skulls and skeletons. The project is concerned with documentary evidence of age and sex not the assessment against physical criteria of age and sex. The main aim was to produce evidence for each individual to the standard of other known age and sex collections such as Christ Church Spitalfields (Molleson and Cox 1993) or St. Bride's Fleet Street (Scheuer and Bowman 1995). Four categories were used to classify the remains.

1. Conclusive evidence to modern standards e.g. birth certificate
2. Clear documented sources such as baptism register, burial register or other official records
3. Possible evidence but not from verifiable sources
4. Tentative or no evidence

Only remains that fall within either of the first two categories were included in the known age and sex collection.

As part of the project a full inventory of the remains was produced, to the level of individual bones. The inventory was developed as part of the NHM data collection project which uses methods based on Buikstra and Ubelaker's (1994) "Standards for data collection from human skeletal remains" and the Institute of Field Archaeologists (IFA) "Guidelines to the Standards for Recording Human Remains" (Brickley and McKinley 2004). These data were recorded using digital recording sheets and entered in to the NHM database KeEMu.

## Challenges

Much of the NHM human remains collection including the potential known age and sex individuals was donated during the nineteenth and early twentieth centuries. The potential known age and sex collection are primarily individuals who lived and died during this period. While some are direct donations to the NHM, others were transferred from the Royal College of Surgeons of England (RCS) and Oxford University (OC) in the late 1940s. This last collection incorporates a series of crania from the Royal Army Medical Corps (RAMC), which was described and catalogued by George Williamson in 1857. The remains therefore have complicated histories and information is often of a variable standard.

*Collectors and Donors Biases*

The 610 potential known age and sex human remains were all collected in a period during which museum curators accepted and solicited the donation of human remains from collectors who came from a variety of backgrounds including colonial administrators, traders, scientists of various disciplines, doctors, soldiers, missionaries etc. (Luyendijk-Elshout 1997; Quigley 2003; Morris 2007). However, other human remains were unsolicited, and donated for the kudos attached to donating to a prestigious institution such as NHM or RCS.

William Henry Flower, in his annual report to the RCS Museum Committee, dated 4$^{th}$ July 1882, about the work carried out during the previous year, remarked that: "[t]*he appeal made a few years ago by Sir Joseph Fayrer to the Medical Officers of the Army serving in India to collect skeletons and crania of various oriental races has been liberally responded to. Among the contributors this year are: Surgeon Major S Coull Mackenzie of the Campbell Hospital, Calcutta (who has forwarded altogether 8 perfect skeletons to the Museum) (...)*" (Flower 1882). Joseph Fayrer's appeal had been received two years earlier by the Office of the Secretary to the Surgeon General, Indian Medical Department. On 27 February 1880, Sergeant Major Nody sent a letter to W H Flower at the RCS in which he writes about a consignment of two cases containing human crania: '*I have to add that the crania have been forwarded in compliance with the request of Sir Joseph Fayrer conveyed in a communication to this office dated London April 1879 in which he states that every effort should be made to procure* <u>*authenticated*</u> *crania of any of the people of India or the neighbouring territories and that these specimens should be despatched to your address.*" (RCS Museum Letter Books Series 2 Volume 4)

These collections were often not collected in any systematic way. As a result, not only were the collections of human remains often assembled by non-professional collectors who subsequently donated them to the institutions of their choice, but also the documentation that accompanied the remains often reflected the collector's and/or donor's biases - especially in relation to the ethnic identity of the remains, this is not to say that there are problems with identifying ethnic origin; rather that some collectors specifically collected from certain areas thus biasing the sample in particular directions. Additionally, the way in which supporting documentation was initially collected, recorded, kept or archived varied greatly from one institution to the other (Quigley 2003; Beck 2007; Morris 2007).

These biases that introduce changes to the records by the collector and/or donor themselves, are epitomized in Barnard Davis' catalogue *Thesaurus Craniorum*, where the author states in his preface that the age of the individual is a result of his direct observation of the remains: "*The sign ♂ indicates a male, and ♀ a female. The sex is for the most part determined by the mere inspection of the cranium, in which there is no infallible rule; hence errors are apt to be made. Doubtful cases are marked as such. The insertion of the age has generally no other foundation, and is therefore marked approximatively, circa, c.*" (Barnard Davis 1867).

*Loss of Historical Information*

Total or partial loss of documentation during the transfer of collections between institutions and limited or no access to historical documentation are two non-negligible biases (Clegg 2009). For example, a series of crania from the Royal Army Medical Corps (RAMC) was described and catalogued by George Williamson in 1857. The RAMC Muniment Collection at the Wellcome Library holds the records of three registers. Other registers quoted by George Williamson (1857) as references for further details about individual human remains in his catalogue could have been lost during the (at least) four recorded transfers of the documentation and collection from one institution to another[2] or be among the unclassified documents in the Archives of the Wellcome Library[3], which are currently not accessible to external researchers. It is therefore possible that some documents currently 'missing' could in future be made available.

With regards to the RCS, this institution lost both specimens and historical documentation when the building was incendiary bombed by the enemy during World War II. A.J.E. Cave (Assistant Conservator) writes in the RCS Scientific Report for the year 1940-1941, about the "*[d]estruction of part of the human osteological collection by bombing during the night of 10 and 11th May 1941 (...). Affected are African, Veddah, Tasmanian and Australian material, the loss of a collection of 150 pelves of known age, sex and race, 80 trephined crania, 30 foetuses*" (Cave 1940-41). He estimates that the numbers of specimens in the Human Anatomy collection fell from 7,500 before the war to 6,065 after the incendiary bombing. Labels and inscriptions on skulls transferred from the RCS to the NHM have also been lost or became illegible as a result of partial damage caused by smoke or fire.

Other major challenges include transcription errors in collection registers, specimen index cards and databases; faded or illegible inscriptions on skulls, labels, historical documents and loss of information recorded on labels now broken or formerly attached to the remains (Clegg 2009). The RCS 1901 Conservator's annual report (written by C. Stewart) records a donation of skulls. He provides a museum reference number for the acquired human remains, but does not mention the donor's name (Stewart 1901). On all the 20 specimen index cards with the same museum reference, the name of the donor "Spitzly" is spelt "*Spitzl**ey***". The name is also recorded as "*Spitzl**ey***" by Arthur Keith, Conservator at the Royal College of Surgeons who received the second part of the collection of human remains in 1913. On one of the twenty index cards (RCS 5.5835) a handwritten addendum mentions that "notes of case in Spitzl**ey** MS Cat. preserved here" (i.e. at the Royal College of Surgeons) (Fig. 3) A search of the RCS database returned no entry for Spitzl**ey**. Yet, there was a handwritten testimony that a catalogue manuscript by the donor was there. Various permutations of the name "Spitsley; Spiztley; Spitzly" were tried until a reference describing a manuscript catalogue by J H Spitzly was found (Spitzly no date).

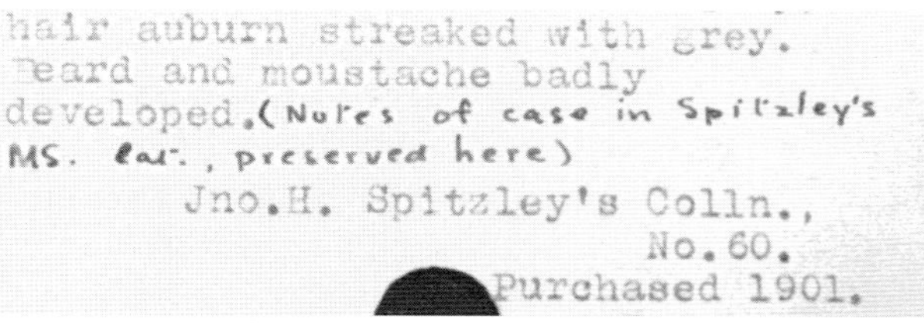
hair auburn streaked with grey.
Beard and moustache badly
developed.(Notes of case in Spitzley's
MS. Cat., preserved here)
Jno.H. Spitzley's Colln.,
No.60.
Purchased 1901.

**Figure 3:** Index card RCS 5.5835 mentions that Spitzley's manuscript catalogue is at the RCS © NHM

*Inscriptions on Skulls*

The vast majority of skulls and/or postcranial elements are marked in ink (Fig. 4). On other remains, the information is recorded on labels glued or attached to the skull and/or postcranial bones.

The nature of the information that is recorded varies from a unique registration number to a name, age, sex, origin, cause of death, date of death and/or occupation of the individual. With time, some inscriptions have partially or totally faded and labels have been lost. Moreover, as well as recording information, inscriptions were possibly intended to increase the value of a skull brought for sale (Lyendijk-Elshout 1997; Quigley 2003). In the assessment of the individuals in the NHM collection, the inscriptions on skulls have only be taken into account as reliable if they are corroborated by reliable historical documentation.

## Results

*Donations of Human Remains to the NHM*

The first recording of a direct donation to the NHM recorded in the Zoological Accessions paper register dates from 15th March 1837. The first human remains to be recorded as a direct donation to the Museum are a series of seven *Homo sapiens* Groenlandica (BMNH 1843.6.23.29 to 35).

A sample of 610 individuals who had donated directly or indirectly to the NHM, RCS and OC by 56 named donors and/or collectors, were initially recorded at the NHM as of potential known age and sex (e.g. on index cards, donation registers). During the 11 months of the study 506 individuals were documented; a further 104 need further study as it was not possible to access the main archive holding the information on these individuals.

According to NHM donation registers and catalogues, the first individuals recorded as being of a known age and sex are a series of five males aged respectively 14, 18, 23, 24 and 28 years old. They were received in 1879 from the India Museum which had received them from Theodore Cantor in 1854. The last donation of six individuals with a recorded known age and sex (other than the dental collection) was received in 1971 from W. C. Osman Hill.

One hundred and nine individuals now form the known age and sex collection in the NHM. Their respective collectors and donors are identified as direct donors to the NHM or the RCS. A total of six named direct donors have been identified. The earliest donation was made by Sorabji Kaikhosri Nariman (Civil Surgeon; Panch Mahals, Doha, India) who sent the crania of a 55 year-old female and 30 year-old male to the RCS, via the office of the Secretary to the Surgeon General of the Indian Medical Department, on 22nd December 1879. The latest, the partial skeleton of a 23-year-old woman was received by the NHM directly from William Charles Osman Hill in 1949. The details, dissection and autopsy of this woman have been published by the donor himself in the *Ceylon Journal of Science* (Osman Hill 1936).

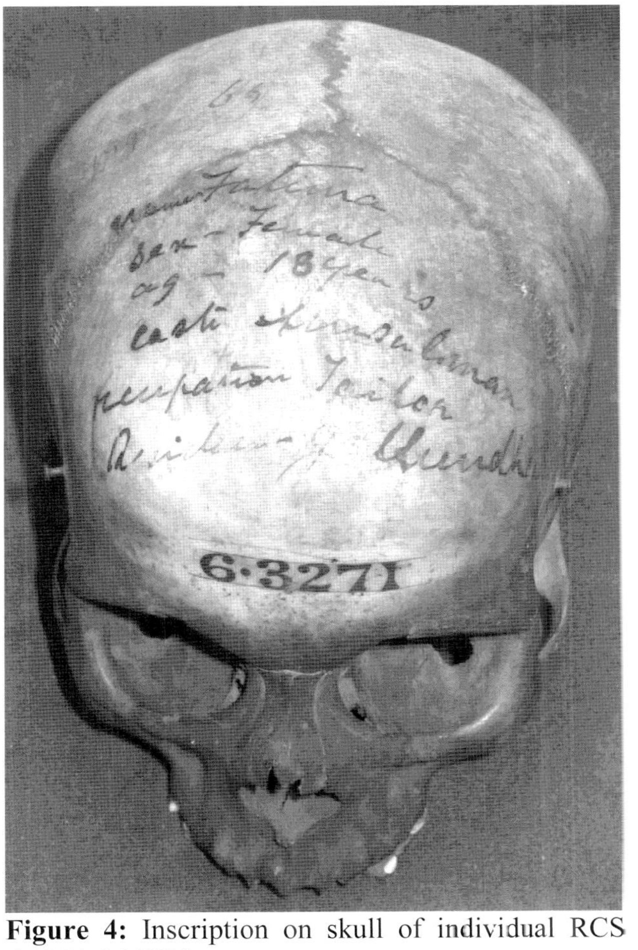


**Figure 4:** Inscription on skull of individual RCS 6.3271 © NHM

The majority of the known age and sex individuals are from Asia (80♂ 16♀). Others were collected in the Americas (9♂ 1♀), Europe (2 ♂) and Africa (1♂). There are no known age and sex individuals from Oceania. However, it should be noted that historical documents demonstrate that the geographical area of collection can sometimes differ from that of the recorded ethnic origin of the individuals. For example, all the 145 individuals whose remains were sold by John Spitzly to the RCS in 1901 and 1913 show diverse origins including Dutch, French, Barbados, Surinamese, Chinese. The human remains were collected by the donor while he was working as Surgeon-in-Chief in the Colonial Hospital in Paramaribo, Surinam. John Spitzly's manuscript notes held in the archives of the Royal College of Surgeons (London) provide the details about the identity, sex and age of the individuals as well as, for some of them, the results of the post-mortems that he carried out. Twelve of the individuals he collected are in the known age and sex collection at the NHM. The transcript of one such entry is below:

> "**60** *Cornelius Bout aet 54 from de Rijp in Holland had been a soldier and a mason in Surinam some 15 years. He had been a great drunkard and had exposed himself much to the influences of climate. On admission on April 1 1886 he was too weak to speak and died soon after the same day. The diagnosis made was pneumonia (very likely he had kidney disease too). He was of a pale greyish complexion, had grey eyes and auburn hair mixed with grey. His beard and moustache were badly developed. The skin of his face was deeply pitted with the scars of smallpox*" (Spitzly no date).

*Age and Sex of the Individuals*

No infants or foetuses were identified as known age and sex. There are no individuals less than 10 years old and there are only four teenagers, three males and one female. The oldest male is 95 and the oldest female is 70. The majority of individuals fall with in the 20 to 50 age group.

*Skeletal and Dental Remains*

For each known age and sex individual, a full inventory of the remains has been carried out. The results are presented in Tables 2 and 3. There are 74 complete crania and no complete postcrania.

**Table 1:** Number of known age and sex individuals

| | Number of Individuals |
|---|---|
| Known age male | 92 |
| Known age female | 17 |
| Known sex male (no age) | 87 |
| Known sex female (no age) | 11 |

**Table 2:** Description of known age and sex human remains

| | Male Adult | Male Juvenile | Female Adult |
|---|---|---|---|
| Cranium complete | 64 | 0 | 10 |
| Cranium incomplete | 27 | 1 | 6 |
| Postcrania complete | 0 | 0 | 0 |
| Postcrania incomplete | 5 | 0 | 2 |

**Table 3:** Dentition of known age and sex remains

| | Male Adult | Male Juvenile | Female Adult |
|---|---|---|---|
| Mandible | 68 | 1 | 13 |
| All teeth missing | 8 | 0 | 2 |
| Complete dentition | 1 | 0 | 0 |

*Geographic Origin of Known Age and/or Sex Collection*

The majority of the individuals are either from Asia, with most from the Indian subcontinent, see Table 4.

**Table 4:** Geographic Origin of the Remains

| Region | Male known age | Female known age | Male | Female |
|---|---|---|---|---|
| Africa | 1 | 0 | 3 | 1 |
| Asia | 80 | 16 | 111 | 23 |
| Europe | 2 | 0 | 53 | 3 |
| Native Americans | 9 | 1 | 12 | 1 |

## Conclusion

The research carried out on documenting a sample of 506 potential known age and sex individuals has set a standard for the methods and criteria that would best assess the historical record. This has shown that the extensive use of archival information and historical documents together with a physical examination of the remains can confirm the age and sex of individuals within a museum collection to standards approaching those for 18th and 19th century archaeological samples.

The examination of historical documentation has allowed for potentially inaccurate records to be identified and to complete the information written on index cards and donation registers. The achievements of this pilot project have resulted in making available to researchers a new collection of 109 individuals of known age and sex and a further

98 individuals of known sex. This provides a total known sex collection of 207 individuals drawn from a more diverse geographic region than other collections. The remains are, however, almost exclusively from the 18th, 19th and early 20th century. Some of these remains are less than 100 years old and held under the provisions of the Human Tissue Act 2004.

**Endnotes**

[1] The NHM's Dental Collection is excluded in its entirety from this project.

[2] The collections were transferred from Fort Pitt/Chatham and Netley to Millbank in 1907 then to Gosport in 1919. The collections and associated documents were then sent to the Oxford University Museum before being presented to the NHM in 1946.

[3] Wellcome Library website (http://www.aim25.ac.uk/cats/20/10876.htm) "*Some archives proper of the College and Fort Pitt Hospital were kept in the RAMC Library and were transferred to the Wellcome Trust with the Muniment Collection: they have never been accessioned with Muniment material and remain uncatalogued*".

**Literature Cited**

Barnard Davis, J. 1867. *Thesaurus craniorum. Catalogue of the skulls of the various races of man.* London.

Beck, L.A. 2007. Documentation systems in human osteology. In: Cassman, V., Odegaard, N. and Powell, J. (eds.) *Human remains. Guide for museums and academic institutions.* Rowan & Littlefield: Lanham. 157-158.

Brickley, M. and McKinley, J. (eds.) 2004. *Guidelines to the standards for recording human skeletal remains.* IFA Paper 7. British Association for Biological Anthropology and Osteoarchaeology and Institute of Field Archaeologists: Southampton and Reading.

Buikstra, J.E. and Ubelaker, D.H. (eds.) 1994. *Standards for data collection from human skeletal remains.* Research Series No.44. Arkansas: Arkansas Archaeological Survey.

Cave, A.J.E. 1941. *Scientific report to the museum committee.* Royal College of Surgeons of England: London.

Clegg, M. 2009. The problem of provenance: inaccuracies, changes and misconceptions. In: Lewis, M.E. and Clegg, M. (eds.) *Proceedings of the ninth annual conference of the British Association for Biological Anthropology and Osteoarchaeology.* Archaeopress: Oxford. BAR International Series 1918: 119-122.

Cox, M. and Mays, S. (eds.) 2000. *Human osteology in archaeology and forensic science.* Greenwich Medical Media: London.

Flower, W.H. 1882. *Annual report of the conservator to the museum committee.* Royal College of Surgeons of England: London.

Hanchant, D. 2004. Practicalities in the return of remains: the importance of provenance and the question of unprovenanced remains. In: Fforde, C. and Hubert, J. (eds.) *The dead and their possessions: repatriation in principle, policy and practice.* Routledge: London. 312-316.

Hoppa, R.D. and FitzGerald, C.M. 1999. From head to toe: integrating studies from bones and teeth in biological anthropology. In: Hoppa, R.D. and FitzGerald, C.M. (eds.) *Human growth in the past. Studies from bones and teeth.* Cambridge Studies in Biological and Evolutionary Anthropology. Cambridge University Press: Cambridge. 1-31.

Luyendijk-Elshout, A.M. 1997. Opening address: the magic of the skull. 'Commercium craniorum' in the nineteenth century. *International Journal of Osteoarchaeology* 7: 571-574.

Molleson, T.I. and Cox, M. 1993. *The Spitalfields Project. Volume 2 – the anthropology. The middling sort.* Research Report 86. Council for British Archaeology: York.

Morris, A.G. 2007. Documentation: history and the sources of skeletons in collections. In: Cassman, V., Odegaard, N. and Powell, J. (eds.) *Human remains. guide for museums and academic institutions.* Rowan & Littlefield: Lanham. 151-161.

Osman Hill, W.C. 1936. Two examples of infantilism. *Ceylon Journal of Science* (D) IV(2): 71-118.

Ousley, S.D., Billbeck, W.T. and Hollinger R.E. 2005. Federal repatriation legislation and the role of physical anthropology in repatriation. *American Journal of Physical Anthropology* 128: 2-32.

Quigley, C. 200. *Skulls and skeletons. Human bone collections and accumulations.* McFarland and Company Inc: Jefferson.

Roberts, C.A. 2009. *Human remains in archaeology: a handbook*. Practical Handbooks in Archaeology No 19. Council of British Archaeology: York.

Roberts, C.A. and Mays, S. 2010. Study and restudy of curated skeletal collections in bioarchaeology: a perspective on the UK and the implications for future curation of human remains. *International Journal of Osteoarchaeology* DOI: 10.1002/oa.1175.

Rogers, T. and Saunders, S. 1994. Accuracy of sex determination using morphological traits of the human pelvis. *Journal of Forensic Sciences* 39(4): 1047-1056.

Royal College of Surgeons of England. *Museum letter books series 2 volume 4.* London.

Scheuer, J.L. and Bowman, J.E. 1995. Correlation of documentary and skeletal evidence in the St Bride's Crypt population. In: Saunders, S.R. and Herring, A. (eds.) *Grave reflections: portraying of the past through cemetery studies*. Canada Scholars' Press: Toronto. 49-70.

Spitzly, J.H. (no date) *Notes on some specimens of skulls collected during my stay in Surinam.* Royal College of Surgeons of England: London.

Stewart, C. 1901. *Annual report of the conservator to the museum committee.* Royal College of Surgeons of England: London.

Volk, C.G. and Ubelaker, D.H. 2002 A test of the Phenice method for the estimation of sex. *Journal of Forensic Sciences* 47(1): 19-24.

White, T. and Folkens, P.A. 2005. *The human bone manual*. Elsevier Academic Press: San Diego.

Williamson, G. 1857. *Observations on the human crania contained in the Museum of the Army Medical Department, Fort Pitt Chatham.* McGlashan and Gill: Dublin.

Wittwer-Backofen, U., Gampe, J. and Vaupel, J.W. 2004. Tooth cementum annulation for age estimation: results from a large known-age validation study. *American Journal of Physical Anthropology* 123(2): 119-29.

Wellcome Institute Library:
http://library.wellcome.ac.uk

Royal College of Surgeons:
http://www.rcseng.ac.uk

# Implementation of Preliminary Digital Radiographic Examination in the Confines of the Crypt of St Bride's Church, Fleet Street, London

Jelena Bekvalac

Centre for Human Bioarchaeology
Museum of London
150 London Wall
London EC2Y 5HN, UK

Email for correspondence: jbekvalac@museumoflondon.org.uk

**Abstract**
St Bride's church in Fleet Street, London was severely bomb-damaged in WWII which ultimately led to the first opportunity for a City of London church to be properly excavated and recorded archaeologically. The archaeological excavations were directed by Professor Grimes and led to interesting discoveries about the history and development of the church as well as the revelation of many burials in and around the church precinct and significantly the individuals buried in the vaults of the crypt. The individuals found in the crypt were associated with their coffin plates, providing valuable biographical data and making them an extremely important assemblage. The 227 individuals in the crypt were analysed and recorded on the Wellcome Osteological Research Database (WORD) and revealed a wide range of dental and bone pathologies of which radiographic analysis would further enhance their interpretation. With the development of palaeopathological analysis radiographic examination can play an important role aiding in a better definition for pathologies and greater clarity for traumata. The location of the assemblage and logistical restrictions meant the viability of radiographic examination had several limitations. Thus the only viable method was to use a portable digital system. The portable system used was direct digital radiography (DDR) and the image process followed DICOM (Digital Imaging and Communications in Medicine) standards. Preliminary examination of the individuals retained in St Bride's crypt highlights the benefits and potential scope for using a portable digital radiographic system and positively overcoming the logistical problems initially encountered.

**Keywords:** St Bride's, Crypt, Biographical, Radiographic, Digital, WORD

## St Bride's Church – Archaeological Background of the Church and the Crypt Assemblage

"St Bride's has watched - and often participated – as English history has been made" (Morgan 1973: 1)

St Bride's church, located in Fleet Street, is synonymous with the history of the printed word and journalism. The church is known as the journalists' church and has over the year's forged close links with the newspapers and journalists alike. One of its most recognisable features and a well-known landmark in the city is its tiered spire (Fig. 1) that remarkably managed to survive the WWII bomb but the intensity of heat did cause the metal of the bell to melt. The spire is noted to have provided inspiration to the baker William Rich to create a tiered wedding cake for his daughter. William Rich died in 1811 and is one of the recorded individuals with biographical information.

St Bride's in its several incarnations had previously faced serious damage to its fabric before being bombed in WWII when it was involved in the maelstrom of the Great Fire of London 1666 and subsequently rebuilt by Wren. Wren's rebuilt design of the church created the vaults in the crypts in which people were able to pay rather handsomely to be buried. The burials in the vaults of the crypt covered a period of about one hundred and eighty years with the last interment taking place in 1853. Following a series of Acts of Parliament during the 1850s, burials were prevented from taking place within the City of London. It was Wren's design, the eighth incarnation of the church that was to be so badly damaged on the worst night of bombing in the City of London on 29$^{th}$ December 1940.

The damage from the WWII bombing destroyed the main body of the church but out of such devastation there was a positive outcome, in that prior to the church once again being rebuilt, there was an opportunity from the excavations to record and gain valuable evidence from the church. The excavations of the church led by Professor Grimes in the early 1950s revealed earlier features and foundations building up a picture of the numerous incarnations of the church over several hundred years. It was in effect the first time that a City of London church had been investigated using archaeological excavations and techniques. The excavations revealed not only ancient historical foundations and artefacts relating to the history and development of the church but also a charnel room with medieval remains and the recovery of 227 individuals with associated biographical information who had been buried in vaults in the crypt.

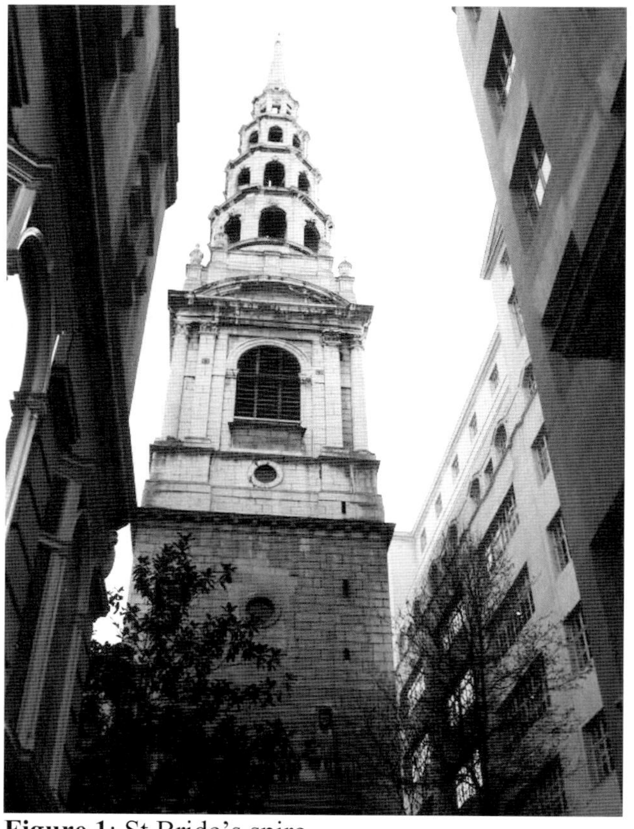

**Figure 1**: St Bride's spire

Professor Grimes produced over his long career a formidable archive of information that provided much of the basis of the details about the development of Roman and Medieval London. The comprehensive publication by Milne in 1997 drew together information from Grime's archaeological archive and latter day *in situ* recording of the church. The information relating to the burials revealed by Grime's excavation within the church aisles and vaults was carefully noted at the time but does not have the degree of detail that is now accorded to burials revealed and recovered in archaeological excavations. William Redpath in his 1958 publication provides important information with some valuable and useful insights to the excavations and the skeletal remains. However, the revelations of the human remains buried within St Bride's that had been long forgotten enabled and continues to enable an invaluable insight into the lives of the people of the parish. They have enriched the field of osteology and continue to do so to the present day.

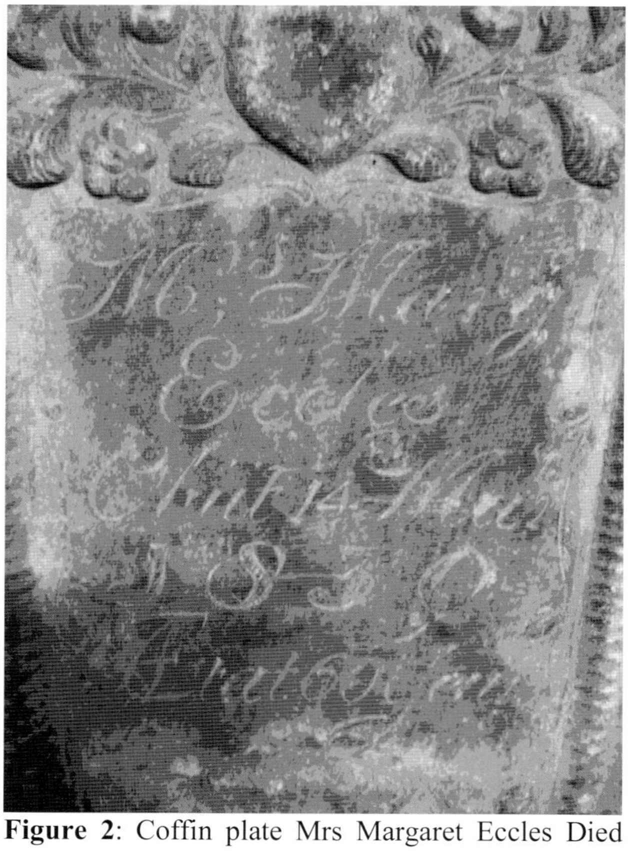

**Figure 2**: Coffin plate Mrs Margaret Eccles Died 1830 Aged 60 Years

Those buried in the vaults were, it seems, all in lead coffins with coffin plates that were kept associated with the remains of the individuals. The legibility of the coffin plates (Fig. 2) varied with corrosion affecting some but was generally good enough to be able to discern the name and date of birth and death. The coffin plates upon later examination by Adrian Miles of Museum of London Archaeology (MoLA) were identified as a combination of outer and inner plates, recognised components of the funereal furnishings of the 18th and 19th century (Adrian Miles *pers. comm.*).

Initially, the individuals discovered and retained from the crypts were placed in ammunition boxes with their respective coffin plates and that at a later date they were then removed from these and placed in to plastic lidded boxes. Although in the most part the individuals were correctly associated with their coffin plates there is one instance, James Blades (d.1788), where there would appear to be a contradiction with respect to the osteological evidence and associated coffin plate.

With the discovery of the charnel remains and individuals retained from the crypts, assessments were made in the 1950s that identified the significance of the biographical assemblage and the immense research potential. Decisions from this point were needed to be taken as to what was to happen to the individuals in the long term, were they to be reburied or kept for research? Writing from the perspective of a present day osteologist looking back, the decision faced at this time by the church and academics was a difficult one, particularly so as the field that we are familiar with now was not yet established. It has to be said that the decision to retain the individuals within the church and allow them to be available for continued research was indeed a decision of considerable foresight and offered myself and others the privilege of being able to closely examine this remarkable assemblage.

Since taking the decision to retain the collection for research a wide-ranging and extensive variety of research has taken place upon the individuals from dental sampling analysis, non metric studies, case studies of interesting individuals to forensic age and sex methods. Other valuable archives of data have also been created including the hand drawn skeletal remains of the crypt assemblage by Rosemary Powers from the Natural History Museum. Latterly, in the 1990s Dr Louise Scheuer & Dr Sue Black (nee MacLaughlin) with funding from the Leverhulme Trust recorded and re-boxed the skeletal remains in conservation cardboard boxes and their associated coffin plates placed in separate containers. The work produced is an invaluable documentary source that provided a rich research foundation which continues to be of benefit to the church and researchers and aided greatly in my own analysis of the individuals on to the WORD database.

The archive relating to the parish records is also an invaluable source as the parish of St Bride's recorded more details than was legally required from 1785, including cause of death and in some instances occupation (Miles and Conheeney 2010). This information in association with the biographical data from the coffin plates makes the individuals such a significantly important assemblage for broadening research parameters in conjunction with the osteological analysis. The individuals from Christ Church Spitalfields are the only other contemporary biographical collection to St Bride's and offer an important prospect for comparative analysis.

**Analysis by the Centre for Human Bioarchaeology**

The Centre for Human Bioarchaeology (CHB) was established in 2003 with funding from the Wellcome Trust to analyse and record the archaeologically derived skeletal remains curated and retained at the Museum of London. The resultant data was to be made available on line through the CHB website with associated cemetery information and links to the London Archaeological Archive Research Centre (LAARC). As part of the three year funded project the individuals excavated from St Bride's Lower Churchyard, Farringdon were analysed and recorded on to the WORD database. With over 600 individuals it is an important post medieval assemblage and provided a broad range of interesting pathologies, traumata, post mortem examinations and a gold filling. It was the burial ground in which the parish poor were buried, with church records and personal letters describing a scene most horrid and foul (Miles and Conheeney 2010).

Leading on from the work in the 1990s by Scheuer and Black and the importance of the assemblage highlighted by Scheuer (Scheuer and Bowman 1995; Scheuer 1998), the Centre decided that it would be of significant research value and potential to be able to record the individuals in the crypt on the WORD database. Fortunately the current Canon David Meara agreed to the project and to bring the project to fruition the Centre was awarded funding from the City of London Archaeological Trust (CoLAT) to enable the recording of the crypt individuals on to WORD. Further funding from the Society of Antiquaries of London enabled collation of the skeletal data for the crypt individuals & individuals from the Lower Churchyard, Farringdon, and in part associated archaeological data and parish records. The collation and comparison of the two skeletal assemblages is of particular interest and significance as they form a group of people from the same parish living in London in the 18$^{th}$ and 19$^{th}$ century but from two very different socio-economic backgrounds.

**Skeletal Biographical Assemblage**

The crypt assemblage comprises 227 individuals with recorded biographical data and included 14 sub-adults and 213 adults, of which there were 122 males and 105 females. The preservation and completeness of the individuals was generally very good but there was some variation depending on which vault they had been in and whether there had been any water ingress or other disturbance. There was often good preservation of hair and in some cases desiccated skin and brain tissue. The demographic profile (Fig. 3) of the individuals was predominantly made up of adults, with more than 50% over 40 years of age and many in their 60s, 70s and 80s. One lady, Agnes Atkinson, was 91 years old when she died in 1821 with a parish record of death being noted as 'Aged'.

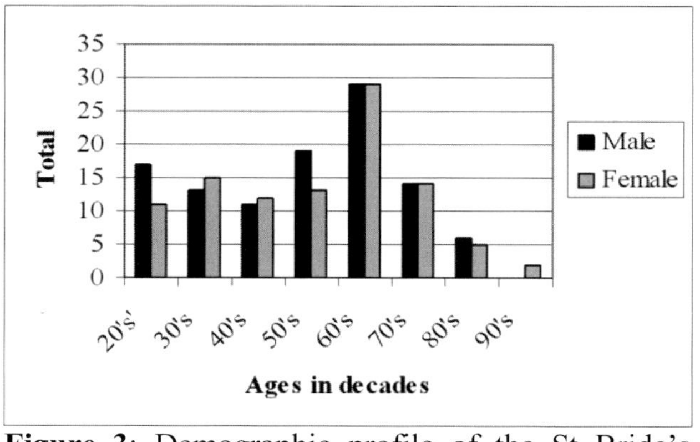


**Figure 3**: Demographic profile of the St Bride's crypt individuals

The analysis of these individuals recorded on to the WORD database revealed a variety of pathologies, traumata and dental interventions including three skilfully worked gold dental plates. It was hoped that following on from the osteological analysis and digital photographs that it would be possible to take x-rays. For certain trauma and pathologies including cancers, infections and Paget's disease, the opportunity to x-ray elements enables greater detail and is a valuable tool in obtaining a more definitive diagnosis.

With the advancement in the imaging field technologies there has been an increase in the application of various techniques to aid with palaeopathological diagnosis. The importance for the utilising of x-rays in relation to archaeological material and comparatively with clinical data has been expressed over the years (Brothwell *et al.* 1968; Lewis 1996; Mays 2008). "Radiography provides a direct link between the changes seen in palaeopathological specimens and those in living people with known diseases. Radiographs from modern patients are useful in aiding palaeopathological interpretation" (Mays 2008: 79).

Transporting any of the individuals from the church to be x-rayed off site would have been problematical and only one of several logistical difficulties faced. IT challenges had already been faced in remotely linking to the Oracle system for recording the individuals *in situ* on to WORD. The confined space of the crypt was also a factor to consider; therefore the only viable option was for a portable and compact digital x-ray system, a system that was robust enough to be able to cope with the conditions of the crypt.

### Preliminary Digital Radiographic Project

The opportunity to take radiographic images of the skeletal assemblage was made possible for the Centre working in conjunction with Jerry Conlogue from the Bioanthropology Research Unit of Quinnipiac University, USA. Jerry Conlogue is an expert in the application of radiographic examination of archaeological material, notably with human remains and has many years expertise. A proposal for funding to the School of Health Sciences, Quinnipiac University was successful to carry out the preliminary digital radiographic investigation of the skeletal remains at St Bride's. The funding made it possible to hire and access with the support of Mark Viner at Inforce and Xograph a portable x-ray machine to initiate a programme of radiographs using a direct digital radiograph (DDR) system. It is a system that has been used in the forensic field and also in part in some commercial archaeological companies. The system, as well as being portable, was able to be set up in the confined and restricted space of the crypt (Fig. 4). The initial phase of the project was to create a digital record of the sub-adults and skulls. From the results obtained and anticipated success, the continuation of the project would be to further x-ray those individuals with recorded pathologies and traumata in the post-cranial skeleton to construct an accessible digital x-ray pathological archive.

### Methods

The application of radiographs is a method of investigation that is desirable for a number of reasons and one of the more important in curatorial terms is it being non-destructive. However, there can be restrictions in availability and access for radiographic examination most notably in many instances cost being a major factor. The funding awarded from the School of Health Sciences, Quinnipiac University enabled the cost of hiring and use of the equipment to be covered. The Direct Digital Radiograph (DDR) system provided by

Xograph through Inforce consisted of component parts and units that were portable in durable travel cases and possible to assemble in the confined space of the crypt.

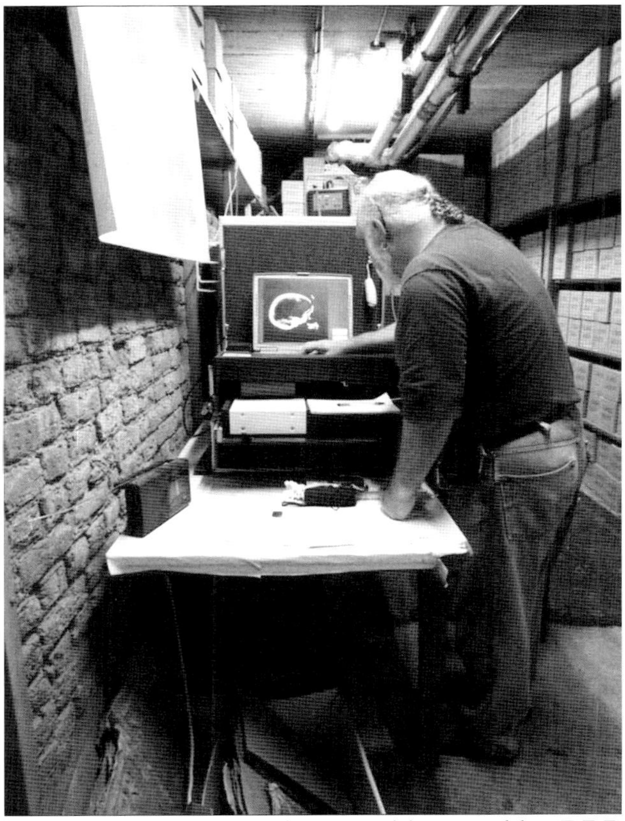

**Figure 4**: Jerry Conlogue with portable DDR system in crypt

The process of the radiographed images followed the guidelines of Digital Imaging and Communications in Medicine (DICOM) – "a global Information- Technology standard, designed to ensure the interoperability of systems and enable medical images to be produced, stored, processed and shared" (Digital Imaging and Communications in Medicine 2010a and b). The elements radiographed were all labelled with the sitecode SB79, an identifying prefix SK=Skull and SUB=Sub-adult, their individual context number and sequential numbers of images taken. The sub-adults were anatomically placed so that it was possible to have an immediate comparison of the elements right and left side. The skulls were supported and positioned with the aid of a foam skull ring and placed in specific positions for radiographs. Skull projections were Waters –PA/AP and Lateral Left/ Right. The skull was also placed for specific maxillae projections, as was the mandible. A detailed list was also compiled in Excel providing the details relating to the individual, the number of images taken and the positions of the images.

**Results**

The initial digital radiographic examinations produced multiple images for all of the 14 sub-adults and over 90 of the skulls and provided the basis of a digital x-ray archive that will hopefully be added to with continued funding support. The benefits of the DDR system were manifold and clearly highlighted the benefits of having a portable system. The results were immediate as it was possible to ascertain details relating to the images instantly from viewing the screen. The overall results of the preliminary project verified the efficiency, speed and versatility of the system and the images demonstrated the clarity of the digital radiographs (Figs. 5-6). The DICOM images produced are easily navigable and can be copied to compact disc where it is also possible to convert the images to tiffs and jpegs.

There were only minor problems encountered with the system, with over heating of the computer but this was soon rectified by improving air flow and Jerry Conlogue will review the method for sequential numbering for each new individual context, as this was found to be a number assigned by the system. The preliminary investigation has already produced a large archive of digital radiographic data and the images are stored by the CHB and Jerry Conlogue on compact discs. The digital x-ray images were firstly copied on to CDs from the hard disk of the portable system. As a further means of safe guarding the images they are stored on an external hard drive with a large capacity for holding more images. Ultimately, after discussions with the museum IT department the x-ray images will be made accessible on line through the CHB website, until this is possible the images can be accessed by students and researchers coming to the CHB lab. These radiographs will, it is hoped, be the beginning of the development of an accessible radiographed pathology and dental archive.

**Discussion**

The WORD database is a valuable research tool and by having the data available on line has enabled greater access to an extensive and unique collection of stratified skeletal assemblages Digital photographs are available in relation to the recorded cemetery sites and as a further development to the archive x-rays will also be available on line for St

Bride's and other curated sites. They will provide an additional means of access to the data and promote a greater insight and means of research into the skeletal assemblages. Following the DICOM (Digital Imaging and Communications in Medicine) standards would also enable access to clinical comparisons. The St Bride's project in this first phase has enabled the initial base to be established so that it can be continued and developed in the future.

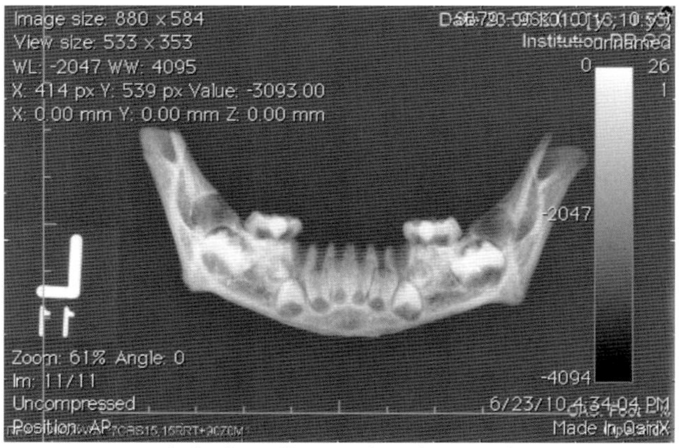


**Figure 5**: Digital radiograph of mandible of Mary Devey (SB79 9) d.1840. Aged 3years 7 months and 9 days

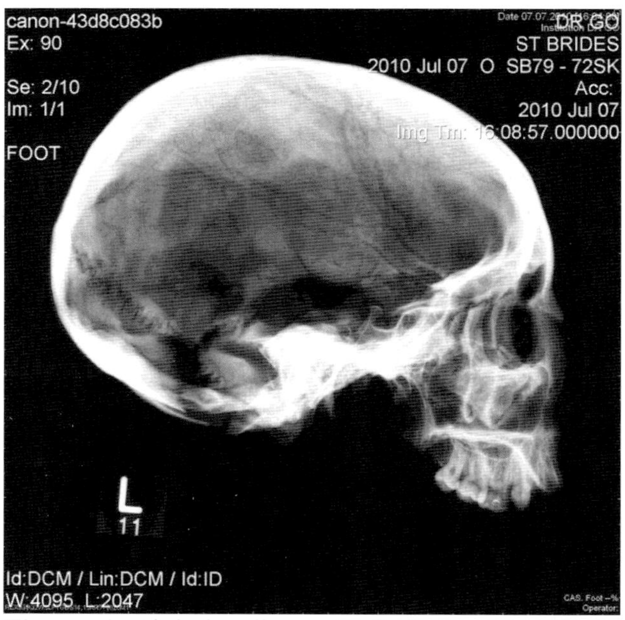


**Figure 6**: Digital radiograph of skull of Mrs Betsy Newman (SB79 72) d.1825 aged 23 years

The benefits of recording the crypt individuals on to WORD and the digital x-ray project are many but in particular that they record a significantly important assemblage using standard recording methods (Buikstra and Ubelaker (eds.) 1994; Connell and Rauxloh 2003; Brickley and McKinley 2004) and provide a searchable archive for researchers. Handling can cause considerable damage over time to skeletal assemblages and the database and x-ray images act as a means of a conservation tool by lessening the amount of times the material has to be handled for research. This does not, however, mean that gaining information about the individuals is limited as detailed searches can be made of the recorded data which will be made available on the CHB website, where it will be possible to download the raw data to enable independent research and refining of searches for selected individuals. The CHB, at the request of the church, acts in a curatorial capacity with regard to the remains and as such research requests on the assemblage can be made through the Centre following the guidelines noted on the Research section of the CHB website. The digital radiographic images so far taken of the St Bride's individuals have already provided a wealth of important data that will add considerable value to the continued research of the crypt individuals. The x-ray data alongside the osteological data can work in tandem both with regard to the crypt individuals but also on a wider scale in the research of other assemblages and hopefully in association with clinical data.

Compared to wet film radiographs this system was much faster and more efficient and enabled a large body of data to be produced and stored with ease of access and potential shared access on line. As another source of data for analysis the images will act as a supporting tool for a more in-depth understanding and diagnosis of the recorded pathologies and traumata. It is hoped that with further funding the project will be expanded enabling the remaining St Bride's skulls to be radiographed, as well as all individuals with traumata and observed gross pathological changes. As such it will produce an invaluable radiographic reference that in following DICOM standards (http://DICOM.nema.org) will provide greater opportunities for broader comparisons to clinical radiographed data.

Although the initial x-ray images are at present limited to the 14 sub-adults and 90 skulls (yet to include the three individuals with dental plates), they have shown that they will be a valuable additional source of data for research. The present images have yet to be utilised for investigation in a specific project in terms of ageing the sub-adults or confirmation of a pathological diagnosis of which, they will at a later date but they have demonstrated the success of the portable digital x-ray system within the confines of the crypt. They represent the beginnings of the digital x-ray archive that will be developed and incorporated in to a variety of research projects and utilised as a means of enhancing research not only of the St Bride's individuals but in association with other assemblages.

There is considerable potential for the addition of the x-rayed post cranial elements to aid and confirm diagnoses of disease. A variety of palaeopathological texts including Aufderheide and Rodríguez-Martín (1998), Ortner (2003), and Roberts and Manchester (2010) incorporate x-rays as a means of assisting in palaeopathological diagnosis and as Mays highlights "have helped to ensure that radiography became a routine aid to description and diagnosis, and a fully integrated core skill in palaeopathology" (Mays 2008: 79). Further investigations in relation to metabolic disorders have also benefitted from the use of x-rays as shown by Brickley and Ives (2008). There is also potential for other research with regard to dental analysis investigating dental development and pathology.

It is hoped that the application of the DDR system will be possible to incorporate other sites curated by the CHB, creating an extensive and unique radiographic archive. It is anticipated that the radiographic data will be possible to access on line through the CHB website alongside the already available downloadable data for analysed cemeteries. Discussions are in place with the CHB, MoLA osteologists and the Museum of London IT section about how best to implement and support such an archive, so that it can be readily accessible as a research tool and added to on a constant basis. The availability of the digital x-ray data will aid in the continued interpretation and research of the St Bride's individuals and other curated skeletal assemblages (as well as sites that have been reburied with only virtual data present) and enable the data to be incorporated as an important facet in future research projects.

**Acknowledgements**

Cannon David Meara of St Bride's and all the team at the church, City of London Archaeological Trust (CoLAT), Society of Antiquaries London, Jerry Conlogue, Bioanthropology Research Institute Quinnipiac University, Mark Viner, Mark Farmer and Deborah Gulliver at Inforce, Kelly Eggleton Forensic student and Xograph www.xograph.com

**Literature Cited**

Aufderheide, A.C. and Rodríguez-Martín, C. 1998. *The Cambridge encyclopedia of human paleopathology*. Cambridge University Press: Cambridge.

Brickley, M. and McKinley, J. 2004. *Guidelines to the standard for recording human remains*. IFA/ BABAO: Reading and Southampton.

Brickley, M. and Ives, R. 2008. *The bioarchaeology of metabolic bone disease*. Academic Press: London.

Brothwell, D.R., Molleson, T. and Metreweli, C. 1968. Radiological aspects of normal variation in earlier skeletons: an exploratory study. In: Brothwell, D.R. (ed.) *The Skeletal Biology of Earlier Human Populations*. Pergamon: Oxford. 149-172.

Buikstra, J.E. and Ubelaker, D.H. (eds.) 1994. *Standards for data collection from human skeletal remains*. Arkansas Archaeological Survey: Arkansas. Research Series No.44.

Connell, B. and Rauxloh, P. 2003. A rapid method for recording human skeletal data. Unpub: Museum of London Report.

Lewis, S. 1996. The osteological use of diagnostic radiographs: further material for osteoarchaeologists. *Organ* 14: 10-12.

Mays. S. 2008. Radiography and allied techniques in the palaeopathology of skeletal remains. In: Pinhasi, R. and Mays. S. (eds.) *Advances in human palaeopathology*. John Wiley & Sons: Chichester. 77-100.

Miles, A. and Conheeney, J. 2010. A post-medieval population from London: excavations in the St Bride's Lower Churchyard, 75–82 Farringdon Street, City of London, EC4. Unpub: MoLAS Studies Series.

Milne, G. 1997. *St Bride's Church London: archaeological research 1952-60 and 1992-5*. English Heritage: London. Archaeological Report 11.

Morgan, D. 1973. *Phoenix of Fleet Street. 2,000 years of St Bride's*. Charles Knight: London.

Ortner, D.J. 2003. *Identification of pathological conditions in human skeletal remains*. 2nd ed. Academic Press: London.

Redpath, W. 1958. *Fleet Street's church restored, 1940-1957. A survey of seventeen eventful years*. Guild of St Bride, Patina Press: London.

Roberts, C.A. and Manchester. K. 2010. *The archaeology of disease*. 3rd ed. Sutton Publishing Ltd: Stroud.

Scheuer, J.L. and Bowman, J.E. 1995. Correlation of documentary and skeletal evidence in the St Bride's Crypt population. In: Saunders, S.R. and Herring, A. (eds.) *Grave reflections: portraying of the past through cemetery studies*. Canada Scholars' Press: Toronto. 49-70.

Scheuer, L. 1998. Age at death and cause of death of the people buried in St Bride's church, Fleet Street, London. In: Cox, M. (ed.) *Grave concerns – death and burial in England 1700-1850*. Council for British Archaeology: York. Research Report 113.

Digital Imaging and Communications in Medicine. 2010a. http://dicom.nema.org/

Digital Imaging and Communications in Medicine. 2010b. http://medical.nema.org/dicom/geninfo/Brochure.pdf

# A Revised Method for Assessing Tooth Wear in the Deciduous Dentition

Anna F Clement* and Alison Freyne

Institute of Archaeology
University College London
31-34 Gordon Square
London WC1H 0PY

*Email for correspondence: a.clement@ucl.ac.uk

**Abstract**
Tooth wear research has almost exclusively focused on the permanent dentition with relatively few studies on deciduous tooth wear. This pilot study investigates macro-wear in the deciduous dentition of three Nubian populations from modern-day Sudan, dating from approximately 13,000 BP until the end of medieval period around the 16th century AD. Unlike the permanent teeth for which a multitude of methods are available for recording wear, a dedicated method has not been developed for the deciduous teeth. For this study tooth wear was measured from digital photographs using image analysis software. A dentine proportion was calculated by dividing the area of exposed dentine by the area of the occlusal surface. The results show that similar to the permanent dentition, the deciduous teeth possess a regular pattern of wear, which largely follows their eruption sequence. The anterior teeth, however, consistently showed higher dentine proportions compared to the posterior teeth from the same jaw. As expected, the overall wear on the deciduous dentition increased with age, but the posterior teeth only showed notable amounts of wear in specimens where the incisors had already been exfoliated. This pilot study highlights the importance of recording deciduous tooth wear and the benefits of using a quantitative method. Deciduous tooth wear has the potential to provide valuable information about both weaning and teething strategies as well as the diet of juveniles in past human groups. Currently very little is known about its variation both within and between different populations.

**Keywords:** Juvenile, Deciduous, Tooth Wear, Sudan

## Introduction

The study of modern human tooth wear in past populations has a long history (Broca 1879), but research has focused almost exclusively on the permanent dentition with deciduous tooth wear receiving relatively little attention. Tooth wear research is motivated by its use in ageing the adult human skeleton and has therefore been fixed on the permanent dentition. Studies of juvenile skeletal and dental growth and development have demonstrated that age can be relatively accurately estimated from both long bone growth and dental development (Scheuer and Black 2004). This means there is little motivation to study deciduous tooth wear as an effective ageing method. Differences in wear patterns between cultural groups, especially agriculturalists and hunter-gatherers have been widely studied (Hinton 1982; Smith 1984; Larsen 1985; Eshed *et al.* 2006; Deter 2009). Again, this research has focused on the diet of adults and their permanent teeth rather than on juveniles with deciduous dentitions.

Despite the lack of focused research into deciduous tooth wear, it has frequently been noted in past populations. It also has the potential to provide valuable information about both weaning and teething strategies in past populations as well as the variability of dental eruption in older children between and within populations. Current research on weaning strategies of archaeological populations is dominated by isotopic analyses, but the lack of precise information regarding bone collagen turnover times makes it difficult to identify the exact age at which weaning took place (Richards *et al.* 2002; Prowse *et al.* 2008). Studies of deciduous tooth wear therefore have the potential to not only compliment these studies, but provide an alternative weaning age, as tooth wear begins as soon as abrasive particles are introduced into the mouth. Unfortunately, a dedicated and standardised system for recording tooth wear in deciduous teeth has not been developed, making it difficult for researchers to record deciduous tooth wear and almost impossible to make comparisons between different sites. This pilot study applies a quantitative method for recording tooth wear to the deciduous dentition and examines the pattern of tooth wear in a sample of 37 juveniles from Sudan.

## Deciduous Tooth Wear

The deciduous teeth begin to develop *in utero* and on average at the time of birth are all partially formed (Lunt and Law 1974; AlQahtani *et al.* 2010). They continue to develop in early infancy and are fully erupted by approximately two-and-a-half years of age (Lunt and Law 1974). They are gradually replaced by the permanent dentition from about six years of age and are normally all exfoliated by 12 years of age (Schour and Massler 1941; Gustafson and Koch 1974; Hillson 1996). Human infants will usually have a total of 20 deciduous teeth, with each quadrant possessing a first and second incisor, a canine and a first and second molar. There are important differences between the structure of deciduous and permanent teeth that will affect the process of tooth wear. Most important is the thickness of the enamel, which is thinner in deciduous teeth than permanent (Wheeler 1965). The dentine, which underlies the enamel on a tooth's occlusal surface, would therefore be exposed earlier in the functional life of a deciduous tooth than a permanent. In addition, the enamel of deciduous teeth is less mineralised and softer than the permanent teeth, again increasing the rate of tooth wear (Fearnhead *et al.* 1982; Johansson *et al.* 2001). In common with the permanent dentition, deciduous tooth wear is also influenced by a number of cultural and biological factors, such as diet, abrasive objects placed within the mouth, tooth morphology, tooth size and palate shape.

Despite the limited amount of research into deciduous tooth wear, a few key studies have demonstrated its potential in providing valuable information about weaning strategies and infant diets in past populations (Davies and Pedersen 1955; Aiello *et al.* 1991; Bullington 1991; Prowse *et al.* 2008). The first detailed study of deciduous tooth wear was made by Davies and Pedersen (1955) and focused on Inuit children from Greenland. They observed that children who subsisted on a traditional diet comprised mostly of fat and meat, which would have required prolonged chewing, showed considerably more tooth wear in their deciduous teeth than those subsisting on a more varied diet that included a high amounts of vegetable foodstuffs.

More recent research into deciduous tooth wear has focused on the information it can provide about weaning practices in archaeological populations, especially the timing of weaning (termination of breastfeeding) and inter-birth spacing. Deciduous teeth erupt into the mouth before the process of weaning has been completed and therefore have the potential to provide information about the average age at weaning, teething practices and inter-birth intervals in different populations. Weaning is the process of transition of an infant from exclusive breastfeeding to exclusive reliance on foods other than breast milk (Sellen and Smay 2001; Sellen 2007). This transition increases the amount of abrasive particles within the mouth which wear away the enamel on a tooth's crown, but is not normally abrupt and often involves an intermediate phase of partial breastfeeding; this phase in an infant's life is known as transitional feeding (Sellen and Smay 2001; Sellen 2007). Abrasive particles introduced through the consumption of harder foodstuff can therefore begin to wear the deciduous dentition before the complete cessation of breastfeeding. Aiello *et al.* (1991) compared the levels of deciduous tooth wear in three ape species and noted that gorillas (*Gorilla gorilla*) showed markedly advanced tooth wear in their deciduous teeth compared to the dentitions of chimpanzees (*Pan troglodytes*) and orang-utans (*Pongo pygmaeus*). They suggested that both the relatively abrasive diet of gorillas compared to chimpanzees and orang-utans, as well as early weaning of their infants and short birth intervals, accounted for these differences.

Research into weaning practices in modern humans has mostly relied upon isotopic evidence (e.g. Richards *et al.* 2002; Clayton *et al.* 2006; Fuller *et al.* 2006), but studies have shown that deciduous tooth wear can also be used (Bullington 1991; Prowse *et al.* 2008). Bullington's (1991) microwear analysis of deciduous tooth wear in a sample of 36 juveniles of between 6 and 27 months of age from the prehistoric period in the Lower Illinois River Valley, showed that the age at the onset of wear can provide valuable information about the weaning strategies of different populations (Bullington 1991). She noted that although the diet differed greatly between the Middle Woodlanders (horticulturists) and Mississippians (agriculturalists), the age at the onset of tooth wear did not. Teething activities were suggested as the primary cause of early wear in both group's deciduous dentition.

Prowse *et al.*'s (2008) study integrated isotopic and tooth wear evidence to provide information on the infant feeding practices of a Roman skeletal sample. The isotopic evidence showed that transitional feeding began by the end of the first year of life and that weaning occurred between two and two-and-a-half years of age. The tooth wear evidence supported this conclusion, suggesting that infants were provided with complimentary foods to breast milk at an early age. However, because a dedicated method for recording deciduous tooth wear has not been developed they scored the stages of tooth wear using methods designed for the permanent dentition: Smith (1984) and Scott (1979). This is problematic as the deciduous teeth not only possess different morphologies to their permanent counterparts, but are smaller in size and possess thinner and softer enamel. In addition, this meant that different scores were generated for the anterior and posterior dentitions making comparisons between these teeth difficult. This is important as previous research has shown how the balance of wear between the front and back of the mouth can be altered through the use of the anterior teeth in cultural practices (Clement 2008; Clement *et al.* 2009).

## Materials

The dental sample used in this pilot study is comprised of 37 specimens from three different sites located in modern day Sudan. Specimens were selected for this study with a stage of dental development between the possession of a fully erupted deciduous dentition, at approximately 18 months old, and complete exfoliation of all deciduous teeth by about 12 years old (Schour and Massler 1941; Gustafson and Koch 1974; Hillson 1996; AlQahtani *et al.* 2010). The dental development ages of the selected specimens were estimated using both Ubelaker's (1978) adaptation of the Schour and Massler (1941) chart and Gustafson and Koch's (1974) chart. These ageing methods were selected as they are both relatively simple to apply and have tested well on known age collections (Miles 1958; Gray and Lamon 1959; Crossner and Mansfield 1983; Liversidge 1994). When different ages were estimated by the two charts an average was taken.

In total, wear was measured in 482 deciduous teeth. The age profile of this dental sample is shown in Table 1. Specimens with a dental development age of between two and four years of age are best represented within the study sample. This was due to both a high number of specimens in this age group as well as the retention of a full deciduous dentition at this age.

**Table 1:** Age profile of the study sample based on dental development stage using an average of the Schour and Massler (1941) and Gustafson and Koch (1974) charts.

| | Dental Development Age (years) | | | | | | | | | |
|---|---|---|---|---|---|---|---|---|---|---|
| | 1-1.9 | 2-2.9 | 3-3.9 | 4-4.9 | 5-5.9 | 6-6.9 | 7-7.9 | 8-8.9 | 9-9.9 | 10-10.9 |
| **No. Teeth** | 32 | 44 | 127 | 102 | 37 | 48 | 28 | 19 | 30 | 15 |

Most of the specimens (n = 23) were recovered during the Sudanese Archaeological Research Society's excavation of the 4th Cataract 3-J-18B site. This cemetery site is located near the modern town of el Tereif. The results of the excavations are currently unpublished, but the cemetery has been dated from the 7th century AD until the 16th century AD and associated with a Christian occupation site, which had an agricultural mode of subsistence (Daniel Antoine 2009, *pers. comm.*). Ten specimens from the cemetery site of Gabati were included in the study sample. This site is located on the east bank of the Nile River near the modern village of Gabati about 260km from Khartoum and is also situated within the 4th cataract. The cemetery was excavated over two seasons between 1994 and 1995 and shown to be a multi-period site, with use spanning from the Meroitic to the Christian period, approximately 300 BC to 1200 AD (Edwards 1998; Filer 1999). The mode of subsistence is reported to have remained mostly unchanged throughout both these periods, with agriculture the primary mode of subsistence and particular reliance on sorghum which was supplemented with vegetables and pulses and occasional meat (Van Gerven *et al.* 1995; Filer 1999). A small number of specimens (n=4) from the cemetery site 117 near Jebel Sahaba met the selection criteria for this pilot study and were included in the sample. This site is located near the northern border of Sudan a few kilometres north of Wadi Halfa and dates to approximately 12,000 - 10,000 years BP (Wendorf 1968). Adult specimens from this site are associated with some of the earliest evidence of warfare, with over half being directly associated with stone projectiles often lodged in the vertebral column or endocranium

(Wendorf 1968; Ferguson 2000). This evidence of violent trauma has been linked to a time of economic and environmental stress where attempts at early agriculture had failed and local groups returned to hunting and gathering (Wendorf 1968; Ferguson 2000).

**Methods**

A wide variety of methods are available for recording tooth wear in the permanent dentition (e.g. Murphy 1959; Molnar 1971; Walker 1978; Mayhall and Kanazawa 1989; Mays *et al.* 1995). The most commonly used for archaeological specimens are the ordinal scales of Smith (1984) and Scott (1979) and for ageing Brothwell (1963) and Miles (1963). Similar methods for recording deciduous tooth wear have not been developed. For this pilot study a quantitative method is used, which has been successfully applied to permanent teeth (Clement 2007; 2008; Clement *et al.* 2009; Deter 2009). The area of exposed dentine within the occlusal surface of a tooth is measured from digital photographs using a simple image analysis program, making it applicable to both deciduous and permanent teeth. It also has the added advantage of producing a continuous measurement which records fine variations in dentine exposure, compared to more simple ordinal methods.

Digital photographs were taken of the occlusal surface of the mandibular and maxillary deciduous teeth, using a Fuji film Finepix camera and tripod. Tooth wear was measured from the digital photograph using image analysis software, Image J. A graphics tablet was used to draw around the margin of the occlusal surface of each tooth (Fig. 1). Image J determined the area by counting the number of pixels enclosed within this perimeter. Calibrated measurements were not needed because the method uses the ratio of areas. The darker area of dentine, often stained brown in archaeological specimens, was then measured using the same method (Fig. 1). If more than one isolated patch of dentine was present on the occlusal surface of a tooth they were measured individually and then added together to calculate the total area of dentine. The summed area of dentine was then divided by the area of the occlusal surface to create a *dentine proportion* for each tooth. Occlusal surfaces that were damaged from heavy chipping, cracking or dental disease were excluded from the analysis.

Before the dentine proportions for the left and right sides of the maxilla and mandible were combined, the possible effect of wear asymmetry was tested on the study sample. A Mann Whitney-U test was applied to each tooth type and no significant differences ($p > 0.05$) between the dentine proportions from the left and right sides of the maxilla and mandible were found. The dentine proportions were therefore combined; where both the left and right teeth were present the average of the two scores was taken, and where only a left or right tooth was present the dentine proportion was recorded for that tooth alone. The repeatability of this method has been tested on the permanent dentition by calculating: the inter- and intra-observer measurement error, and the effect of the angle of the camera in relation to the occlusal surface of teeth (Clement 2007; 2008). The measurement error in each case was less than 2%.

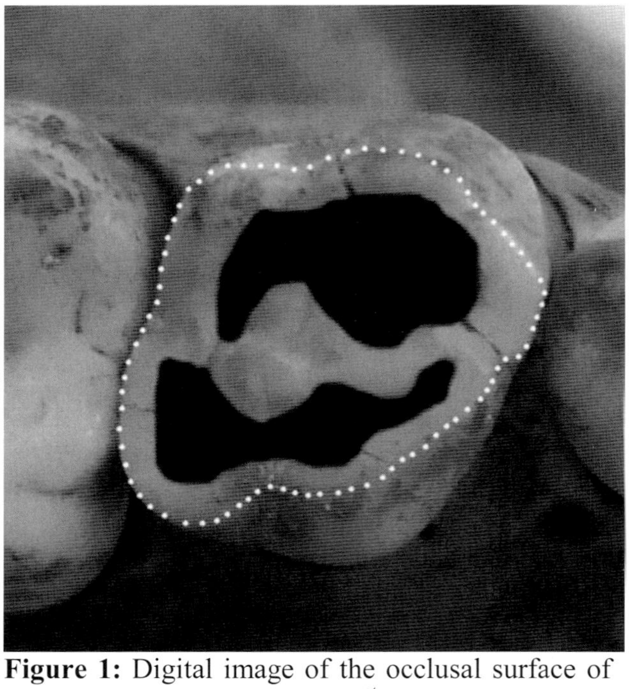

**Figure 1:** Digital image of the occlusal surface of an upper right deciduous 1st molar where the occlusal surface has been outlined and the dentine highlighted.

*Tooth Wear and the Eruption Sequence*

Dental development and more specifically dental eruption sequences have been widely studied in modern humans (Schour and Massler 1941; Hurme 1949; Dahlberg and Menegaz-Bock 1958; Gustafson and Koch 1974; Jaswal 1983; Smith and Garn 1987). This interest has been fuelled by their importance in ageing juveniles and young adults from both archaeological and forensic contexts. While the deciduous teeth exhibit some variation in the sequence and timing of their eruption, these teeth are normally in full occlusion by two-and-a-half-years after birth (Hillson 1996). The average eruption sequence is the same for the maxillary and mandibular teeth: dI1, dI2, dM1, dC, dM2 (M denotes molar, I incisor, and C canine) (Liversidge and Molleson 2004).

The dental eruption sequence is an important consideration when interpreting tooth wear patterns because it dictates the amount of time each tooth is exposed to wear. The first incisor, for example, is normally the first deciduous tooth to erupt, between approximately eight and 16 months old, whereas the deciduous second molar erupts significantly later in a juvenile's life, between about 24 and 36 months (Liversidge and Molleson 2004). This difference in eruption times means that the deciduous first incisor is exposed to considerably more wear than the second molar until it is exfoliated at approximately six years of age. If we assume a constant rate of wear for all deciduous teeth then at any age it follows that the teeth which erupt first will exhibit more advanced wear than those that follow until they are exfoliated. For example, the deciduous incisors should show higher amounts of wear than the second molars as these teeth erupt between approximately eight and 18 months apart. If the rate of tooth wear is not constant for all teeth, then the degree of wear will not reflect the expected eruption sequence. This is the fundamental principle of the interpretations of wear patterns in this study.

Mean eruption times, such as those provided by Liversidge and Molleson (2004), can be used to suggest the expected wear pattern for an individual. Figure 2 illustrates the differences in months between the eruption of the deciduous first incisor and the other deciduous teeth within the maxillary and mandibular dentitions. The first incisor is normally the first deciduous tooth to erupt in both the maxilla and mandible and all other teeth fall below this dashed line, which represents the eruption of the deciduous first incisor. This expected wear pattern graph can be used to suggest the relative exposure to wear of different teeth. Due to its early eruption it is expected that the deciduous first incisor would be the most heavily worn tooth within the deciduous dentition, closely followed by the second incisors and first molars. The canine and the second molar demonstrate slightly later eruption times than the incisors and first molars and would therefore be expected to be less worn.

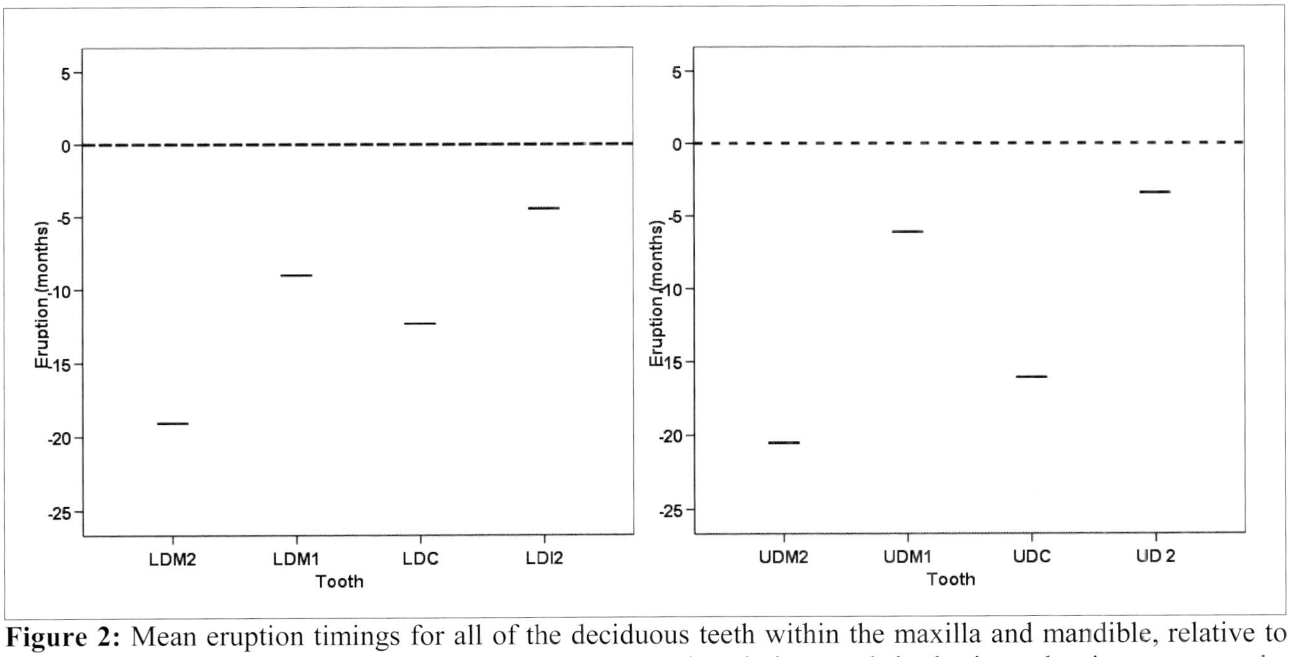


**Figure 2:** Mean eruption timings for all of the deciduous teeth within the maxilla and mandible, relative to the first incisor. The y-axis represents the average eruption timings and the horizontal axis represents the tooth type. The first incisor is not shown as it is being used as the reference tooth, but is represented by a horizontal dashed line passing through 0 on the y-axis. As the pattern of wear through the dentition strongly reflects relative eruption timing, this represents the expected pattern of wear. Mean eruption times from Liversidge and Molleson (2004).

Tooth wear is usually recorded as an overall amount, such as a dentine proportion or wear stage (e.g. Walker 1978; Hinton 1982; Kieser *et al.* 1985; Lovejoy 1985; Buikstra and Ubelaker *et al.* 1994). Tooth wear, however, normally increases with age and this often obscures the pattern of wear within a population or sample. When examining patterns of wear age therefore needs to be removed as a major factor. This is achieved by presenting the dentine proportion of each deciduous tooth as a ratio of the dentine proportion for one particular reference tooth in the dentition. For this study, the first incisor was selected as it is usually the first deciduous tooth to erupt and therefore expected to be the most heavily worn. The dentine proportions of the other deciduous teeth were then divided by the dentine proportion of the first incisor from the same jaw to create a *wear ratio*. Those deciduous teeth with a similar wear state to the first incisor should therefore have a wear ratio near 1. Those with more wear should have a wear ratio greater than 1, and those with less wear should have a wear ratio of less than 1.

This method was previously applied to two archaeological collections of medieval monks from London (Clement 2007). Their permanent tooth wear pattern closely followed the average eruption sequence of the permanent dentition. Departures from the eruption sequence pattern have been noted amongst groups of hunter-gatherers such as Australian Aborigines and Inuit of Canada (Clement 2008; Clement *et al.* 2009), who show relatively high amounts of wear in their anterior teeth. These studies suggest that this difference was the result of the use of the front teeth as tools. The wear pattern for the deciduous dentition has, however, never been previously studied.

## Results

### *The Deciduous Tooth Wear Pattern*

The wear ratios (relative to the deciduous first incisor) for the Sudanese deciduous maxillary teeth demonstrate a clear pattern of wear (Fig. 3). The median wear ratios of all the maxillary teeth fall below the first incisor line. In fact, only the molars of specimen 14 and the second incisor of specimen 17 are more are more heavily worn than the first incisor from the same jaw. The canine and second incisor possess the highest median wear ratios of 0.75 and 0.3, respectively. The maxillary canines also show the largest inter-quartile range. Low median wear ratios, relative to the first incisor, are observed in both molars, with the second molar being relatively unworn. This is not what would be expected if the wear merely reflects the eruption sequence (Fig. 2). Whilst the first and second incisors show the highest amounts of wear, as expected from the eruption sequence, the canine and molars do not follow the expected wear pattern. If all the deciduous teeth were exposed to a constant amount of wear then the canines should be less worn, compared to the first incisor, than the first molar, as it normally erupts later. In addition, the relative wear ratios of the first molar would be expected to be much higher at a similar level to the second incisor.

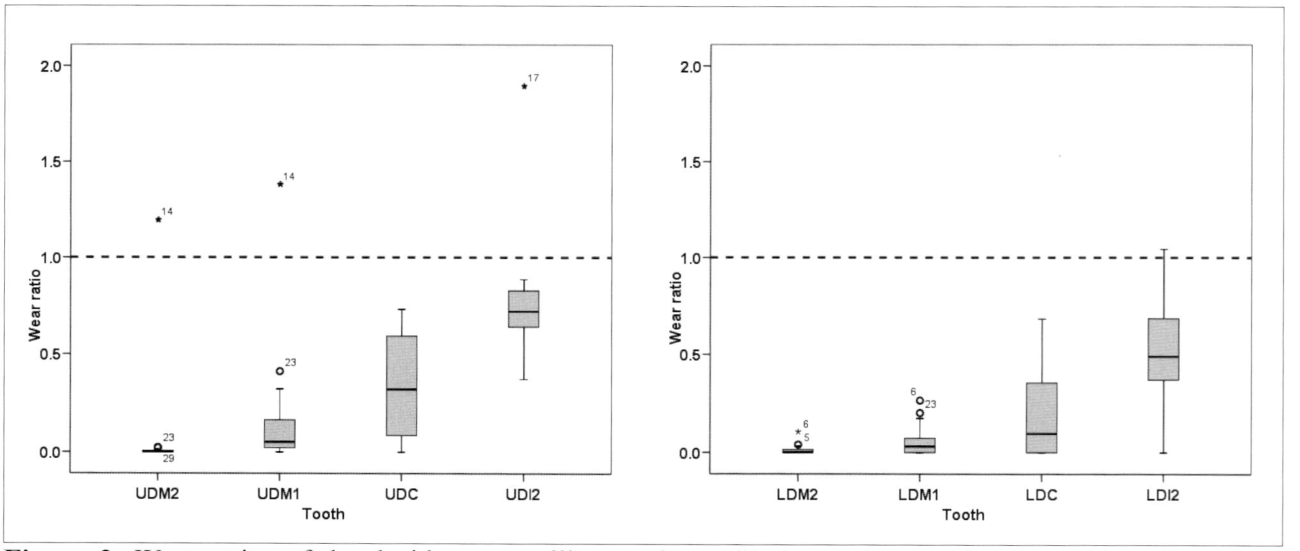


**Figure 3:** Wear ratios of the deciduous maxillary and mandibular teeth. Percent of occlusal surface area occupied by dentine, for each tooth in the maxillary dentition, expressed as ratios of this wear measure in the first incisor. This box plot (and the following ones) represents each individual tooth, starting with the back of the mouth (second molars) following through to the front (second incisors) – the first incisor is not included as it is the reference tooth for these ratios. The top and bottom of each box represent the upper and lower quartile values, and so the height of the box represents the inter-quartile range. The bar inside each box represents the median, and the 'whiskers' represent the overall range of values. Outliers are represented by 'O' and '*' symbols: 'O' indicates values which are separated from the upper or lower quartile by more than 1.5 times the inter-quartile range; '*' indicates values separated by more than 3 times the inter-quartile range.

The deciduous mandibular teeth show a similar wear pattern to their maxillary counterparts, but all possess lower median wear ratios (Fig. 3). The mandibular second incisor shows the highest median wear ratio, relative to the first incisor, as is expected from the eruption sequence, but is only 0.5 compared to 0.75 for the maxillary second incisor. This tooth does, however, show the widest range of wear values, and for some specimens rises above the first incisor line. As with its maxillary counterpart the mandibular canine possesses the largest inter-quartile range, but has a much lower median wear ratio of 0.1. Lower wear ratios than would be expected from their position within the eruption sequence are shown by both mandibular molars, being relatively unworn compared the first incisor.

*Deciduous Tooth Wear and Age*

The tooth wear pattern for the deciduous dentition, described above, only includes specimens with complete dentitions; specimens above the dental development age of seven are not represented in Figure 3. The pattern of deciduous tooth wear can also be illustrated by presenting the average dentine proportions of each tooth type against dental development age category (Fig. 4). Specimens were allocated an age category based on estimations of their dental development stage. These were rounded to the nearest whole number, for example an individual of 6.3 years was rounded down to six, while an individual aged 6.5 years was rounded up to seven.

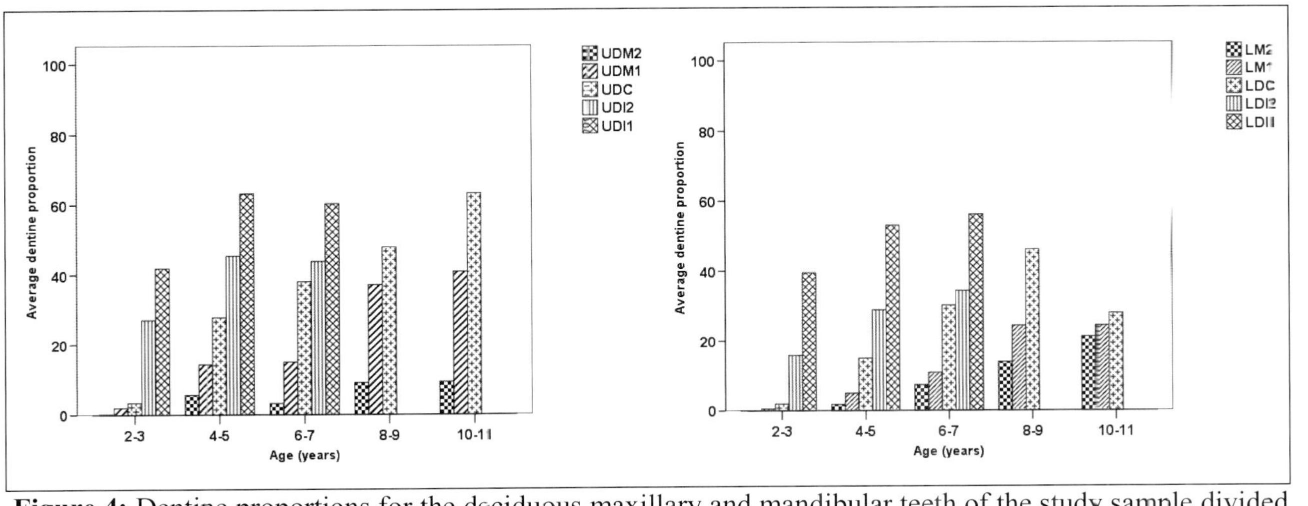


**Figure 4:** Dentine proportions for the deciduous maxillary and mandibular teeth of the study sample divided into dental development age groups.

All of the deciduous teeth, apart from the lower deciduous canine, show an increase in their dentine proportion with age. A decrease in the average dentine proportion of the lower deciduous canine is observed in the ten to eleven year age category and is probably the result of the small sample size for this group. The results also confirm that for the first three age categories (two to seven years) the deciduous first incisors are the most heavily worn tooth type, followed by the second incisors, canines, first molars and lastly the second molars. The average dentine proportions for the maxillary and mandibular first incisor in the two to three year age category are already at a high level of approximately 40% dentine. These increase to an average of almost 60% in the six to seven year age category. This is in contrast to the deciduous molars which possess average dentine proportions of less than 5% in the two to three year age category. However, the dentine proportions for the maxillary and mandibular first molars are substantially higher in the eight to nine and ten to eleven year age categories, where the deciduous incisors have been exfoliated. The average dentine proportions of the deciduous maxillary second molars remain below 10% for each age category. In contrast, the average dentine proportions of the mandibular second molars increase with each successive age category, rising to over 20% in the ten to eleven year age group. Despite this increase, the maxillary and mandibular canines continue to show higher average dentine proportions than the molars, with an average of over 60% in the maxillary ten to eleven year group.

## Discussion

The results of this pilot study show that the deciduous teeth from the Sudanese sample possess a clear pattern of wear. As expected from the eruption sequence the first incisor was the most heavily worn of the deciduous teeth closely followed by the second incisor. The deciduous canine also possessed a high wear ratio, relative to the first incisor; higher than expected from its position within the eruption sequence. In addition, the deciduous molars showed relatively low dentine proportions, compared to the first incisor. The dentine proportions of the first molar were, however, much higher in specimens above the dental development age of seven, when the incisors had been exfoliated. This departure from the expected wear pattern suggests that the deciduous teeth were not exposed to a constant level of wear throughout their functional life. The levels of tooth wear in the different dental development age categories (Fig. 4) imply that within the study sample the anterior teeth were exposed to heavier amounts of wear during the first years of life than the molars. While interpretations of this wear pattern remain speculative until further research into deciduous tooth wear has been made, some interesting explanations can be offered.

If dentine exposure in the deciduous dentition is the result of abrasive food particles, as suggested by previous studies (Davies and Pedersen 1955; Prowse *et al.* 2008), then information can be gathered about weaning strategies in the Sudanese sample. Exposed dentine is observed from the developmental age of 18 months and indicates the weaning process began long enough before this age to wear away the layer of enamel and reveal the underlying dentine. Interestingly, differences were not observed in the commencement times of dentine exposure in the three different groups. There is a large increase in the dentine proportions of the first molar at approximately eight years of age, suggesting a more abrasive diet is being consumed.

In addition, this information about weaning activities can also be used to make suggestions about the inter-birth period and general fecundity of a population. Breastfeeding acts as a natural contraceptive, suppressing the mother's fertility and therefore reducing the chance of a subsequent early pregnancy (Sellen and Smay 2001; Kennedy 2005). The longer a child is breastfed the longer the period of suppressed fertility in the mother and larger the inter-birth interval. The presence of tooth wear at an early age would suggest a short inter-birth period, while the lack of tooth wear may represent an extended period of breastfeeding and a longer inter-birth spacing. However, this is a rather simplistic interpretation of a complex process because while breastfeeding reduces the fertility of the mother it is not a totally reliable form of contraception and a mother may continue to breastfeed for several years even after the introduction of alternative foods.

Previous work on tooth wear in the permanent dentition has demonstrated that factors other than diet can affect the pattern of wear, such as the use of the front teeth as tools (Clement 2008; Clement *et al.* 2009). For the deciduous dentition the use of teething implements, such as such as leather, rags, wood or bones, as noted by Prowse *et al.* (2008), could explain the high levels of tooth wear in the anterior teeth compared to the molars. The use of vessels, such as ceramic bottles to feed the younger infants would also affect the anterior teeth more than the molars and may also have contributed to their higher dentine proportions.

The standard pattern of tooth wear can also be disrupted as shown by specimens 14 and 17 (Fig. 3). Observations of the tooth wear in specimen 14 confirm the presence of an unusually large amount of tooth wear on the deciduous mandibular right molars. The distribution of dentine on the occlusal surface of these two teeth is indicative of an abrasive object being placed within the right side of the mouth and habitually chewed. The opposing maxillary molars show evidence of highly destructive carious lesions and it seems reasonable to suggest that the chewing of an object may have alleviated the discomfort of this ailment.

## Conclusions

This pilot study demonstrates that a quantitative method measuring the dentine proportions on the occlusal surface of a tooth can be successfully applied to the deciduous dentition as well as the permanent teeth. It also highlights the need to develop and test methods for recording deciduous tooth wear to enable a wealth of information to be gathered on the variation in deciduous wear patterns between and within different populations. A quantitative approach can be used, but this is more time consuming than simple ordinal methods and requires access to digital images and a computer system. The development of an ordinal paper-based system for recording tooth wear in the deciduous dentition is therefore paramount and would allow deciduous tooth wear to be recorded relatively rapidly in large skeletal collections. While the sample size for this pilot study was small the results indicate the potential information that can be gained about the diets, weaning, teething and feeding practices of past populations from the study of their deciduous tooth wear.

**Acknowledgements**

The authors wish to thank Dr Daniel Antoine and the Department of Ancient Egypt and Sudan at the British Museum for granting access to their collection of human remains. Thanks are also given to Professors Simon Hillson and Tony Waldron for their advice and encouragement.

**Literature Cited**

Aiello, L.C., Montgomery, C. and Dean, C. 1991. The natural history of deciduous tooth attrition in hominoids. *Journal of Human Evolution* 21: 397-412.

AlQahtani, S.J., Hector, M.P. and Liversidge, H.M. 2010. The London atlas of human tooth development. *American Journal of Physical Anthropology* 142: 481-490.

Broca, P. 1879. Instructions relatives à l'étude anthropologique due système dentaire. *Bulletin et Memoires de la Societe d'Anthropologie de Paris* 2: 128-152.

Brothwell, D.R. 1963. *Digging up bones*. British Museum of Natural History: London.

Buikstra, J.E. and Ubelaker, D.H. 1994. *Standards for data collection from human skeletal remains*. Arkansas Archaeological Survey: Fayetteville.

Bullington, J. 1991. Deciduous dental microwear of prehistoric juveniles from the lower Illinois River Valley. *American Journal of Physical Anthropology* 84: 59-73.

Clayton, F., Sealy, J. and Pfeiffer, S. 2006. Weaning age among foragers at Matjes river rock shelter South Africa, from stable nitrogen and carbon isotope analyses. *American Journal of Physical Anthropology* 129: 311-317.

Clement, A.F. 2007. A new method for recording tooth wear. In: Zakrzewski, S.R. and White, W. (eds.) *Proceedings of the seventh annual conference of the British Association for Biological Anthropology and Osteoarchaeology, Oxford, UK*. Archaeopress: Oxford. British Archaeological Reports International Series 1712: 72-81.

Clement, A.F. 2008. *Tooth wear patterns in Neanderthal and early Modern Humans*. Unpublished PhD thesis: University College London.

Clement, A.F., Hillson, S.W., de la Torre, I. and Townsend, G. 2009. Tooth use in Aboriginal Australia. *Archaeology International* 11: 37-40.

Crossner, C.G. and Mansfield, L. 1983. Determination of dental age in adopted non-European children. *Swedish Dental Journal* 7: 1-10.

Deter, C.A. 2009. Gradients of occlusal wear in hunter-gatherers and agriculturalists. *American Journal of Physical Anthropology* 138:247-254.

Dahlberg, A.A. and Menegaz-Bock, R.M. 1958. Emergence of the permanent teeth in Pima Indian children. *Journal of Dental Research* 37:1123-1140.

Davies, T.G.H. and Pedersen, P.O. 1955. The degree of attrition of the deciduous teeth and first permanent molars of primitive and urbanised Greenland natives. *British Dental Journal* 99: 35-43.

Edwards, D.N. 1998. *Gabati: A Meroitic, Post-Meroitic and Medieval Cemetery in Central Sudan*. Sudan Archaeological Research Society Publication no. 3: London.

Eshed, V., Gopher, A. and Hershkovitz, I. 2006. Tooth wear and dental pathology at the advent of agriculture: new evidence from the Levant. *American Journal of Physical Anthropology* 130: 145-159.

Ferguson, R.B. 2000. The causes and origins of 'primitive warfare': on evolved motivations for war. *Anthropological Quarterly* 73: 159-164.

Fearnhead, R.W., Kawasaki, K. and Inoue, K. 1982. Comments on the porosity of human tooth enamel. *Journal of Dental Research* 61: 1524-1531.

Filer, J. 1999. The Gabati cemetery: new work in Ancient Nubia. In: Anderson, S. (ed.) *Current and recent research in osteoarchaeology 2: proceedings of the fourth, fifth and sixth meetings of the Osteoarchaeological Group held in York on 27th April 1996, Cardiff on 16th November 1996, and Durham on 7th June 1997*. Oxbow Books: Oxford. 17-22.

Fuller, B.T., Fuller, J.L., Harris, D.A. and Hedges, R.E.M. 2006. Detection of breastfeeding and weaning in modern human infants with carbon and nitrogen stable isotope ratios. *American Journal of Physical Anthropology* 129: 279-283.

Gray, S.W. and Lamon, F.P. 1959. Skeletal development and tooth eruption in Atlanta children. *American Journal of Physical Anthropology* 45: 272-277.

Gustafson, G. and Koch, G. 1974. Age estimation up to 16 years of age based on dental development. *Odontologisk Revy* 25: 297-306.

Hillson, S. 1996. *Dental anthropology*. Cambridge University Press: Cambridge.

Hinton, R.J. 1982. Differences in interproximal and occlusal tooth wear among prehistoric Tennessee Indians: implications for masticatory function. *American Journal of Physical Anthropology* 57: 103-115.

Hurme, V.O. 1949. Ranges of normalcy in the eruption of the permanent teeth *Journal of Dentistry for Children* 16: 11-15.

Jaswal, S. 1983. Age and sequence of permanent-tooth emergence among Khasis. *American Journal of Physical Anthropology* 62:177-186.

Johansson, A.K., Sorvari, R., Birkhed, D. and Meurman, J.H. 2001. Dental erosion in deciduous teeth- an in vivo and in vitro study. *Journal of Dentistry* 29: 333-340.

Kennedy, G.E. 2005. From the ape's dilemma to the weanling's dilemma: early weaning and its evolutionary context. *Journal of Human Evolution* 48: 123-145.

Kieser. J.A., Groeneveld, H.T. and Preston, C.B. 1985. Patterns of dental wear in the Lengua Indians of Paraguay. *American Journal of Physical Anthropology* 66:21-29.

Larsen, C.S. 1985. Dental modifications and tool use in the Western Great Basin. *American Journal of Physical Anthropology* 67:393-402.

Liversidge, H.M. 1994. Accuracy of age estimation from developing teeth of a population of known age (0 to 5.4 years). *International Journal of Osteoarchaeology* 4: 37-46.

Liversidge, H.M. and Molleson, T. 2004. Variation in crown and root formation and eruption of human deciduous teeth. *American Journal of Physical Anthropology* 123: 172-180.

Lovejoy, C.O. 1985. Dental wear in the Libben population: its functional pattern and role in the determination of adult skeletal age at death. *American Journal of Physical Anthropology* 68:47-56.

Lunt, R.C. And Law, D.B. 1974. A review of the chronology of calcification of deciduous teeth. *Journal of the American Dental Association* 89: 599-606.

Mayhall, J.T. and Kanazawa, E. 1989. Three-dimensional analysis of the maxillary first molar crowns of Canadian Inuit. *American Journal of Physical Anthropology* 78:73-78.

Mays, S., de la Rua, C. and Molleson, T. 1995. Molar crown height as a means of evaluating existing dental wear scales for estimating age at death in human skeletal remains. *Journal of Archaeological Science* 22:659-670.

Miles, A.E.W. 1958. The assessment of age from the dentition. *Proceedings of the Royal Society of Medicine* 51: 1057–1060.

Miles, A.E.W. 1963. The dentition in the assessment of individual age in skeletal material. In: Brothwell, D.R. (ed.) *Dental Anthropology*. Pergamon Press: Oxford. 191-209.

Molnar, S. 1971. Human tooth wear, tooth function and cultural variability. *American Journal of Physical Anthropology* 34: 175-190.

Murphy, T. 1959. The changing pattern of dentine exposure in human tooth attrition. *American Journal of Physical Anthropology* 17:167-178.

Prowse, T.L., Saunders, S.R., Schwarcz, H.P., Garnsey, P., Macchiarelli, R. and Bondioli, L. 2008. Isotopic and dental evidence for infant and young child feeding practices in an imperial Roman skeletal sample. *American Journal of Physical Anthropology* 137: 294-308.

Richards, M.P., Mays, S. and Fuller, B.T. 2002. Stable carbon and nitrogen isotope values of bone and teeth reflect weaning age at the medieval Wharram Percy site, Yorkshire, UK. *American Journal of Physical Anthropology* 119: 205-210.

Schour, I. and Massler, M. 1941. The development of the human dentition. *Journal of the American Dental Association* 28:1153-1160.

Scheuer, L. and Black, S. 2004. *The juvenile skeleton.* Elsevier: London.

Scott, E.C. 1979. Dental wear scoring technique. *American Journal of Physical Anthropology* 51: 213-217.

Sellen, D.W. and Smay, D.B. 2001. Relationship between subsistence and age at weaning in 'preindustrial' societies. *Human Nature* 12: 47-87.

Sellen, D.W. 2007. Evolution of infant and young child feeding: implications for contemporary public health. *Annual Review of Nutrition* 27: 123-148.

Smith, B.H. 1984. Patterns of molar wear in hunter-gatherers and agriculturalists. *American Journal of Physical Anthropology* 63: 39-56.

Smith, B.H. and Garn, S.M. 1987. Polymorphisms in eruption sequence of permanent teeth in American children. *American Journal of Physical Anthropology* 74: 289-303.

Ubelaker, D.H. 1978. *Human skeletal remains: excavation, analysis, interpretation.* Aldine: Chicago.

Van Gerven, D.P., Sheridan, S.G. and Adams, W.Y. 1995. The health and nutrition of a medieval Nubian population: the impact of political and economic change. *American Anthropologist* 97: 468-480.

Walker, P.L. 1978. A quantitative analysis of dental attrition rates in the Santa Barbara Channel area. *American Journal of Physical Anthropology* 48: 101-106.

Wendorf, F. 1968. Site 117: a Nubian final Paleolithic graveyard near Jebel Sahaba, Sudan. In: Wendorf, F. (ed.) *The prehistory of Nubia, V. II.* Southern Methodist University Press: Dallas. 954-995.

Wheeler, R.C. 1965. *Dental anatomy, physiology and occlusion.* WB Saunders: Philadelphia.

# A Study of Interobserver Variation in Cranial Measurements and the Resulting Consequences when Analysed using CranID

Richard J. Slater* and Martin J. Smith

Bournemouth University
School of Applied Sciences
Christchurch House
Talbot Campus
Fern Barrow, Poole
Dorset, BH12 5BB

*Email for correspondence: rich_slater@hotmail.co.uk

**Abstract**

In Biological Anthropology, as with many sciences, the potential for corruption of data due to interobserver differences is ever present. This article presents results of an experiment in which 11 observers analysed a single cranium using CranID. These user data were then compared using Degrees of Variation to proportionally represent the degree of disparity in results on the assumption that no single set could purport to be more accurate than any other without further study. MANOVA analysis was also applied to see if any of the cranial measurements were more consistent than others. Finally the data were subjected to CranID analysis and the results for each of the 11 observers compared to see what effect interobserver variation would have on identifying ancestry.

Each observer showed both positive and negative variation, seemingly randomly, with only 3 of the 11 observers achieving an average lower than 5 Degrees of Variation across all measurements. When accounting for experience it was discovered that the two most experienced observers' measurements differed significantly from each other. Seven measurements exhibited extremely high levels of variation between observers. Worryingly only one measurement had no significant difference, one had minimal difference, the rest showed increasingly significant variation. Although there was some evidence of correlation between the results, there was still a high enough degree of variation to prove disconcerting. This small study highlights a justified need for independent methods of testing observers' accuracy.

**Keywords:** Interobserver Error, Interobserver Variation, Craniometric, CranID

## Introduction

"Ancestry is defined as the biogeographic population to which a particular individual belongs, by virtue of his or her genetic heritage" (Barker *et al.* 2007: 322)

It has been clearly demonstrated that it is possible to infer ancestry through osteological analysis, especially craniometry. The work of Giles and Elliot (1962), and Howells (1969, 1973, 1989) has demonstrated significant correlation between metric cranial attributes and population diversity. Developing upon this, Wright (1992) and Ousley & Jantz (1996) have formatted computer programs which perform complex computations to this end. The uptake of CranID and Fordisc has allowed for faster and simpler analysis of cranial population assessment, however these remain computer programs and the computing maxim of 'Rubbish In, Rubbish Out' applies, therefore one should consider the accuracy of one's measurements before considering the validity of the results.

A number of studies have examined the reliability of interobserver measurements, Heathcote (1981) and others (Utermohle & Zegura 1982, Utermohle *et al.* 1983, Palmeirim 1998) have pointed out there is a wide scope for corruption of data between observers, referring to 'Interobserver Error', however whilst this suggests the degree to which one or other observer is right or wrong their studies have not defined what they consider to be 'correct'.

Firstly this study analyses the differences in measurements recorded between multiple observers, but without making assumptions of accuracy, and so will refer to 'interobserver variation' or the degree to which a group of observers vary from the mean average of their collective scores. Secondly this study analyses the effects that this variation has upon population studies, especially when applied to CranID analysis. As the range of measurements used in CranID differ substantially in size, the effect of a few millimetres difference alters between measurements; this study shall utilise Degrees of Variation (°V) to enable comparable analysis of variation.

## Method

Participants were invited personally to take part in this experiment; all being either Forensic Science students, or faculty staff from the school of Applied Sciences at Bournemouth University. The skull used for measuring was collection number 1021 from the Quaker burial ground at Kingston-upon Thames, which is recorded as being a female aged 23 (Cox 1998). It was selected for having a known history, whilst at the same time having proved to be an interesting example for CranID analysis having previously produced unexpected results.

Participants were presented with the skull, a set of spreading callipers, a set of sliding callipers, and an alternative to coordinate callipers in the form of a short ruler section to be used in combination with sliding callipers in order to measure subtenses. The latter has been recommended by Richard Wright as both cheaper and less damaging to bone than coordinate callipers. Subjects were also supplied with data recording sheets and pages 36-56 of the CranID manual (Wright 2009) that describe and illustrate the relevant landmarks and measurements. Additional training was given in the use of the alternative to coordinate callipers by the researcher, however this training was not demonstrated on any of the required measurements so as not to influence readings unduly, but it was felt that clarification was required in order to accurately assess interobserver variation in measurement as opposed to error due to misinterpretation of the instructions.

CranID analysis was performed using version 6 (CRa6IND), as per the instructions in the accompanying manual (Wright 2009). Results were collated using the top five results for both Linear Discriminant Analysis (LDA), and Nearest Neighbour Discriminant Analysis (NNDA); both statistical tests of pattern, in this case looking at relatedness between populations using cranial measurements. Also included in the results were any warnings regarding individual measurements, any cautions highlighted in the CranID results, and the actual nearest neighbour.

Results were prepared for analysis by calculating the mean average result for each measurement, individual observer results were then compared to the mean result for variation. In order to compare the variation between results Degrees of Variation (°V) were used, these calculate the mean result for each measurement from all observers (ɱ), and then calculate individual variation from the mean (¥) and express it as a percentage of the mean ( [100÷ɱ]×¥).

The original data were further submitted to multivariate analysis of variance (MANOVA) using PASW statistics (v18) as recommended by Field (2009), to test for significant statistical differences between observers for each of the 29 measurements.

## Results

MANOVA analysis resulted in a Wilks' Lambda probability distribution critical-F value of 199380.429, when compared to the F values of the 29 measurements taken by all observers (see Table 1) only GOL (Glabello-Occipital Length) showed no significant difference, and only NOL (Nasio-Occipital Length) showed a minimal significant difference. Of the remainder a staggering 16 measurements showed a variation in excess of 10% in either a positive or negative bias, and of these 4 were greater than 10% average variation in both directions, Figure 1 illustrates the collective negative and positive variation from the mean. Figure 2 identifies OCS (Lambda-Opisthion Subtense) as the measurement with the greatest total variation, followed by SSS (Zygomaxillary Subtense) and NAS (Nasio-Frontal Subtense), NLH (Nasal Height) is the non-subtense measurement with the highest Degree of Variation.

Of the 11 observers that took part only two had consistently low Degrees of Variation across all measurements, whilst three demonstrated a clear positive bias in their variation, including Observer-11 who could arguably be one of the more accurate observers (by reason of experience). Only one had a consistent negative bias to their data. Observer-3 proved to be consistently close to the mean for the group, recording the smallest average Degree of Variation across all measurements at 4.4%, with a maximum Degree of Variation of 10.5%. It is important to remember that this is not a measure of accuracy however.

Despite the high levels of variation between users in a number of measurements, CranID analysis demonstrates a higher degree of concurrence in results of both LDA and NNDA analysis. Figure 6 clearly shows that although a number of potential populations are presented for the 11 observers' data, there is a close grouping to the relatedness of these populations, especially when looking at the LDA analysis illustrated on the left of the diagram. NNDA analysis shows a wider variation when accounting for the top five results, however summation of the Actual Nearest Neighbour results demonstrates an even tighter range of results. Both LDA and NNDA analysis identified the most likely population between all observers as EGYPT_26-30_DYN_F.

Of all the LDA results there is a clear inference that the skull is of a female (Figure 5), though this is far from conclusive and is shown to be highly population dependent.

**Discussion**

Looking at individual observer results there are alarming degrees of variance, with no observer achieving a set of results that lack high Degrees of Variation in multiple measurements. Of the 11 observers tested only three achieved an average of less than 5 Degrees of Variation across all measurements. Accounting for experience Observer-11 is likely to prove the most accurate observer; it is interesting to note that Observer-11 is the only observer that has an almost exclusively positive bias in variation compared to the mean for the group suggesting a general tendency to underestimate. However on the same assumptions Observer-1 would be expected to be the next most accurate and we would expect to see greater collusion in results between these two observers, yet there is considerable variation, the largest being almost 39%, and on average there was an 8.5% variation across all measurements.

The lack of consistency between all observers could be explained by levels of training; however it is apparent that the two measurements GOL and NOL do have a degree of accuracy, effectively acting as control measurements further highlighting the excessive degree of variation elsewhere. As stated this study simply observes the levels of variation from the mean per observer, and does not presume to represent accuracy.

As alarming as the collective high levels of variation, are the substantial levels of variation within specific measurements, in fact aside from NOL and GOL none of the other 27 measurements achieve a high consistency between observers. MANOVA analysis highlights the excessive levels of variation found in 7 of the 29 measurements raising further questions as to why. Given the high level of variation detected in measurements it is unsurprising that there should be an effect when these results were subjected to CranID analysis. Indeed when the top five results for all observers are collated there are 20 different populations represented by LDA analysis and 23 by NNDA analysis. What is surprising is when we consider these results in relation to each other. Figure 6 identifies the top results by weighting on the CranID dendrogram and the results are not as randomly distributed as might be expected. These results show that although there is a high degree of variation found between observers that in CranID analysis these variations do not affect results randomly, a definite grouping of results is evident, and although the populations differ, their relatedness cannot be ignored.

It should also be noted that in the results from the CranID analysis none of the user data were identified as being within an acceptable number of standard deviations from the nearest neighbour, and many had warnings flagged on a number of measurements. In this instance it is believed that this is due to the unusual shape of the skull analysed, yet this shows that CranID has a number of inbuilt precautions which should not be ignored.

These results do suggest the need to view results of any comparisons in terms of context. How these results would compare to a full CranID analysis performed by Richard Wright is unknown, and may prove an interesting point of comparison, offering a measure of accuracy that is unachievable with Degrees of Variation. What we have seen is that between 11 observers, all with some degree of training, there is little concurrence in results and a high level of variation, it would be interesting to see if the same degree of variation exists amongst more experienced craniometrists.

**Conclusion**

Utermohle and Zegura (1982: 302) concluded "we hope that other investigators who use craniometric measurements to study population affinities… will include some kind of measurement error analysis as an important baseline for the interpretation of the biological significance of their results"; advice that is not always followed, and which, on evidence of

**Table 1**: Results showing measurements recorded by each observer, Degrees of Variation, and MANOVA test results.

| | Observer 1 | | Observer 2 | | Observer 3 | | Observer 4 | | Observer 5 | | Observer 6 | |
|---|---|---|---|---|---|---|---|---|---|---|---|---|
| | Result | °V | Result | °V | Result | °V | Result | °V | Result | °V | Result | °V |
| GOL | 177 | 0.57 | 176 | 0.00 | 176 | 0.00 | 176 | 0.00 | 176 | 0.00 | 177 | 0.57 |
| NOL | 174 | 0.37 | 176 | 1.52 | 171 | -1.36 | 174 | 0.37 | 171 | -1.36 | 174 | 0.37 |
| BNL | 93 | -5.01 | 92 | -6.04 | 92 | -6.04 | 90 | -8.08 | 116 | 18.48 | 93 | -5.01 |
| BBH | 118 | -2.26 | 118 | -2.26 | 118 | -2.26 | 119 | -1.43 | 124 | 2.71 | 118 | -2.26 |
| XCB | 136 | 7.78 | 136 | 7.78 | 130 | 3.03 | 137 | 8.57 | 123 | -2.52 | 137 | 8.57 |
| XFB | 106 | -1.10 | 108 | 0.76 | 110 | 2.63 | 106 | -1.10 | 135 | 25.95 | 107 | -0.17 |
| AUB | 109 | 3.01 | 108 | 2.06 | 108 | 2.06 | 109 | 3.01 | 109 | 3.01 | 108 | 2.06 |
| ASB | 98 | 3.16 | 101 | 6.32 | 96 | 1.05 | 96 | 1.05 | 94 | -1.05 | 100 | 5.26 |
| BPL | 86 | -5.31 | 90 | -0.90 | 86 | -5.31 | 86 | -5.31 | 97 | 6.81 | 86 | -5.31 |
| NPH | 56 | -1.91 | 60 | 5.10 | 57 | -0.16 | 56 | -1.91 | 53 | -7.17 | 56 | -1.91 |
| NLH | 43 | 10.00 | 43 | 10.00 | 40 | 2.33 | 41 | 4.88 | 42 | 7.44 | 40 | 2.33 |
| OBH | 32 | 4.76 | 32 | 4.76 | 30 | -1.79 | 30 | -1.79 | 30 | -1.79 | 29 | -5.06 |
| OBB | 32 | -6.38 | 38 | 11.17 | 32 | -6.38 | 32 | -6.38 | 33 | -3.46 | 34 | -0.53 |
| JUB | 101 | 2.02 | 105 | 6.06 | 95 | -4.04 | 97 | -2.02 | 96 | -3.03 | 100 | 1.01 |
| NLB | 21 | 7.94 | 21 | 7.94 | 19 | -2.34 | 19 | -2.34 | 18 | -7.48 | 18 | -7.48 |
| MAB | 56 | 7.32 | 56 | 7.32 | 48 | -8.01 | 53 | 1.57 | 52 | -0.35 | 52 | -0.35 |
| ZMB | 78 | -8.43 | 79 | -7.26 | 94 | 10.35 | 78 | -8.43 | 86 | 0.96 | 79 | -7.26 |
| SSS | 19 | -15.00 | 22 | 1.63 | 21 | -6.10 | 22 | -1.63 | 24 | 7.32 | 15 | -32.90 |
| FMB | 89 | -1.11 | 88 | -2.22 | 86 | -4.44 | 89 | -1.11 | 92 | 2.22 | 87 | -3.33 |
| NAS | 18 | -11.60 | 19 | -6.70 | 19 | -6.70 | 15 | -26.34 | 22 | 8.04 | 18 | -11.60 |
| EKB | 86 | -0.32 | 89 | 3.16 | 91 | 5.48 | 83 | -3.79 | 91 | 5.48 | 81 | -6.11 |
| DKB | 17 | 8.72 | 17 | 8.72 | 14 | -10.47 | 16 | 2.33 | 16 | 2.33 | 11 | -29.60 |
| WMH | 18 | 5.88 | 17 | 0.00 | 16 | -5.88 | 15 | -11.70 | 19 | 11.76 | 10 | -41.18 |
| FRC | 101 | -1.51 | 104 | 1.42 | 100 | -2.48 | 100 | -2.48 | 108 | 5.32 | 99 | -3.46 |
| FRS | 24 | 3.53 | 25 | 7.84 | 21 | -9.41 | 21 | -9.41 | 24 | 3.53 | 24 | 3.53 |
| PAC | 106 | -1.77 | 106 | -1.77 | 105 | -2.70 | 104 | -3.62 | 121 | 12.13 | 105 | -2.70 |
| PAS | 19 | -4.13 | 18 | -9.17 | 18 | -9.17 | 16 | -19.20 | 24 | 21.10 | 23 | 16.06 |
| OCC | 98 | 3.95 | 98 | 3.95 | 95 | 0.77 | 96 | 1.83 | 86 | -8.78 | 97 | 2.89 |
| OCS | 34 | 19.87 | 31 | 9.29 | 27 | -4.81 | 29 | 2.24 | 19 | -33.01 | 34 | 19.87 |
| Ave °V | | 5.34 | | 4.94 | | 4.40 | | 4.97 | | 7.40 | | 7.89 |
| Max °V | | 19.87 | | 11.17 | | 10.47 | | 26.34 | | 33.01 | | 41.18 |

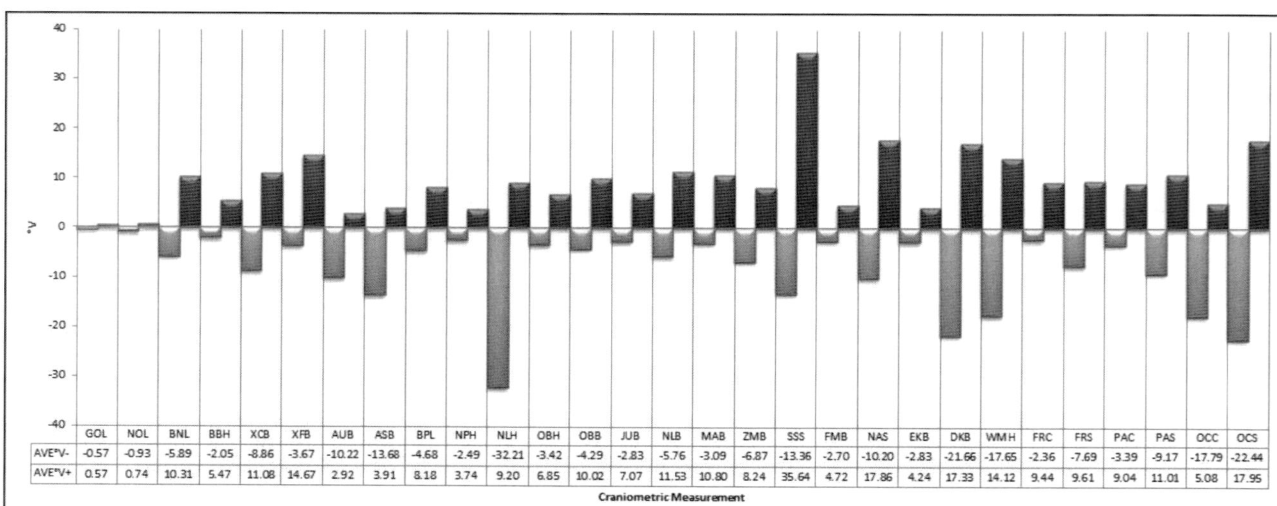


**Figure 1**: Collective Degrees of Variation between users identified by measurement and divided into both positive and negative variation from the mean.

**Table 1 cont.**

| Observer 7 | | Observer 8 | | Observer 9 | | Observer 10 | | Observer 11 | | Mean | Mean | Standard | MANOVA |
|---|---|---|---|---|---|---|---|---|---|---|---|---|---|
| Result | °V | Result | °V | Result | °V | Result | °V | Result | °V | Result | °V | Deviation | F Value |
| 175 | -0.57 | 176 | 0.00 | 175 | -0.57 | 176 | 0.00 | 176 | 0.00 | 176 | 0.21 | 0.633 | 851840.00 |
| 174 | 0.37 | 172 | 0.79 | 173 | -0.21 | 174 | 0.37 | 174 | 0.37 | 173 | 0.68 | 1.502 | 146639.07 |
| 110 | 12.35 | 92 | -6.04 | 107 | 9.29 | 93 | -5.01 | 99 | 1.11 | 98 | 7.5 | 8.927 | 1323.21 |
| 128 | 6.02 | 118 | -2.26 | 130 | 7.68 | 118 | -2.26 | 119 | -1.43 | 121 | 2.98 | 4.474 | 8009.01 |
| 115 | -8.86 | 126 | -0.14 | 102 | -19.10 | 109 | -13.60 | 137 | 8.57 | 126 | 8.06 | 12.545 | 1112.97 |
| 106 | -1.10 | 105 | -2.04 | 95 | -11.30 | 96 | -10.40 | 105 | -2.04 | 107 | 5.34 | 10.342 | 1181.41 |
| 109 | 3.01 | 106 | 0.17 | 102 | -3.61 | 88 | -16.80 | 108 | 2.06 | 106 | 3.72 | 6.258 | 3145.07 |
| 96 | 1.05 | 97 | 2.11 | 70 | -26.30 | 98 | 3.16 | 99 | 4.21 | 95 | 4.98 | 8.532 | 1363.67 |
| 105 | 15.62 | 84 | -7.51 | 92 | 1.30 | 88 | -3.10 | 99 | 9.01 | 91 | 5.95 | 6.750 | 1991.22 |
| 60 | 5.10 | 58 | 1.59 | 58 | 1.59 | 56 | -1.91 | 58 | 1.59 | 57 | 2.72 | 2.023 | 8764.09 |
| 45 | 15.12 | 31 | -20.70 | 43 | 10.00 | 22 | -43.72 | 40 | 2.33 | 39 | 11.71 | 6.730 | 371.14 |
| 32 | 4.76 | 28 | -8.33 | 30 | -1.79 | 31 | 1.49 | 32 | 4.76 | 31 | 3.73 | 1.369 | 5480.39 |
| 35 | 2.39 | 33 | -3.46 | 36 | 5.32 | 33 | -3.46 | 38 | 11.17 | 34 | 5.46 | 2.272 | 2489.01 |
| 96 | -3.03 | 99 | 0.00 | 97 | -2.02 | 99 | 0.00 | 104 | 5.05 | 99 | 2.57 | 3.286 | 9982.50 |
| 20 | 2.80 | 18 | -7.48 | | -7.48 | 21 | 7.94 | 21 | 7.94 | 19 | 6.29 | 1.369 | 2223.11 |
| 55 | 5.40 | 52 | -0.35 | 51 | -2.26 | 48 | -8.01 | 51 | -2.26 | 52 | 3.93 | 2.750 | 3960.05 |
| 94 | 10.35 | 84 | -1.39 | 87 | 2.13 | 78 | -8.43 | 100 | 17.40 | 85 | 7.49 | 7.821 | 1304.95 |
| 29 | 29.67 | 18 | -19.50 | 19 | -15.00 | 19 | -15.00 | 38 | 69.92 | 22 | 19.44 | 6.329 | 137.35 |
| 86 | -4.44 | 88 | -2.22 | 93 | 3.33 | 99 | 10.00 | 93 | 3.33 | 90 | 3.43 | 3.924 | 5735.71 |
| 24 | 17.86 | 19 | -6.70 | 20 | -1.79 | 25 | 22.77 | 25 | 22.77 | 20 | 12.99 | 3.233 | 436.31 |
| 86 | -0.32 | 84 | -2.63 | 83 | -3.79 | 88 | 2.00 | 87 | 0.84 | 86 | 3.08 | 3.319 | 7430.70 |
| 22 | 40.70 | 10 | -36.05 | 14 | -10.40 | 18 | 15.12 | 17 | 8.72 | 16 | 15.75 | 3.325 | 243.29 |
| 19 | 11.76 | 18 | 5.88 | 15 | -11.70 | 22 | 29.41 | 18 | 5.88 | 17 | 12.83 | 3.066 | 338.19 |
| 101 | -1.51 | 98 | -4.43 | 115 | 12.15 | 100 | -2.48 | 102 | -0.53 | 103 | 3.43 | 4.947 | 4726.54 |
| 19 | -18.00 | 23 | -0.78 | 27 | 16.47 | 23 | -0.78 | 24 | 3.53 | 23 | 6.99 | 2.183 | 1240.94 |
| 112 | 3.79 | 120 | 11.20 | 98 | -9.18 | 104 | -3.62 | 106 | -1.77 | 108 | 4.93 | 7.007 | 2609.20 |
| 19 | -4.13 | 22 | 11.01 | 21 | 5.96 | 18 | -9.17 | 20 | 0.92 | 20 | 10.01 | 2.442 | 724.45 |
| 101 | 7.14 | 97 | 2.89 | 69 | -26.80 | 102 | 8.20 | 98 | 3.95 | 94 | 6.47 | 9.339 | 1120.88 |
| 28 | -1.28 | 32 | 12.82 | 14 | -50.64 | 30 | 5.77 | 34 | 19.87 | 28 | 16.32 | 6.439 | 213.47 |
| | 8.23 | | 6.22 | | 9.64 | | 8.76 | | 7.7 | | | | |
| | 40.70 | | 36.05 | | 50.54 | | 43.72 | | 69.9 | | | | |

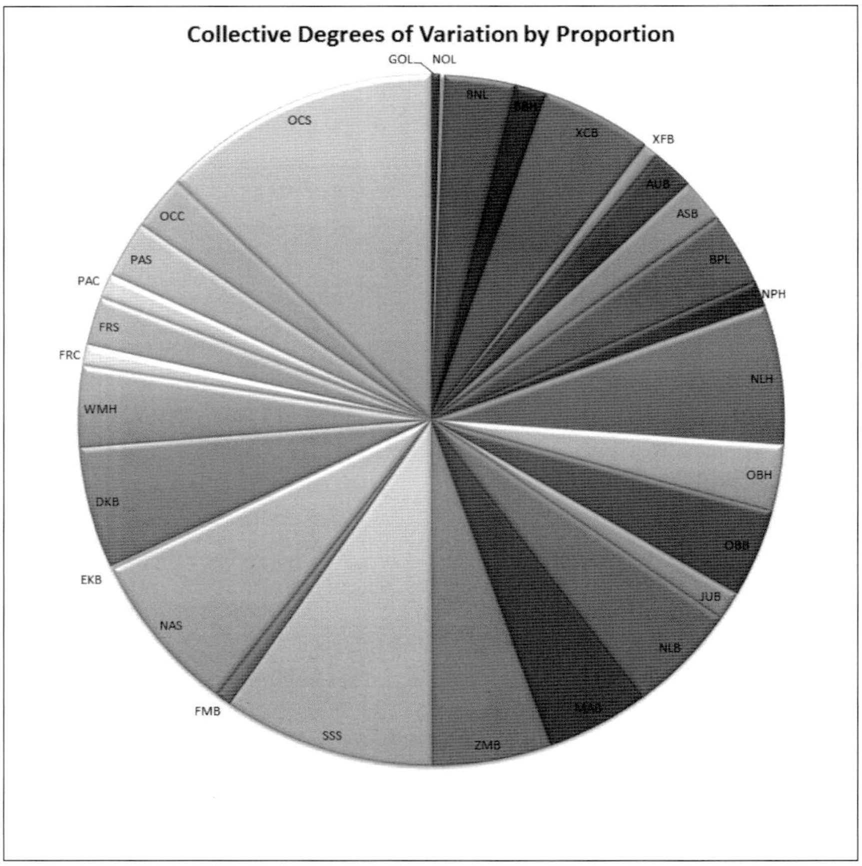


**Figure 2**: The collective Degrees of Variation for each measurement represented as a proportion of the total variation found in the study, indicating the differences in proportional variation between measurements.

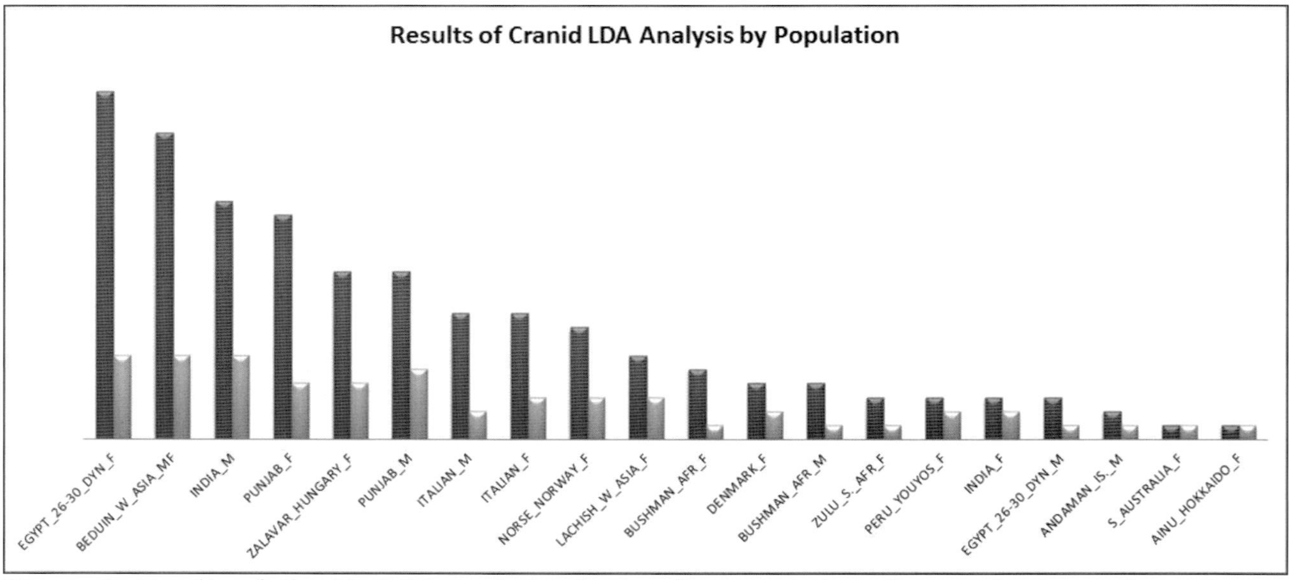


**Figure 3**: Results of CranID LDA analysis, the top five populations from each observer's results are displayed; the dark bar representing the weighted results by position within the top five, the lighter bar representing the number of times it appeared within all the observer's results.

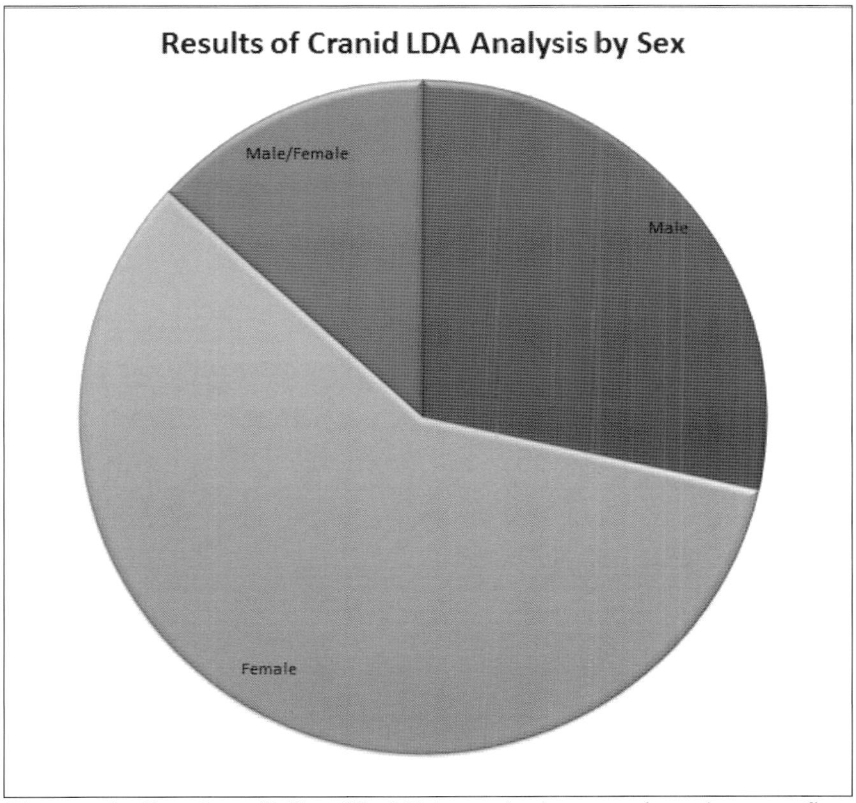


**Figure 4**: Results of CranID LDA analysis grouping the top five results for each observer by sex, demonstrating a clear inference of the specimen being female in the results.

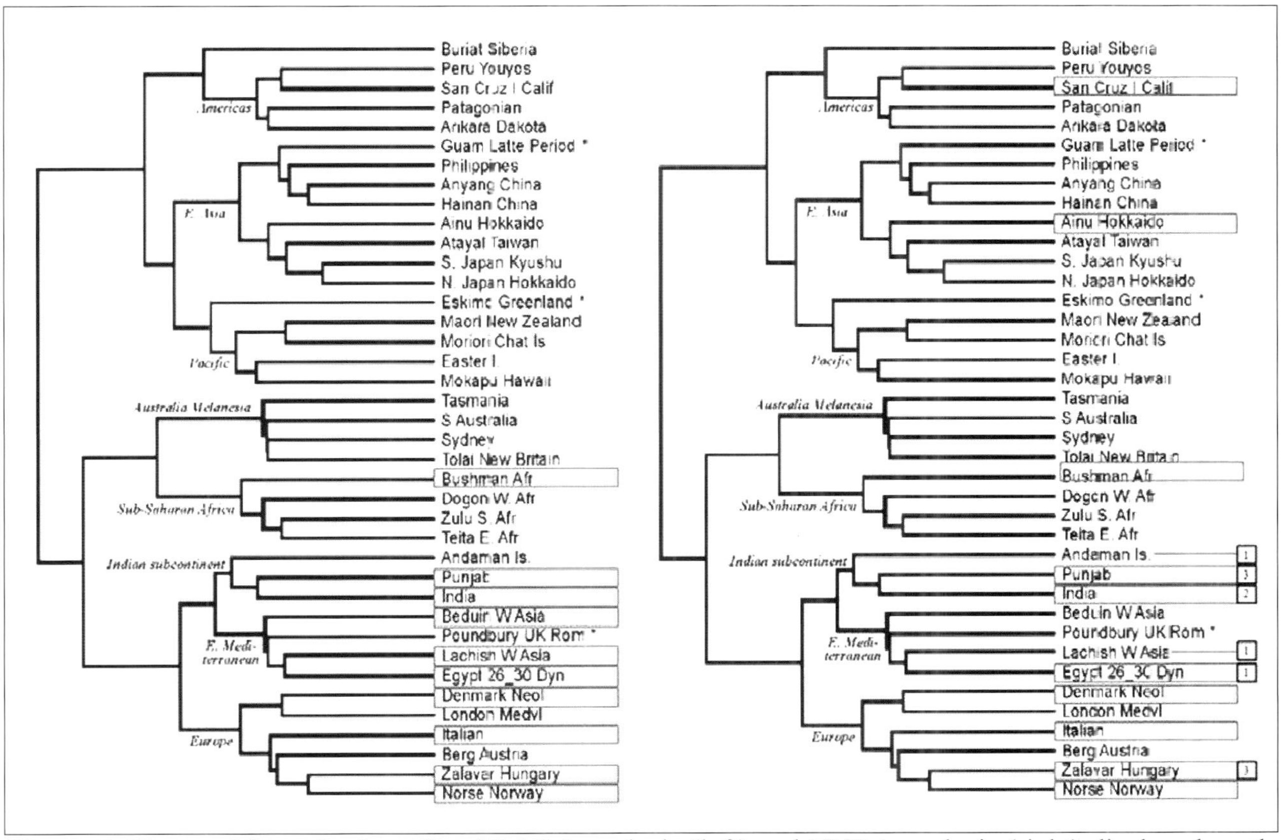

**Figure 5**: The top 10 results from CranID LDA analysis (left) and NNDA analysis (right) displayed on the CranID dendrogram of population relatedness, actual Nearest Neighbour results are also noted on the right (Dendrogram © R.Wright 2009).

such a high degree of variation as seen in this study, is a proposal that should be re-considered. The problem of any metric analysis lies with the reliability of the individual observer, the variation found between observers in this study is in accordance to that observed in previous studies (Heathcote 1981, Utermohle & Zegura 1982, Utermohle *et al.* 1983, Palmeirim 1998), although the level of variation detected is considerably higher. Whether this is down to higher expertise of observers in other studies, or whether it is simply that this study utilised more observers than previous is unclear.

MANOVA analysis showed significant levels of variation in 28 of the 29 measurements required for CranID. Closer inspection of individual results showed worryingly high degrees of variation for 10 of 11 observers. Although Degrees of Variation do not account for accuracy they do highlight a lack of congruence between observers, indicating that at most only one observer may have a high degree of accuracy. Given their experience it would be expected that either Observer-1 or Observer-11 would prove the most accurate, however given the variation found between these two it is impossible to define any level of accuracy within the group without further testing. Further studies would be advised to form a measure of accuracy for comparison, however it is not clear how best to decide on a set of definitive results.

The results of CranID analysis were less disheartening than the results of interobserver variation. Whilst there was still a range to the ancestry results given it was not as wide a range as may have been expected given the levels of variation detected, inspection of collective CranID results through the weighted analysis shows a relatedness of results according to the CranID populations dendrogram.

The science supporting ancestry determination through craniometric measurement is sound, however we must allow for our own fallibility and that of others. There are undoubtedly irreconcilable causes of interobserver variation; however it is the recognition and analysis of this that is important. Making allowances in our planning, and taking measurement of variation in our experiments will aid in increasing the reliability of our findings and validate our science.

**Acknowledgements**

Thanks to Richard Wright for his assistance throughout and his permission to use diagrams from the CranID manual, to Martin Smith for his supervision, and to Lisa always.

**Literature Cited**

Barker, C., Cox, M., Flavel, A., Laver, J. and Loe, C. 2007. Mortuary procedures II - skeletal analysis I: basic procedure and demographic assessment. *In:* Cox, M., Flavel, A., Hanson, I., Laver, J. and Wessline, R. (eds.) *The scientific investigation of mass graves.* Cambridge University Press: Cambridge.

Cox, M. 1998. *Grave concerns: death and burial in England 1700-1850.* Council for British Archaeology: York.

Field, A. 2009. *Discovering statistics using SPSS (and sex and drugs and rock 'n' roll)* 3rd ed. SAGE Publications: London.

Giles, E. and Elliot, O. 1962. Race identification from cranial measurements. *Journal of Forensic Sciences* 7: 147-157.

Heathcote, G.M. 1981. The magnitude and consequences of measurement error in human craniometry. *Canadian Review of Physical Anthropology* 3: 18-40.

Howells, W.W. 1969. The use of multivariate techniques in the study of skeletal populations. *American Journal of Physical Anthropology* 31 (3): 311-314.

Howells, W.W, 1973. Cranial variation in man: a study by multivariate analysis of patterns of difference among recent human populations. In: *Papers of the Peabody Museum of Archaeology and Ethnology, Vol. 67.* Harvard University Press: Cambridge.

Howells, W.W. 1989. Skull shapes and the map: craniometric analyses in the dispersion of modern Homo. In: *Peabody Museum of Archaeology and Ethnology, Vol. 79.* Harvard University Press: Cambridge.

Ousley, S.D. and Jantz, R.L. 1996. *Fordisc 2.0: personal computer forensic discriminant functions.* The University of Tennessee: Knoxville.

Palmeirim, J.M. 1998. Analysis of skull measurements and measurers: can we use data obtained by various observers? *Journal of Mammology* 79 (3): 1021-1028.

Utermohle, C.J. and Zegura, S.L. 1982. Intra- and interobserver error in craniometry: a cautionary tale. *American Journal of Physical Anthropology* 57: 303-310.

Utermohle, C.J., Zegura, S.L. and Heathcote, G.M. 1983. Multiple observers, humidity, and choice of precision statistics: factors influencing craniometric data quality. *American Journal of Physical Anthropology* 61: 85-95.

Wright, R.V.S. 1992. Correlation between cranial form and geography in *Homo sapiens*: CRANID – a computer program for forensic and other applications. *Archaeology Oceania* 27: 105-112.

Wright, R.V.S. 2009. *Guide to using the CRANID programs CR6aInd: for linear and nearest neighbours discriminant analysis*. Available from: http://www.box.net/shared/static/n9q0zgt-1y.EXE. Accessed 30 October 2009.

# Early Bronze Age *Busta* in Cambridgeshire? On-Site Experiments to Investigate the Effects of Fires and Pyres on Pits.

Natasha Dodwell

Cambridge Archaeological Unit
Department of Archaeology
University of Cambridge
Downing Street
Cambridge CB2 3DZ, UK

Email for correspondence: nd207@cam.ac.uk

**Abstract**

Small scorched Bronze Age pits, containing cremated human bone and pyre debris are a phenomenon which has been encountered on archaeological sites in Cambridgeshire. There appears to be no satisfactory explanation for them in the literature. They seem too small to be true *bustum* style burials, a type of burial practiced in the Roman period where the pyre site (often built over a pit) is also the final place of burial. In addition, their stratigraphy is not always compatible with a *bustum*, which usually has charred wood at the base of the pit overlain by cremated bone. By constructing experimental pyres/bonfires above a pit, in the manner of a *bustum,* and within a pit, and recording the temperatures reached and the pattern and degree of scorching, the interpretation of these cremation features can be based on objective criteria.

Two small pits were dug through silty subsoil and gravels. In each pit, thermocouple probes were positioned at the base of the cut, half way up and at the top of the feature. A 'pyre' of native wood species was constructed *over* the first pit and *within* the second pit. Both were lit and temperatures recorded at regular intervals. Later they were excavated and recorded as though they were archaeological features.

The maximum temperature recorded in the fire of the *bustum* style pit was almost 1000 $^0$C , more than 300$^0$C higher than that in the bonfire in the pit. The sides of both pits showed evidence of scorching, although the *bustum* style pit was more evenly and heavily scorched particularly at the surface. Far less charcoal and charred timber was recovered from the *bustum* style pit than the bonfire pit. The experiment established that the scorched sides of the Bronze Age cremation features are most likely the result of a pyre being constructed over a pit.

**Keywords:** *Bustum*, Early Bronze Age, Experiment, Cremation, Burial

## Contextualising the Experiment

In the last ten years or so, archaeologists working in the commercial sector in Cambridgeshire have been encountering a type of burial feature which has provoked much discussion. The features, which date to the early Bronze Age (*c.* 1800-1500 BC) are small pits with bright, salmon-pink sides, suggestive of *in situ* burning and containing cremated human bone and pyre debris (Fig. 1).

The majority of these features have been associated with barrows or ring ditches *e.g.* at the Cambridgeshire sites of Butcher's Rise, Barleycroft (Dodwell 1998), Diddington (Evans 1995), Haddenham (Evans and Hodder 2006), Over Quarry (Dodwell 2010 and in prep.) and Brigg's Farm, Thorney (Pickstone and Mortimer 2011). Two seemingly isolated pits with heavily scorched sides and containing cremated bone were also recorded at Bradley Fen, Whittlesey near Peterborough (Gibson and Knight 2006).

The pits are oval or sub-circular in plan and range in size from *c.* 0.35 x 0.50m to *c.* 0.90 x 1.00m, with the majority *c.* 0.45 x 0.75m (Table 1). Most

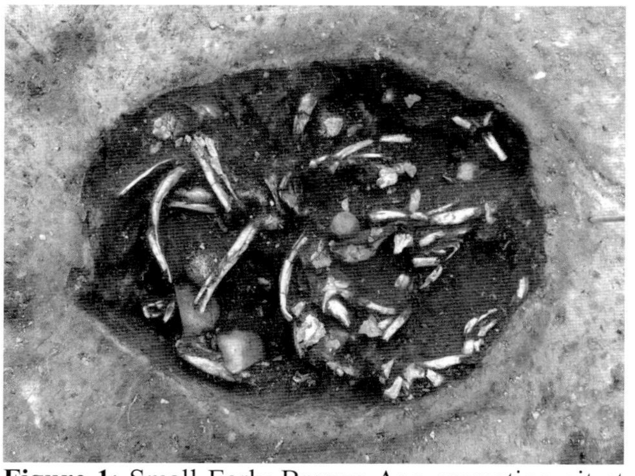

**Figure 1**: Small Early Bronze Age cremation pit at Bradley Fen with evidence of *in situ* burning

appear to be untruncated, with little or no bone lost, and survive to depths between 0.18-0.83m, with the majority around 0.35m deep. The edges of all of the pits have a bright red or salmon-pink colour which extends to 0.01-0.08m beyond the cut into the natural silts and gravels. The stratigraphy within the pit can vary between features but has the following basic organisation; the basal fill is usually a layer of charcoal-rich silt and ash, with lots of burnt wood fragments, sometimes with fragments of orange/red burnt soil and burnt flint, which ranges in thickness from just 0.01 to 0.25m. More rarely, the basal fill is just charcoal-stained and contains very few fragments of charred wood. Above this basal fill is the cremated bone which is usually mixed with charcoal-rich silts. In most instances the cremated bone is spread evenly across the pit but in some cases it appears to form a concentration. In some instances evidence of articulated skeletal elements has been observed during excavation. At Haddenham, for example, several articulated vertebrae were recognised (Evans and Hodder 2006: 27), at Butcher's Rise, Barleycroft, a tibia and fibula were recorded as being articulated (Dodwell 1998: 58) and at Over a calcaneus and talus were fused with iron pan in anatomically correct position (Dodwell 2010 and in prep.). Indeed, slow, meticulous excavation of these features at Butchers Rise (ibid), Over (Dodwell 2010 and in prep.) and Brigg's Farm (Pickstone and Mortimer 2011), where individual elements or small groups of bones have been planned, labelled and lifted, has shown at the analysis phase that in many instances there is a pattern to the position of the elements beyond the articulation recorded on site. When skeletal elements are plotted the cremation can appear as a fragmented, tightly crouched inhumation.

**Table 1**: Dimensions of pits with evidence of *in situ* burning and weight of cremated bone

| Site name | Feature No. | Depth (m) | Diameter (m) | Age | Bone weight |
|---|---|---|---|---|---|
| Butchers Rise, Barleycroft | F.691 | 0.25 | 0.25 x 0.80 | A | 1661g |
| | F.718 | 0.23 | 0.37 x 0.50 | A | 1026g |
| Bradley Fen | F.1279 | 0.18 | 0.41 x 0.54 | A | 1242g |
| | F.1024 | 0.38 | 0.40 x 0.52 | I/A | 547g |
| Diddington | F.503* | 0.55 | 0.70 x 0.70 | A | 756g |
| Snow Farm, Haddenham | F.76 | 0.62 | 0.90 x 1.06 | A | 1889g |
| Over (2000 training excavation) | F.519 | 0.83 | 0.90 x 0.90 | A + I | 2332g |
| Over Godwin Ridge (2008) | F.392 | 0.21 | 0.78 x 0.65 | A | 1429g |
| Over Barrows (2008) | F.1007 | 0.50 | 0.78 x 0.80 | I | 221g |
| | F.1034 | 0.28 | 0.80 x 0.60 | A + I | 1876g |
| | F.1037 | 0.48 | 0.62 x 0.80 | I | 134g |
| | F.1053 | 0.51 | 0.62 x 1.04 | A | 1902g |
| | F.1084 | 0.35 | 0.41 x 0.54 | A | 1588g |
| | F.1087 | 0.32 | 0.46 x 0.64 | A | 1946g |
| | F.1098 | 0.32 | 0.56 x 0.81 | A | 1986g |
| | F.1099 | 0.35 | 0.31 x 0.45 | I | 7g |
| Over (2010) | F.2011 | 0.31 | 0.38 x 0.52 | A | 1835g |
| Brigg's Farm, Thorney | F.2067 | 0.46 | 0.71 x 0.70 | A + I | 2647g |
| | F.2710 | 0.48 | 0.88 x 0.88 | A | 1712g |

Abbreviations: A = adult, I = immature, I/A = older subadult/young adult, * = truncated/disturbed (*i.e.* all of the bone originally deposited is unlikely to be present).
With the exception of the published sites at Diddington and Haddenham, the weights of the cremated bone are those calculated in the assessment phase of the osteological analysis and may alter slightly upon publication.

The weight of cremated bone collected from undisturbed scorched pits that contain one adult ranges from 1026-1986g (Table 1) and this is consistent with what one would expect from an adult cremation; McKinley's observations at modern crematoria found that the weight range of bone expected from an adult cremation lies between 1000 and 2400g with an average of *c.* 1650g (McKinley 1993). The bone in several of these features is sometimes poorly fired and there is often evidence of differential oxidisation; the patella, distal femur and femur shaft are the elements most frequently being black/blue in colour. Several of the pits have had, within and above their upper fills, large charred planks or logs, sometimes running parallel to each other and to the sides of the pit.

Both pyre goods and grave goods have been recovered from these scorched cremation pits. Burnt bone pins and pointed implements, flint knives and barbed and tanged arrow heads, animal bone and collared urns are amongst the objects that would have been placed on the pyre either adorning the body or accompanying it. These finds are similar to those found with other types of cremation deposits i.e. urned and unurned burials. Fragments of animal bone, a bone belt hook and a small fragment of open weave textile (preserved as a result of a waterlogged burial environment) are the unfired artefacts that have been recovered from the scorched cremation pits. None of them appeared to have been deliberately or carefully placed within the deposit. Whether they were added to the deposit once the pyre had burnt out or had simply escaped incineration by where they were positioned on the pyre is unclear.

**Potential Interpretations**

The process of cremation, the nature of cremated bone and examples of historical and ethnographic pyre cremation have been described in detail elsewhere (e.g. McKinley 1994a: 72-81).

Several interpretations have been proffered as to what these scorched pits represent and these will be discussed in turn. Could the scorched edges of these early Bronze Age cremation pits (and the semi-articulated nature of the cremated bone) be the result of:

*Placing Hot Pyre Debris and Cremated Bone into the Open Pit*

The suggestion that the scorching is a result simply of placing a hot deposit of cremated bone and pyre debris into a pit seems unlikely. Previous experiments, placing hot deposits, with temperatures ranging from 500-900 °C, have been found not to have altered the appearance of the soil (McKinley 1997: 65 and *pers. comm.*, Marshall 2011:36).

*A Body Cremated within the Pit*

Some authors have suggested that the body was cremated *in* the pit (e.g. Gibson 2004: 188, Evans and Hodder 2006: 27). However, most of the scorched pits are far too small to place a body into, even a tightly bound one, and still leave room for pyre material. Both fires and bodies need oxygen to burn and, although it could be argued that a body could fit into some of the larger scorched pits, such as the pit at Snow's Farm barrow, Haddenham 0.90 x 1.06 x 0.62m deep) or the primary cremation burial beneath one of the Over barrows (0.90 x 0.90 x 0.83m deep), there would be a very limited supply of oxygen within the pit. In addition, any covering of the body with fuel would reduce the supply of oxygen still further resulting in highly inefficient cremation. The majority of the cremated bone recovered from the scorched pit at Haddenham is indeed described as a colour 'approaching that of unburnt bone' (Lee 2006: 29), and bone from one of the Over cremations had far more blue/black and charred fragments than others associated, perhaps suggesting less efficient cremation (Dodwell in prep.). However, whilst the bone might not show full oxidation, the transformation of the cut sides to a bright salmon pink does suggest oxidising conditions.

*Dismembered Body Parts being Placed into a Fire*

Where scorched pits containing cremated bone have been smaller, it has been suggested that some degree of dismemberment could have occurred with bones being dropped into a fire set within the pit (Evans 1996: 21, Gibson 2004: 188). By its very nature cremated bone is fragmentary and exhibits splits, fissures and cracks, but no evidence of butchery or de-fleshing cut marks has been observed by the author during the analysis of some 10 or so of these smaller cremation burials. McKinley (1994b) has successfully demonstrated that there are many factors which result in cremated bone fragmenting, none of which involve deliberate breakage of the bone prior to burial. Analysis of the cremated bone from the barrows at Over (Dodwell 2010 and in prep.) and the ring ditch at Butcher's Rise, Barleycroft (Dodwell 1998) have shown that the bone fragment size is in fact slightly larger in the burials within scorched pits than in other unurned cremation burials on those sites.

*A Fire having been Lit within the Pit to 'Seal' the Edges, the Cremation Taking Place Elsewhere*

It is also possible that the cremation took place elsewhere and that the reddened sides are the result of fires being lit within the pits to 'seal' the edges. The reddened upper profiles of the pits are often hard and almost ceramic-like, as though the fire has deliberately transformed the cut itself into a 'ceramic vessel' prior to the cremated bone and pyre debris being deposited within it. This is argued to be the case in several examples of burnt funerary pits at the Roman cemetery of Matrica in Hungary, where it is postulated that fires were lit in pits to seal or purify them (Topál 1981: 75-77). In these cases the pits have been cleaned out and cremated bone deposited with unfired grave goods. Similarly heavily scorched pits, with unfired grave goods and cremated human bone contained within vessels or concentrated in small piles (possibly originally contained within an organic container such as a bag), were excavated in 1990 at the Roman cemetery at Porta Palaeo, Verona, Italy (*pers. obs.*). In the early Bronze Age examples from Cambridgeshire, however, there is no evidence for the fills of the burnt pit having being cleaned out, or of the cremated bone having been interred as a secondary rite.

*A Body Placed on Top of a Pyre Set over the Pit*

Another possible explanation is that the reddened edges of the pits result from pyres being constructed above the pits in a manner similar to the Roman *busta* or more specifically the *Grubenbusta* described by Struck (1993: 92-3). Definitions of *busta* vary slightly but they are essentially pyre sites which also function as the place of burial. Struck (ibid) describes two different types; *Flächenbustum* where the cremation takes place on the ground surface (and is only found beneath barrows) and *Grubenbustum* where the cremation takes place above a pit. In the latter, the body would be placed on top of a pyre which was itself built over a relatively deep pit. The upper margins of the pit are burnt *in situ* and reddened by oxidation and both the pyre and the cremated body collapse into the pit. With no further movement or manipulation one would expect to find considerable quantities of fuel ash in the lower levels of the pit as well as large fragments of charred logs, since the finer fuel ash would not blow away and the oxygen supply would be insufficient for complete combustion (McKinley 2000a: 40). Presuming that the body was placed on top of the pyre, as most sources suggest (McKinley 1994a: 81), the cremated bones should lie above the thick deposit of charred wood and fuel ash.

As mentioned above, the thickness of the basal charcoal-rich deposits in the early Bronze Age pits varies considerably and many of the features have large, charred planks or logs in their *upper* fills, or covering the top of the cut, rather than at their base. *Grubenbusta* appear to be confined to the Roman period, at least in Britain (McKinley 2000a: 39; Struck 1993: 91) and even then are relatively uncommon.

In order that these burnt funerary features could be interpreted objectively, rather than through untested assumptions, a simple experiment was conducted focusing on how the architecture of a pyre/bonfire, specifically a pyre lit *over* a pit and a fire lit *in* a pit, affected the temperatures that could be obtained, altered the colour of the cut edges and affected the quantity of fuel ash that was produced and that was preserved within the pit. The number of variables was deliberately kept to a minimum and this experiment is seen as the first of a series.

## The Experiment

*Background*

The experiment was conducted in May 2010 to the northwest of Cambridge at Hanson's Needingworth Quarry, close to the village of Over, Cambridgeshire. The area chosen for the experiment was adjacent to the site of a group of 5 Bronze Age barrows, where 8 of these small, scorched pits were excavated by the Cambridge Archaeological Unit in 2008 (Dodwell 2010 and in prep.). A sixth barrow was excavated close by in 2010 and a further small scorched pit containing cremated bone was identified (Dodwell in prep.). The geology at the experiment site, calcareous silts and gravels, was identical to that where the early Bronze Age scorched pits had been identified.

*Methodology*

The topsoil over an area measuring $10m^2$ was stripped by mechanical excavator. Two small (0.75 x 0.50 x 0.35m), vertically sided, rectangular pits with flat bases were then hand dug through the silty subsoil into natural gravels. Three thermocouple probes were positioned on the edge of each of the cuts to measure the temperature within the pits at regular intervals; at the surface of the cut, halfway up the cut and at its base. In the first pit (Pit A) a criss-cross frame work of wood, measuring *c.* 1.20m in length, was constructed *over* the cut. In the second pit (Pit B) a wigwam structure of short, thick sticks and poles was constructed *within* the cut with larger logs measuring *c.* 0.7m placed around the wigwam. In both pyres/fires, straight logs and poles of native wood species (oak, birch, ash and hazel) with diameters ranging from 0.01-0.15m were used for the main structures. Small brushwood and handfuls of couch and goose grass in-filled the main frameworks and bark chips were used as kindling. Because of the architectural differences in the pyre/bonfire structures, the volume of wood used in each framework was different; above Pit A *c.* 0.4m$^3$ of wood was used, with just *c.* 0.1m$^3$ in Pit B. It is acknowledged that the differences in the quantities of wood used in and over the pits will have affected the temperatures that the fires reached, and the lengths of time that they would have burnt for. No additional fuel was added once the fires had been lit and neither was tended in any way.

## Results

### *Combustion Temperatures*

Both of the fires/pyres burnt very quickly with maximum temperatures being reached between 20 and 30 minutes after ignition.

In pit A, where the timber framework was constructed *above* the pit, the maximum temperature recorded was 942°C, reached after nearly 30 minutes (Fig. 2a). This was almost 300°C higher than the maximum temperature recorded in Pit B, where 648°C was reached after just over 20 minutes (Fig. 2b). This difference will be due both to the draft effect of the pit below the pyre and the difference in the quantity of wood that could be burnt in each pyre.

In Pit A, the highest temperature was recorded at the top of the cut with the maximum temperature at the base of the cut reaching only 308°C, one third of the temperature reached just 0.3m higher. This is in marked contrast to Pit B where the temperature at the pit base increased, reaching a maximum of 445°C after almost 45 minutes, some 70% of the highest temperature reached at the upper level. The basal temperature dropped slightly but hovered between 320-400°C until the recording finished (after *c.* 1.5 hours).

### *Effects on Pyre Architecture*

In Pit A the timber framework began to collapse into the pit 1 hour and 10 minutes after it was set alight, although burning brushwood and grasses that had slipped through the structure were alight at the base of the pit after about 25 minutes.

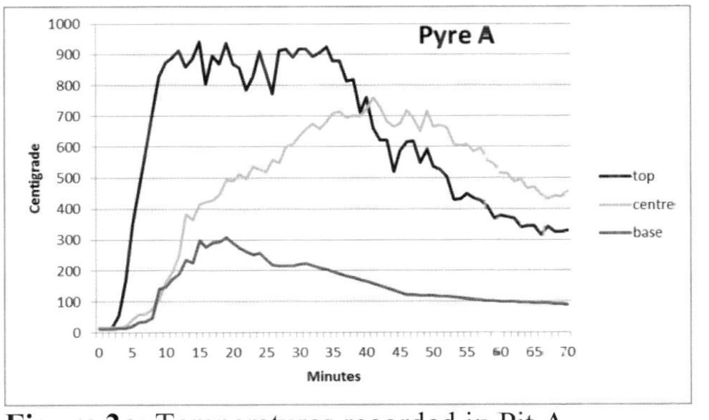


**Figure 2a**: Temperatures recorded in Pit A

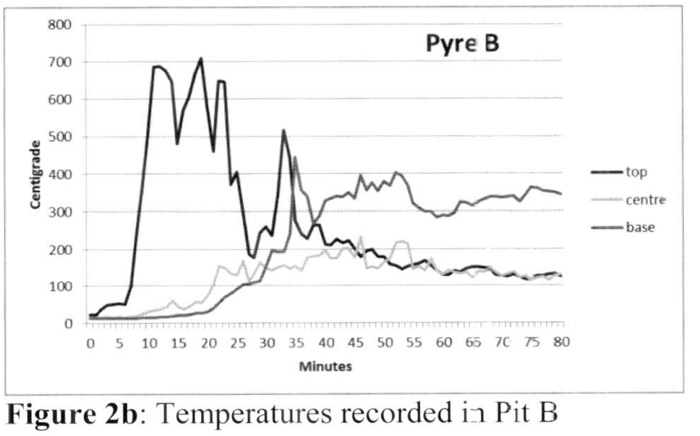


**Figure 2b**: Temperatures recorded in Pit B

### *Recording the Features*

The following day, the pits and their fills were recorded as though they were archaeological features, with plan and section drawings being made during and after excavation.

Both pits had a layer of charcoal fragments mixed with fine, pale grey wood ash covering their base; this was much deeper in Pit A (0.09m at the pit centre to a maximum of 0.21m in one of the corners) than in Pit B (0.02-0.06m) but this may simply reflect the different quantities of wood burnt in each pyre (Figs. 3 and 4).

There was a very clear outline of where the pyre had lain around pit A; on the surface there were patches of wood ash over areas of red (oxidized) and black (reduced) subsoil up to 0.17-0.37m beyond the edge of the cut (Fig. 5). Beyond these were the very ends of charred and unburnt logs. Once these had been removed, a distinct margin of deep salmon-pink/red oxidised soil was recorded in plan around the top of the pit, extending *c.* 40-70mm back from the cut edge.

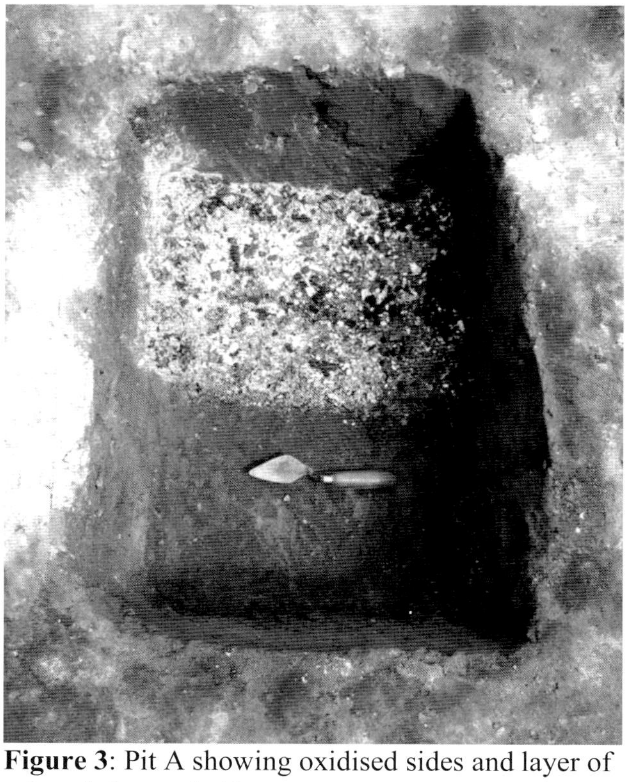

**Figure 3**: Pit A showing oxidised sides and layer of ash and charcoal at base.

The sides of Pit A were also scorched a deep salmon-pink except for the lower 5-10mm, which lay below the level of the wood ash. This scorched, oxidised soil was uniform around the cut edges. The sides of Pit B were sooted black and when this was troweled away there were only small patches of scorched pink/red natural on the cut sides and these were towards the base and middle of the cut sides where hot temperatures had been prolonged and more constant.

*Sampling Methodology*

The wood ash that had accumulated at the base of the pits was 100% sampled with subdivision between the western and eastern halves. The samples were processed by hand using bucket flotation, with flots collected in 300µm sieves and residues in 1mm sieves. All fractions were dried prior to analysis.

*Analysis and Interpretation of Results*

A correspondingly greater volume of charcoal was recovered from Pit A than Pit B (Table 2).

When adjusted to a percentage of the original wood fuel (Fig. 6), Pit A contained charcoal equivalent to 1.7% of the original wood volume, whilst Pit B contained charcoal equivalent to 3.3% of the original wood volume.

This suggests that the combustion in Pit A was more efficient, with a greater proportion of the wood converted to carbon dioxide and silica ash. Approximately 90% of the charcoal recovered from each of the pits was >4mm in size, but the difference in the temperatures reached and degrees of combustion means that there is a greater quantity of large charcoal fragments in Pit B.

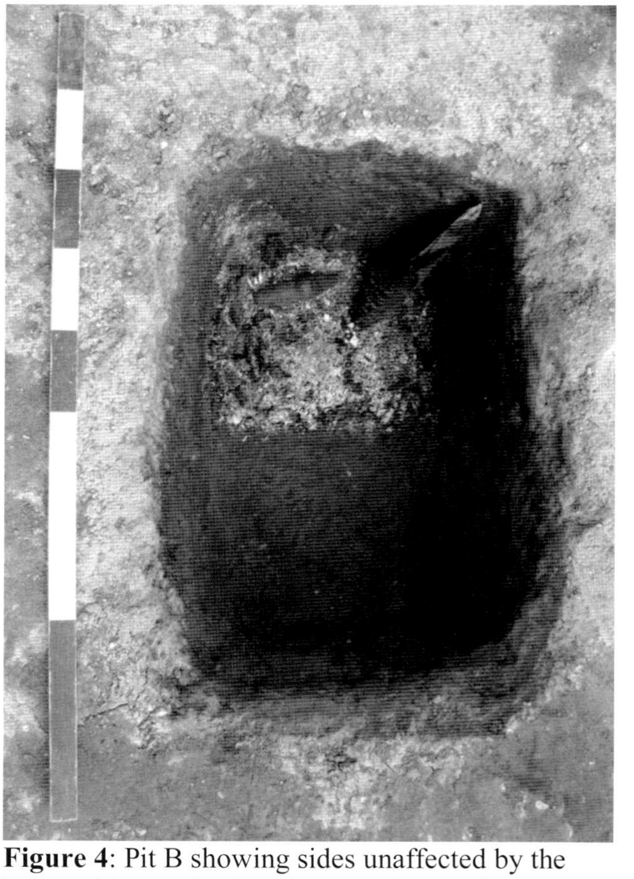

**Figure 4**: Pit B showing sides unaffected by the heat and layer of ash and charcoal at the base.

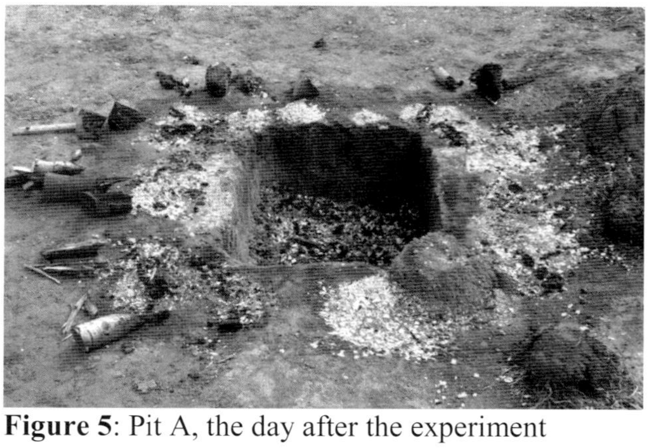

**Figure 5**: Pit A, the day after the experiment

**Table 2**: Composition of the bulk ash samples

| Pit | A | | | B | | |
|---|---|---|---|---|---|---|
| **Context** | **West half** | **East half** | **Overall** | **West half** | **East half** | **Overall** |
| Wood fuel used/litres | 150 | 150 | 300 | 30 | 30 | 60 |
| Unprocessed ash volume/litres | 2.2 | 4 | 6.2 | 1.5 | 2 | 3.5 |
| >4mm charcoal/litres | 2 | 2.5 | 4.5 | 0.6 | 1.2 | 1.8 |
| 1-4mm charcoal/litres | 0.15 | 0.05 | 0.2 | 0.1 | 0.02 | 0.12 |
| 0.3-1mm charcoal/litres | 0.2 | 0.1 | 0.2 | 0.04 | 0.01 | 0.05 |
| Gravel>1mm | 0.3 | 0.3 | 0.6 | 0.25 | 0.25 | 0.05 |

Traits in the gravel recovered from the heavy residues further suggest oxidising conditions predominated in Pit A, where *c.* 30% of the gravel is found as heat-whitened flint fragments. In contrast, reducing conditions appear to have predominated in Pit B, where blackened earth and gravel fragments form *c.* 10% of the heavy residue.

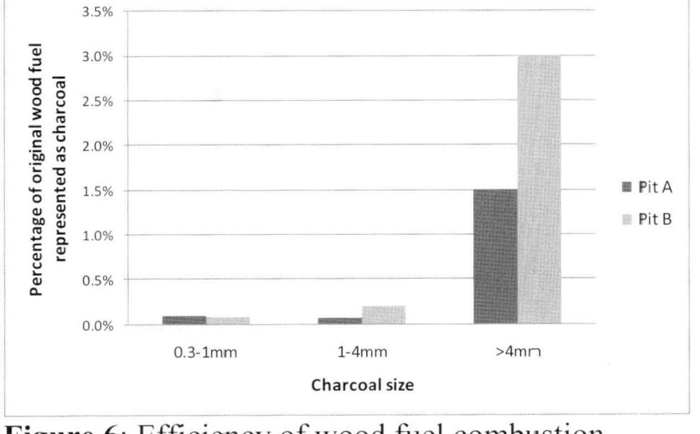


**Figure 6**: Efficiency of wood fuel combustion within the pits.

Two important caveats are, firstly, that different volumes of wood were used in the two fires and this will have affected the size and intensity of the resultant pyres. Secondly, a percentage of the fuel for Pit A fell to the ground surface around the pit edges and was not collected as ash from the pit. The latter is thought unlikely to have contributed greatly to the different combustion efficiencies for Pits A and B since the surface ash was almost entirely smoke-borne silica ash and unburnt fuel that had fallen from the pyre.

### Discussion and Future Work

This simple experiment demonstrates that the scorched edges observed in the small, early Bronze Age cremation features in Cambridgeshire are *not* the result of fires within pits but of fires built *over* pits. In the former, the size of the pits means that only a small quantity of fuel can be used and that the circulation of oxygen within the feature is insufficient to allow temperatures sufficient to oxidise the edges of the cut.

Prior to this experiment it was thought that the small size of the pits and the nature of their fills suggested that they could not be *bustum* style burials; Roman *bustum* burials are relatively large with pits ranging in size from *c.* 1.10-1.75m by 0.60-0.70m, and 0.50-0.70m deep (McKinley 2000b: 62) and have a thick layer of fuel ash and charred timbers at their base overlain by the cremated bones (McKinley 2000a: 40). Early Bronze Age inhumations were generally tightly crouched and it appears that cremation burials were similarly arranged, thus requiring both a smaller pyre and a smaller pit than those seen in the Roman period. Here, relatively little wood ash or charcoal accumulated at the base of the pit with the pyre constructed over it, and there were no large fragments of charred wood at the base of the cut, both in contrast to Roman *Busta.* It is possible that the charred timbers which remained beyond the edge of the pit at the end of the cremation were incorporated into the feature; in several of the cremation features with scorched edges at Over and Thorney large pieces of charred timber were recorded in the upper fills or on the surface of the features (Dodwell 2010 and in prep., Pickstone and Mortimer 2011).

McKinley's experimental pyre work has demonstrated not only the shallow depth to which the effects of a pyre penetrate (*c.* 0.1m) but also how the corpses (in her experiments, sheep) maintain their position in relation to the rest of the pyre throughout the cremation process; the cremated bones remaining in roughly the correct anatomical position on a bed of wood ash (1997: 65-8 and fig. 46). Her experiment in 1999 reconstructing a Roman *bustum* cremation (McKinley 2000a: 40) again demonstrated how the cremated bones were recovered from above and within the upper layers of fuel ash in roughly the correct anatomical order.

This experiment has shown that the early Bronze Age scorched cremation pits identified in Cambridgeshire were almost certainly the result of a cremation process that involved the construction of a pyre above the burial pit. Furthermore, the spatial distribution of the skeletal elements, and the degree of articulation recorded, suggests that the body was placed on the pyre in a tightly crouched position directly over the pit.

The majority of the archaeological data referenced in this paper is to date unpublished, being part of the ever expanding collection of information accumulated as 'grey literature'. It is thus in large part based upon personal knowledge of the archaeology of the Eastern Region. It is hoped that the publication of this experiment will not only better our understanding of the processes involved in this funerary tradition but that it will lead to further discussion as to whether this is a distinctly regional or more widespread early Bronze Age funerary practice.

**Acknowledgements**

I would like to thank the BABAO committee (2009) for awarding me the small research project grant which enabled me to conduct this experiment. Rachel Ballantyne and Simon Timberlake helped with the experiment. Both of them worked on site and Simon's technical knowledge and input was invaluable; Rachel also processed and analysed the environmental samples. I would also like to thank Chris Evans, director of the CAU for helping me to facilitate the experiment on site and for allowing me to use unpublished data. Chris Gregory at West Stow and Peter Hobbs and Lee Pearce at Hinchingbrooke Country Park helped to source the timber for the pyres. Finally I would like to thank Richard Mortimer of OA East and my colleagues at the CAU for all the useful discussions over the years on the subject of pits and pyres.

## Literature Cited

Dodwell, N. 1998. Human Bone Assessment Report. In: Evans, C. and Knight, M. (eds.) *Butcher's Rise ring ditches, Barleycroft.* Unpublished Cambridge Archaeological Unit report no. 283.

Dodwell, N. 2010. Human bone assessment report. In: Evans, C. and Tabor, J. (eds.) *The Over Narrows (Pt IV;2008): archaeological investigations in Hanson's Needingworth Quarry. The Low Grounds barrows.* Unpublished Cambridge Archaeological Unit report no. 940.

Dodwell, N. in prep. Report on the human bone. In: Evans, C. with Tabor, J. and Vander Lindon, M. (eds.) *Twice-crossed River: prehistoric and palaeoenvironmental investigations at Barleycroft Farm/Over, Cambridgeshire.* The Archaeology of the Lower Ouse Valley, Volume III. McDonald Institute Monograph: Cambridge.

Evans, C. 1996. The excavation of a ring-ditch complex at Diddington, near Huntingdon, with a discussion of second-millennium BC pyre burial and regional cremation practices. *Proceedings of the Cambridge Antiquarian Society* LXXXV: 11-26.

Evans, C. and Hodder, I. 2006. *Marshland communities and cultural landscapes from the Bronze Age to present day.* McDonald Institute Monograph: Cambridge.

Gibson, A. 2004. Burials and beakers: seeing beneath the veneer in late Neolithic Britain. In: Cebreszuk, J. (ed.) *Similar but different: Bell Beakers in Europe.* Adam Mickiewicz University: Poznań. 173-192

Gibson, D. and Knight, M. 2006. *Bradley Fen excavations Whittlesey, Cambridgeshire 2001-2004.* Unpublished Cambridge Archaeological Unit report no. 733.

Lee, F. 2006. The human bone. In: Evans, C. and Hodder, I. (eds.) *Marshland communities and cultural landscapes from the Bronze Age to present day.* McDonald Institute Monograph: Cambridge. 28-30.

Marshall, A. 2011. *Experimental archaeology: 1. Early Bronze Age cremation pyres 2. Iron Age grain storage.* British Archaeological Reports British Series 530. Archaeopress: Oxford.

McKinley, J.I. 1993. Bone fragment size and weights of bone from modern British cremations and its implications for the interpretation of archaeological cremations *International Journal of Osteoarchaeology* 3: 283-287.

McKinley, J.I. 1994a. *The Anglo-Saxon cemetery at Spong Hill, North Elmham Part 8: the Cremations.* East Anglian Archaeology 69. Norfolk Archaeological Unit: Gressenhall.

McKinley, J.I. 1994b. Bone fragment size in British cremation burials and its implications for pyre technology and ritual. *Journal of Archaeological Science* 21: 339-342.

McKinley, J.I. 1997. The cremated human bone from burials and cremation-related context. In: Fitzpatrick, A.P. (ed.) *Archaeological excavations on the route of the A27 Westhampnett Bypass, West Sussex, 1992. Volume 2: the late Iron Age, Romano-British, and Anglo-Saxon cemeteries*. Wessex Archaeology Report No. 12: Salisbury: 55-72, 244-252.

McKinley, J.I. 2000a. Phoenix rising; aspects of cremation in Roman Britain. In: Pearce, J., Millett M. and Struck, M. (eds.) *Burial society and context in the Roman world.* Oxbow: Oxford. 38-44.

McKinley, J.I. 2000b. Funerary practice. In: Barber, B. and Bowsher, D. (eds.) *The eastern cemetery of Roman London. Excavations 1983-1990.* MoLAS Monograph 4. Museum of London Archaeology Service: London. 60-81.

Pickstone, A. and Mortimer, R. 2011. *The archaeology of Brigg's Farm, Prior's Fen, Thorney, Peterborough.* Unpublished Oxford Archaeology East Report No. 1094.

Struck, M. 1993. *Busta* in Britannien und ihre verbindungen zum Kontinent. Allgemeine Überlegungen zur Herleitung der Bestattungssittee. In: Struck, M. (ed.) *Römerzeitliche Gräber als quellen zu Religion Bevölkerungsstruktur und Sozialgeschichte.* Archäologische Schriften des Instituts für Vor-und Frühgeschichte der Johannes Gutenberg-Universität Mainz. Band 3: 81-93.

Topál, J. 1981. *The southern cemetery of Matrica (Százhalombatta-Dunafüred).* Fontes Archaeologici Hungariae. Akadémiai Kiadó: Budapest.

# Archaeological Insights into the Disarticulation Pattern of a Human Body in a Sitting/Squatting Position

Karina Gerdau-Radonic

Bournemouth University
School of Applied Sciences,
Christchurch House, Talbot Campus
Fern Barrow, Poole, Dorset, BH12 5BB, UK

Email for correspondence: kgradonic@bournemouth.ac.uk

**Note:** This paper is the English revised version of an article published in Spanish by *Antípoda. Revista de Antropología y Arqueología*, Bogotá, Colombia, no.13, Julio-Diciembre 2011, 75-94.

**Abstract**
Archaeological contexts constitute an unparalleled source of information on skeletal disarticulation patterns and taphonomical events. Cultural as well as personal preferences dictate how, when and where the remains of the deceased will be laid to rest, all of which are factors that affect decomposition and, consequently, skeletal disarticulation. Understanding the latter helps reconstruct the original layout of the remains as well as identify any post-depositional events that may have altered the original context. This study looks at a set of pre-Columbian collective burials from Tablada de Lurín (Lurín Valley, Peru; A.D. 1-200). Through careful excavation and *in situ* anatomical and taphonomical observations recommended by the French school of *Archéothanatologie*, the author aimed to study the disarticulation pattern of individuals in a sitting/squatting position within a funerary bundle. It was possible to identify the disarticulation pattern as well as reconstruct the original burial position and the preparation of the bundles, which included placing the individuals upon a basket and wrapping them in at least one shroud. Moreover, the study also provided information on the order of dislocation of certain joints during decomposition, within the context of a funerary bundle. It appears that in such contexts the ankle and hip joints decompose more rapidly than the knee joint. Also, the shoulder joint is more persistent than the claviculo-sternal one and the anatomical connection between the scapula and the posterior ribcage.

**Keywords**: Decomposition, Disarticulation Process, Taphonomy, Pre-Columbian Archaeology, Funerary Bundle

Archaeological excavation of human remains provides information on the decomposition process, and on how the burial environment and burial practices can affect decomposition and skeletal disarticulation. Understanding decomposition, the sequence of disarticulation and how different skeletal elements can shift once soft tissue no longer holds them together is crucial in reconstructing events since death up to the moment archaeologists unearthed a body or rather, its remains. Post-mortem treatment of the body, original body placement and subsequent post-depositional events affect the decomposition process, the degree of disarticulation and the final layout of the remains. It is therefore possible to reconstruct original context and even post-mortem treatment through detailed analysis of disarticulated and sometimes partial remains as well as their surrounding environment (see *inter alia*: Duday 1986; 1987; Boddington 1987; Brothwell 1987; Duday *et al.* 1990; Haglund and Sorg 1997; 2002; Duday 2005; 2006; Andrews and Bello 2006; Duday and Guillon 2006).

In terms of mortuary treatment and taphonomic events, archaeological contexts are an unparalleled source of information and can enrich our understanding of taphonomy in diverse situations, whether culturally or environmentally different. Funerary practices as well as the timing of these vary according to the beliefs and preferences of the deceased and his or her kin. Moreover, certain situations as well as geographic and environmental context, among other factors, can also influence decisions on funerary proceedings and their timing.

The present paper aims, on the one hand, to explain

the disarticulation pattern of individuals buried in a flexed sitting/squatting position and as funerary bundles, by discussing the archaeological evidence from the pre-Columbian site of Tablada de Lurín, in the Peruvian central coast. On the other hand, it also aims to enrich the discussion on which joints are more labile or persistent during the decomposition process.

A brief summary of the archaeological findings pertaining to the site is followed by a description of the sample available for analysis and the methods used to analyse and interpret the findings. The sequence and pattern of skeletal disarticulation inside a funerary bundle as gleaned from the remains at Tablada are then described. Finally, the observations and findings are discussed.

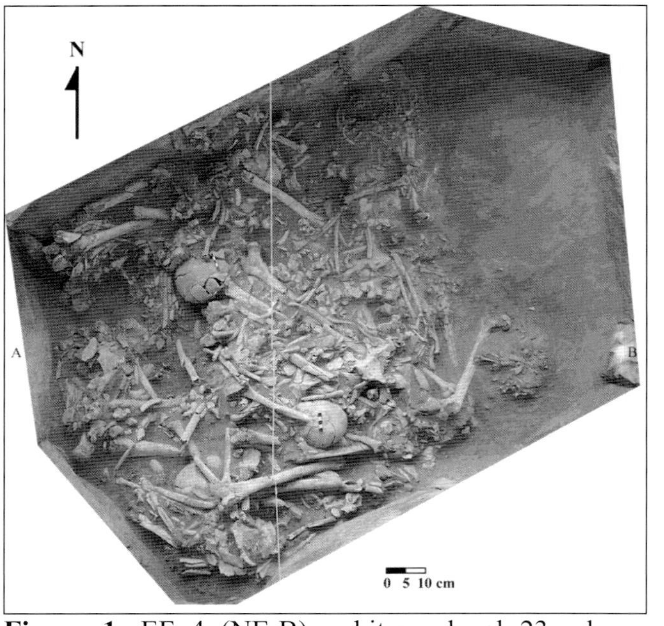


**Figure 1**: EF 4 (NE-B), arbitrary level 23, plan view.

## Tablada de Lurín

The archaeological site of Tablada de Lurín is located in the Lurín valley, in the Peruvian central coast. It is 20 km south of the historic centre of the city of Lima, within the new southern suburbs. Two teams have excavated the site over four decades during the latter half of the 20th century (Cárdenas and Vivar 1999; Makowski 2002; 2009a; 2009b). The main pre-Columbian occupation was a large necropolis (estimated at 52 ha) dating to the first half of the Early Intermediate Period (EIP; B.C. 200 – 200 A.D.), with two consecutive yet very distinct funerary phases (Makowski 2002; 2009a; 2009b).

The first phase dates from the second and first centuries B.C. and was characterised by pit burials, mostly single (Makowski 2002; 2009a; 2009b). This phase was immediately followed in time by a second phase with a different funerary pattern. Currently, it is not understood why or how this break occurred; the author, together with Makowski and other colleagues, is undertaking further research to elucidate this question.

The second funerary occupation dates from the first two centuries A.D. Burial pits from the first occupation were destroyed to make way for the new funerary architecture: semi-subterranean funerary structures used for collective burials. The content from these single pit burials was treated with little respect. During the excavations, the remains of some of the individuals were found within the fill used to bury the semi-subterranean burial chambers, once these structures were no longer in use (Balbuena 1996: 41; Gerdau 2007: 62).

In total, thirty-five collective burial chambers were excavated by the two teams having worked on the site (Cárdenas and Vivar 1999; Makowski 2002; 2009a; 2009b). The author conducted anthropological analysis on the remains excavated by Makowski's team from five such burial structures (the material from the previous team's excavations was not available). The method used to estimate the Minimum Number of Individuals (MNI) was the one detailed by Gallay and Chaix (1984: doc. 154), which gives the MNI based on bone frequency. Juveniles were tabulated separately from adults. These five funerary chambers contained between 20 to 55 individuals (Table 1), mostly adults, constituting either primary or secondary funerary deposits. Bone frequencies showed the remains of most individuals were incomplete, in particular missing the smaller bones, especially, vertebrae, hand and foot bones (Gerdau 2007: 176-200), which are more difficult to recover and can be left behind when the remains are being taken from one place to another as in the case of secondary funerary rituals (Duday *et al.* 1990: 43; Duday 2006: 46).

Detailed field observations, together with refitting and bone pairing analyses during post-excavation studies indicated that the remains had been subjected to multiple displacements and manipulations while the tombs had been in use, as the interior had had to be re-organised (Gerdau 2007). Notwithstanding, a few individuals had remained intact, or almost, and in their original location (Figs. 1-3).

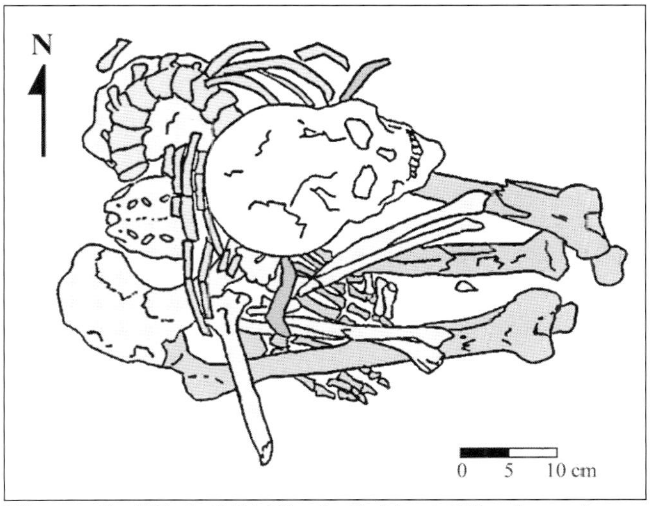


**Figure 2**: EF 4 (NE-B), Individual VI, plan view (rendering artist: Karla Gerdau).

From the works of Balbuena (1996), the author (Gerdau 2007) and Makowski (2002; 2009a; 2009b; Gerdau and Makowski 2011), it has been possible to ascertain that the individuals within these chambers had originally been wrapped into simple funerary bundles, without mummification. They were seated or placed in a squatting position upon baskets, with both the upper limbs flexed and crossed over the chest, the lower limbs flexed, with the knees drawn up to the chin, and the heels tucked underneath or just in front of the pubis. They were then wrapped in one or more pieces of cloth, '*mantos*', in order to constitute a simple and small funerary bundle. Small grave goods were placed within the bundle, whereas larger items were placed outside the bundle, within the burial chamber. This burial position can be seen, for example, in the photographs and radiographic images of the South American mummies housed at the *Museum für Völkerkunde* in Berlin (now the *Ethnologisches Museum*; Herrmann and Meyer 1993).

The remains at Tablada presented no signs of mummification in the shape of desiccated soft tissue or as evidence of a paradoxical disarticulation sequence. In natural conditions, when the body has not been mummified, the first joints to disappear are the 'labile' ones, like those within the hands, i.e. the interphalangeal, metacarpophalangeal, carpo-metacarpal, and intercarpal joints, which tend to have little soft tissue. The 'persistent' joints last longer (e.g., the knee; see Duday *et al.* 1990: 31; Duday 2005: 167; 2006: 33). It is therefore possible in the case of secondary deposits or remains that have been displaced to find an intact knee or other persistent joint, whereas the multiple joints within the hands, the feet and the neck may be entirely disarticulated and 'unrecognisable', i.e., they have lost their anatomical order. On the contrary, in cases of mummification, whether natural or artificial, which decomposed, Maureille and Sellier (1996) have described a disarticulation sequence which is inverted. It is those areas of the body with little soft tissue (e.g. interphalangeal joints) that persist and do not decompose, whereas more persistent joints with more soft tissue decompose more rapidly as they provide more nutrients to the bacteria and other decomposing agents. This is why decomposed mummified individuals are said to present a paradoxical disarticulation sequence (Duday *et al.* 1990: 33).

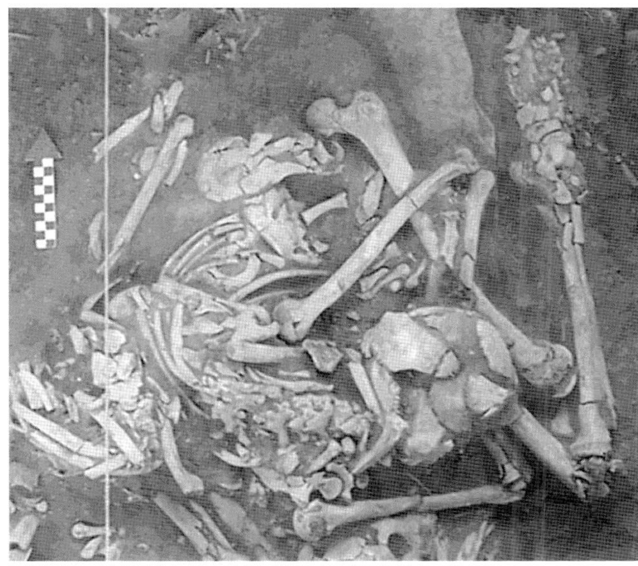

**Figure 3**: EF 4 (NE-B), Individual X, plan view, scale 10 cm.

## Materials and Methods

The disarticulation pattern described below was observed during excavations conducted by the Proyecto Arqueológico – Taller de Campo "Lomas de Lurín", research project directed by K. Makowski of the Pontificia Universidad Católica del Perú. Though this project studied both funerary occupations at Tablada de Lurín, the present author only participated in the study of the second phase of occupation of the cemetery. Therefore, the observations presented here stem from the excavation of one collective mortuary structure (EF 4 (NE-B)) and were complemented by information from the reports, dissertations and visual excavation records of preceding field seasons (García 1994; Atalaya 1996; Balbuena 1996; Makowski *et al.* 1996). Observations of osteological relationships of the first order (Duday 2006: 50) were made directly in the field and were also sought within the visual excavation records produced by other team members.

*Excavation Techniques and Site Recording*

As stated above, Makowski's team excavated five collective burial structures. Excavation and site recording techniques were in line with the guidelines recommended by the French school of *Archéothanatologie* (see Duday 1986; 1987; Duday *et al.* 1990; Duday 2005; 2006; Duday and Guillon 2006), which specifies that detailed observations and records should be made and kept in the field.

Due to the density of remains enclosed within each structure, after the roof of the chamber was dismounted, excavation progressed by lifting one layer of remains at a time. It must be stressed that these layers did not represent different depositional events. On the contrary, they were delimited by the extent of material that could be identified, recorded and lifted within a single photographic plan view of the whole structure (Fig. 1). For example, in structure EF 4 (NE-B), a total of 64 plan views were required to record all specimens (osteological or otherwise) within the structure. The first represented the top-most layer of remains, the last the bottom layer of remains lying directly upon the chamber's floor. Drawn plan views were based on these photographs.

The location of each osteological specimen (as defined by Grayson 1984 cited in Lyman 1994: 100) lifted was recorded on these photographic plan views. Additionally, the depth at which each specimen lay was also recorded from a known datum point. For the excavation of EF 4 (NE-B), the author recorded the depth of long bones at both the proximal and distal ends in order to assess whether they lay flat on the surface or at an incline. This provided a record of the location of each specimen within three-dimensional space. This visual record enabled the assessment of spatial relationships of all specimens recovered.

During the excavation of structure EF 4 (NE-B) by the author, every specimen over 1 $cm^2$ in size was identified *in situ* in as much detail as possible; however, whole anatomical elements smaller than that size, such as foot phalanges, were also identified and recorded. Previous excavations of the other four structures by other persons in the team had proceeded in a similar manner, though smaller elements had not been recorded in as much detail as for EF4 (NE-B). Notwithstanding, it was still possible to retrieve the location of most specimens and to assess their spatial relationship as well as the degree of disarticulation of certain individuals and of isolated skeletal parts through the excavations' visual and written records of the other burial structures. Osteological relationships of the first order had been noted in the field by all members of the team, and despite the commingling within all structures, it was possible to individualise certain remains. Associated material was also recorded within three-dimensional space.

*Sample Size*

The minimum number of individuals (MNI) varied within each structure (Table 1). As mentioned above, within each burial chamber, the excavators were able to individualise certain groups of remains (Table 1). As shown in Table 1, within all five structures only five of these individuals were complete and appeared as primary intact deposits. However, a more substantial number (39) were incomplete and to date it is difficult to ascertain whether they were primary disturbed deposits or secondary ones, due to the multiple displacements and reductions the individuals had undergone (Gerdau 2007).

These intact individuals (Table 1) were able to provide information on mortuary treatment, including post-mortem preparation of the body for burial, the original body position of the remains, and, finally, the sequence of skeletal disarticulation within a funerary bundle. Sample size is small; there are only 4 adult individuals and one juvenile within 5 structures that have been positively identified as primary deposits (Table 1). These four adult individuals did not all show exactly the same pattern, but a general trend, described below, can be gleaned. Moreover, incomplete individuals served to corroborate certain patterns observed. Table 2 presents the joints that could be observed and the individuals displaying those features.

Finally, it is important to emphasise that the disarticulation sequence detailed in this paper only applies to adult individuals who were buried as funerary bundles in a flexed sitting/squatting position, and who were deposited within an empty space (not a filled grave). Juveniles whose epiphyses have not yet fused may show a different pattern of disarticulation, but further research needs to be conducted on this topic.

**Table 1**: Minimum Number of Individuals (MNI)

| | MNI (Gerdau 2007) | Individuals identified as primary deposits | Other individuals (adults and juveniles) identified (can be primary disturbed or secondary deposits) |
|---|---|---|---|
| EF 1(NE-B) | 36 | 0 | 11 |
| EF 2 (NE-B) | 38 | 0 | 2 |
| EF 3 (NE-B) | 29 | 1 adult | 8 |
| EF 4 (NE-B) | 55 | 3 adults (and 1 juvenile) | 15 |
| EF 6 (NE-A) | 20 | 0 | 3 |

Number of individuals positively identified as primary deposits and number of other identified individuals (disturbed) within each collective funerary structure excavated by Proyecto Arquelógico - Taller de Campo "Lomas de Lurín". Notice there is a large discrepancy between the MNI and the actual number of individuals identified. This is because only a small number of individuals could be identified as such within each structure; all other individuals were commingled and not readily identifiable as individuals (after García 1994; Atalaya 1996; Balbuena 1996; Gerdau 2007).

**Table 2**: Individuals upon which the above listed joints could be observed. See Gerdau (2007) for a detailed description of each individual.

| Joint Appearance | Individuals Observed |
|---|---|
| Head slumped on torso | EF 3 (NE-B): inds. I<br>EF 4 (NE-B): inds. VI, X, XIII (juvenile) |
| Persistence of shoulder girdle with dislocation of scapula-thoracic connection and claviculo-sternal joint | EF 4 (NE-B): inds. X |
| Spine articulated up to cervical vertebrae | EF 3 (NE-B): inds. I<br>EF 4 (NE-B): inds. VI; X, XIII (juvenile) |
| Persistence of elbow | EF 3 (NE-B): inds. I, III<br>EF 4 (NE-B): inds. I, V, VI, VIII, X |
| Dislocation of wrist and joints within hand | EF 3 (NE-B): inds. I, IV, V<br>EF 4 (NE-B): inds. I, II, VI, VIII, X, XIII (juvenile) |
| Persistence of lower spine | EF 1 (NE-B): ind. I<br>EF 2 (NE-B): inds. I, II<br>EF 3 (NE-B): inds. III<br>EF 4 (NE-B): inds. I; II, XIV (juvenile), XVI, XVI |
| Persistence of pelvis | EF 2 (NE-B): inds. I, II<br>EF 3 (NE-B): inds. I, III<br>EF 4 (NE-B): one set of pelvis and feet, inds. I; II, V, VI, VIII, X, XIII (juvenile), XIV (juvenile), XVI, XVII |
| Persistence of feet | EF 1 (NE-B): ind. I<br>EF 2 (NE-B): inds. I, II<br>EF 3 (NE-B): inds. I, III, IV, V<br>EF 4 (NE-B): one set of pelvis and feet; inds. VI (dislocation of sacrum), X, XIII (juvenile), XVII |
| Persistence of knee | EF 1 (NE-B): ind. I<br>EF 3 (NE-B): inds. III, IV, V<br>EF 4 (NE-B): inds. V; VI, VIII, X, XIII (juvenile), XVI |
| Displacement of lower limb bones with no tarsal dislocation | EF 3 (NE-B): inds. I<br>EF 4 (NE-B): inds. VI, X, XIII (juvenile) |

## Skeletal Disarticulation within a Funerary Bundle

As stated above, original body position was upright sitting or squatting with both upper and lower limbs flexed in front of the chest. Individuals had been placed in baskets and wrapped in at least one textile wrapping. Textiles and organic materials do not preserve well in Tablada and these were progressively replaced by the sediment used to fill in the structures when they were definitely closed, or by sediment that had progressively infiltrated itself over time within the structure (see Balbuena 1996 and Gerdau 2007). It is the position of skeletal elements, as described below, as well as some organic fibres found among the remains that provide evidence for the basket and textiles.

*Axial Skeleton*

Given the upright position of the torso, the upper half, as well as the long bones of the limbs, were destabilised as the process of decomposition advanced. Once the internal organs liquefied and disappeared, there was an empty space within the thoracic, abdominal and pelvic cavities. The upper half of the thoracic cage fell within these cavities and most anatomical connections were lost. The cephalic skeleton settled itself upon the remains of the thorax, but the head kept its original orientation.

The bundle helped preserve the anatomical connections of the lower spine (Figs. 2 and 3). The textile wrappings appear to have provided some kind of support upon which the column could lean against without the vertebrae dislocating. Contiguous funerary bundles also served as a support to the remains of individuals buried beside or in front of them. For example, in Figure 3, one can distinguish individual X leaning partially against individual XIII.

The upper half of the ribs fell in anatomical disorder within the abdominal and pelvic cavities. The lower half, however, settled itself on either side of the lumbar vertebrae, dislocating from the thoracic vertebrae, yet maintaining their natural anatomical order (Figs. 2-4).

*Shoulder Girdle and Upper Limbs*

The movement of the bones in the upper limb and the shoulder girdle was dependent on the space available around the body within the bundle. If the body had been placed with a straight upright back and if the bundle had had some kind of posterior support, then the scapula slid downward toward the innominate of same laterality and appeared behind it and in superior view. If the person's torso had been oriented or slumped forward, then the scapula appeared above the ribs and the pelvis, in posterior view (Fig. 3). The humerus and the clavicle followed the scapula in its fall, and were found in close proximity to it.

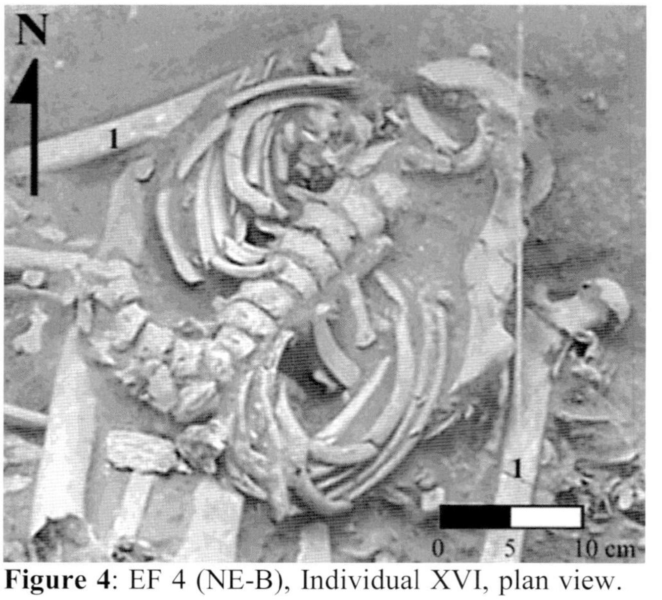


**Figure 4**: EF 4 (NE-B), Individual XVI, plan view. Long bones numbered '1' do not belong to this individual.

The exact position of the hands was difficult to ascertain. All individuals placed in an upright sitting/squatting position within the '*cistas*' were found with their carpals, metacarpals, and phalanges heavily disarticulated within the abdominal and pelvic cavities. As previously mentioned, forearms were crossed in front of the chest and this meant that the hands could have been in one of four positions: covering the face, at chin height, on either shoulder, or upon the chest. These positions have been recorded in pre-Columbian Peruvian mummies (Herrmann and Meyer 1993). In any one of these positions, the hand bones would have been destabilised as decomposition progressed and empty spaces were generated within the body.

*Pelvic Girdle and Lower Limbs*

Depending on the original position of the lower limbs, these fell on either side of the body. The hips and the ankle suffered minor dislocations (Figs. 2 and 3). It appears that the knee is a more persistent joint than the ankle and hip. Once nothing could hold the femur in place at the hip, it fell to one side but remained articulated to the tibia, fibula and patella. The leg did not pull the tarsals into the fall, but the feet remained articulated (Fig. 3).

Thanks to their position within the basket base of the bundle, both the pelvis and the feet maintained full articulation or almost. The shape of the pelvis should render it unstable once there is no connective tissue holding the bony elements together. The ossa coxae should open up laterally and posteriorly, and the sacrum should fall either forwards or backwards (Duday 2005: 170; 2006: 35). Yet, within Tablada's funerary bundles, the sides of the basket provided a support to the coxal bones and sacrum, holding them in articulation despite the loss of connective soft tissue. Furthermore, as the feet lay flat on their soles within the basket, they dislocated only slightly as this position was stable.

## Discussion

The sample of complete individuals within each structure is very limited (Table 1). Nevertheless, even though more observations certainly need to be collated, a pattern is discernible. In Tablada, the vertical position of the individual buried in a sitting/squatting position increases the degree of disarticulation of the upper half of the skeleton as once decomposition advances there is nothing to hold the skeletal elements together. These will then naturally fall. The textile wrapping and the inferior support/container, a basket, provide stability to the lower half of the thorax, the pelvis and the feet, maintaining them in full or partial articulation.

When an individual is found whose thoracic cage, spine and pelvis are still in correct anatomical position, this may be due to two possibilities:

(1) the progressive replacement of decomposing soft tissue by sediment infiltrating the burial deposit (in the case of burials in 'fluid' soil (Duday 2005: 185-186; 2006: 41)); or,

(2) because the bony elements are held together by some kind of exterior support (in the case of deposits in an empty space, as is the case of the burial chambers in Tablada). In two individuals in structure EF 4 (NE-B), the column remained in almost full articulation because of the support provided by the textile wrappings and the contiguous remains (Figs. 2 and 3).

## Labile vs. Persistent Joints

### *Joints within the Neck*

Some observations made in Tablada also corroborate observations made elsewhere about labile and persistent joints (Table 3). For example, the atlas was found directly underneath the base of the cranium of individual X (EF 4 (NE-B)). Duday and colleagues (1990: 31) state that the atlanto-occipital joint is more persistent than the cervical intervertebral joints. Duday (2006: 35) writes that 'initial disarticulation' at the neck occurs at the level of the atlas-axis or axis-third cervical intervertebral joint. Andrews and Bello (2006: 17) also list the neck as a labile joint. It is therefore possible that some joints within the neck are more labile (atlas-axis or axis-third cervical joint) than others (atlanto-occipital joint). Moreover, within the funerary bundles, the cervical vertebrae were found in anatomical disarray within the thoracic and abdominal cavities.

### *Shoulder Joint*

In Tablada, the shoulder joint presented evidence of being much more persistent and decomposed more slowly that the claviculo-sternal joint and scapulo-thoracic anatomical connection. When the scapula disarticulates from the ribcage, the clavicle and humerus follow suit. On the other hand, the joint between the sternum and clavicle becomes undone. Duday (Duday *et al.* 1990: 31; Duday 2005: 167; 2006: 33) also lists the scapulo-thoracic connection as labile.

### *Wrist and Hand Joints*

The joints within the hand, including the wrist, are listed in the literature as labile (Duday *et al.* 1990: 31; Duday 2005: 167; 2006: 33; Andrews and Bello 2006: 17). Within these funerary bundles these same joints also appear as labile. Notwithstanding, the wrist is likely to decompose after the interphalangeal, metacarpophalangeal, carpometacarpal and intercarpal joints. Within the bundles, fully articulated hands did not appear to fall from the wrist, but rather the hand bones had tumbled down separately.

### *Lower Spine and Pelvis*

The pelvis and lower spine appear as persistent within Tablada's funerary bundles, and are listed as such in the literature (Duday *et al.* 1990: 31; Duday 2005: 167; 2006: 33). Nevertheless, it should be noted that in this case, it might be a product of funerary pattern. Indeed the pelvis and lower spine are held together by the basket and wrappings used to form the bundle.

**Table 3**: List of labile and persistent joints as listed in the literature.

| Labile | Persistent | Reference | Tablada* |
|---|---|---|---|
| Cervical intervertebral joints | | Duday et al. 1990; Duday 2005, 2006; Andrews and Bello 2006 | X |
| Joints within the hand | | Duday et al. 1990; Duday 2005, 2006; Andrews and Bello 2006 | X |
| Wrist less labile than joints within hand | | | X |
| Distal joints of the feet | | Duday et al. 1990; Duday 2005, 2006; Andrews and Bello 2006 | |
| Costo-sternal joints | | Duday et al. 1990; Duday 2005, 2006; Andrews and Bello 2006 | |
| Scapulo-thoracic connection | | Duday et al. 1990; Duday 2005, 2006; Andrews and Bello 2006 | X |
| Claviculo-sternal joint | | Duday et al. 1990; Duday 2005, 2006; Andrews and Bello 2006 | X |
| Hip | | Duday 2005, 2006 | |
| | Atlanto-occipital joint | Duday et al. 1990; Duday 2005, 2006 | X |
| | Shoulder joint | Duday et al. 1990; Duday 2005, 2006 | X |
| | Lumbar spine, sacro-lumbar joint, sacro-iliac joint | Duday et al. 1990; Duday 2005, 2006 | X |
| | Knee, ankle, tarsals | Duday et al. 1990; Duday 2005, 2006 | X |
| | Knee more persistent than hip and ankle | Pereira 1996 | X |

*The Tablada box is only checked if the taphonomic evidence pointed towards the joints as being either labile or persistent; it does not indicate whether the joints were observable (see Table 2).

### *Hip, Knee and Ankle Joints*

The degree of persistence of the knee appears stronger than the hip and the ankle joints. Within the funerary bundles, once the hip joint decomposed, the femur could no longer be held in its vertical or slightly inclined position, therefore, the thigh, patella and leg bones fell to one side. Yet, they fell together and remained articulated at the knee. The ankle joint became slightly undone due to the fall of the leg bones; but the tibia and fibula did not pull any of the tarsal bones with them in the fall. The feet remained in full articulation. These observations on the knee and ankle confirm those made by G. Pereira (1996) at the Mexican archaeological site of Potrero de Guadalupe (Michoacán). It should be noted that Duday (Duday *et al.* 1990: 31; 2005: 167; 2006: 33) lists the knee and ankle as persistent joints. The evidence from Tablada and Michoacán do not contradict this. They only point to the knee being more persistent than the ankle joint.

## Conclusions

As demonstrated above, detailed excavation and observation of body and skeletal layout of archaeological human remains can provide information on the order of disarticulation of some anatomical joints within the human body. For example, in this particular case, it appears that the knee joint is more persistent than the ankle joint, and confirms observations made elsewhere (Pereira 1996). Similarly, the data from Tablada also points to a persistent shoulder joint and a labile scapulo-thoracic anatomical connection and claviculo-sternal joint (also recorded in Duday *et al.* 1990: 31; Duday 2005: 167; 2006: 33). However, as sample size is small, this needs to be further investigated.

Information on labile and persistent joints can help with the interpretation of primary vs. secondary deposits, and possibly reveal the presence of decomposed mummified remains. Furthermore, close observation of the remains and their surrounding context can also reveal the presence or absence of wrappings, supports or other grave goods and burial artefacts that may have decomposed and disappeared over time (see Duday 1986; Boddington 1987; Duday 1987; Duday *et al.* 1990; Duday 2005; 2006; Duday and Guillon 2006;). It is unlikely that such detailed observations can be made in the context of contract/rescue archaeology as this branch of the discipline has limited time and is confined to a clearly delimited space. However, research archaeology in Europe and elsewhere can pursue this line of investigation and be a source for some kinds of information: e.g., conditions that preserve soft tissue, disarticulation patterns, understanding and excavating commingled remains.

## Acknowledgements

The author would like to thank H. Duday and K. Makowski for their kind support, guidance and insightful comments throughout her research. She also extends many thanks to G. Oré, M. Jiménez, P. Castro de la Mata, E. Tomasto, R. Luna, A. Zamora, J. Rodríguez, E. Chonlón, L. Watson, as well as the members of Laboratoire d'anthropologie des populations du passé (UMR 5199 – PACEA, U. Bordeaux I), of Proyecto Arqueológico Taller de Campo « Lomas de Lurín » (Departamento de Humanidades, PUCP), and the PhD examiners. She is also very grateful to her family and friends for their kind and generous support throughout her research, in particular Alex, Tadeo, Silvia, Kati, Karla (rendering artist), Milena, Eliana and Greg. Finally, thanks are due to the reviewers for their insightful comments and to H. Schutkowski for our discussion on this topic.

This work was financed by the Ministère de l'Enseignement Supérieur et de la Recherche (France), Cementos Lima, S.A. (Peru), and PATL-PUCP (Peru).

## Literature Cited

Atalaya Huerta, E. 1996. *Informe. Sector Noreste. Unidad de exposición A. Unidad de excavación N 123-126, E 127-131.* Unpub: Proyecto Arqueológico Tablada de Lurín, Pontificia Universidad Católica del Perú: Lima.

Andrews, P. and Bello, S. 2006. Pattern in human burial practice. In: Gowland, R. and Knüsel, C. (eds.) *Social archaeology of funerary remains.* Oxbow Books: Oxford. 14-29.

Balbuena Cotlear, L. 1996. *Entierros múltiples en Tablada de Lurín: una aproximación al ritual funerario.* Undergraduate thesis, Pontificia Universidad Católica del Perú: Lima.

Boddington, A. 1987. Chaos, disturbance and decay in an Anglo-Saxon cemetery. In: Boddington, A., Garland, A.N., and Janaway, R.C. (eds.) *Death, decay, and reconstruction: approaches to archaeology and forensic science.* Manchester University Press: Manchester. 27-42

Brothwell, D.R. 1987. Decay and disorder in the York Jewbury skeletons. In: Boddington, A., Garland, A.N., and Janaway, R.C. (eds.) *Death, decay, and reconstruction: approaches to archaeology and forensic science.* Manchester University Press: Manchester. 22-26.

Cárdenas Martín, M. and Vivar Anaya, J. 1999. *Tablada de Lurín: excavaciones 1958-1989; patrones funerarios.* Pontificia Universidad Católica del Perú - Instituto Riva-Agüero: Lima. 2 vols.

Duday, H. 1986. Contribution des observations ostéologiques à la chronologie interne des sépultures collectives. In: Duday, H. and Masset, C. (eds.) *Anthropologie physique et archéologie. Méthodes d'étude des sépultures : actes du colloque de Toulouse, 4, 5 et 6 novembre 1982.* CNRS: Paris. 51-59.

Duday, H. 1987. La quantification des restes humains. Application à l'étude des sépultures à incinérations ou des différentiels autres que la conservation. In: *Méthodes d'études des sépultures, compte-rendu de la 2e table ronde de la R.C.P. 742 du CNRS, St. Germain-en-Laye (16 et 17 mai 1987),* R.C.P. 742 du CNRS: Paris. 17-22

Duday, H. 2005. L'archéothanatologie. In: Dutour O., Hublin, J.-J., and Vandermeersch B. (eds.) *Objets et méthodes en paléoanthropologie.* Comité des travaux historiques et scientifiques : Paris. 153-215.

Duday, H. 2006. Archaeothanatology or the archaeology of death. In: Gowland, R. and Knüsel, C. (eds.) *Social archaeology of funerary remains.* Oxbow: Oxford. 30-56.

Duday, H., Courtaud, P., Crubézy, E., Sellier, P. and Tillier, A.-M. 1990. L'anthropologie de terrain. *Bulletins et mémoires de la Société d'Anthropologie de Paris*, n.s. 2 (3-4): 29-50.

Duday, H. and Guillon M. 2006. Understanding the circumstances of deposition when the body is skeletonised. In: Schmitt A., Cunha, E. and Pinheiro, J. (eds.) *Forensic anthropology and forensic medicine: complementary sciences from recovery to cause of death.* Humana Press: Totowa New Jersey. 117-158.

García Malpartida, R. 1994. *Informe de la segunda práctica pre-profesional: la estructura funeraria 2 en Tablada de Lurín.* Unpub: Proyecto Arqueológico Tablada de Lurín. Pontificia Universidad Católica del Perú: Lima.

Gallay, A. and Chaix, L. 1984. *Le site préhistorique du Petit Chasseur (Sion, Valais), 5 et 6. (Le dolmen MXI).* Département d'anthropologie de l'Université de Genève. Bibliothèque historique vaudoise: Lausanne. Cahiers d'archéologie romande, nos. 31 and 32.

Gerdau-Radonic, K. 2007. *Les tombes collectives de Tablada de Lurín (Vallée de Lurín, Pérou ; Ier - IIIe s. ap. J.C.).* Unpublished PhD thesis. Université Bordeaux I, Bordeaux.

Gerdau-Radonic, K. and Makowski, K. 2011. Las sepulturas colectivas de Tablada de Lurín: una perspectiva desde la antropología biológica. In: Vetter, L., Téllez, S. and Vega-Centeno, R. (eds.) *Arqueología peruana. Homenaje a Mercedes Cárdenas.* Pontificia Universidad Católica del Perú: Lima. 145-176.

Grayson, D.K. 1984. *Quantitative zooarchaeology: topics in the analysis of archaeological faunas.* Academic Press: Orlando, FL.

Haglund, W.D. and Sorg, M.H. (eds.).1997. *Forensic taphonomy: the postmortem fate of human remains.* CRC Press: Boca Raton, FL.

Haglund, W.D. and Sorg, M.H. (eds.). 2002. *Advances in forensic taphonomy. Method, theory and archaeological perspectives.* CRC Press: Boca Raton, FL.

Herrmann, B. and Meyer, R.-D. 1993. *Südamerikanische Mumien aus vorspanischer Zeit: eine radiologische Untersuchung.* Staatliche Museen zu Berlin--Preussischer Kulturbesitz: Berlin.

Lyman, R.L. 1994. *Vertebrate taphonomy.* Cambridge University Press: Cambridge.

Makowski, K. 2002. Power and social ranking at the end of the Formative Period. The Lower Lurin Valley cemeteries. In: Isbell, W.H. and Silverman, H. (eds.) *Andean archaeology I: variations in sociopolitical organization.* Kluwer Academic/ Plenum Publishers: New York. 89-120.

Makowski, K. 2009a. Poder y estatus social a fines del Periodo Formativo: los cementerios del valle bajo de Lurín. In: Burger, R.L. and Makowski, K. (eds.) *Arqueología del período formativo en la cuenca baja de Lurín.* Fondo Editorial Pontificia Universidad Católica del Perú: Lima. 209-236.

Makowski, K. 2009b. Tablada de Lurín: aspectos cronológicos de la ocupación de lomas costeras de Atocongo. In: Burger, R.L. and Makowski, K. (eds.) *Arqueología del período formativo en la cuenca baja de Lurín.* Fondo Editorial Pontificia Universidad Católica del Perú: Lima. 237-282.

Makowski, K., Vega Centeno, R., Amaro, I., Carillo, H., León, E., Rodríguez de March, C., Castro de la Mata, P., Dulanto, J., Tomasto, E., Balbuena, L., Atalaya, E., Gorriti, M., Santos, I., Salcedo, L., Escajadillo, G., and Arana, E. 1996. *Proyecto arquelógico - Taller de Campo PUCP "Tablada de Lurín": informe de las temporadas 1993/1994 y 1994/1995.* Unpub : Instituto Nacional de Cultura: Lima.

Maureille, B. and Sellier P. 1996. Dislocation en ordre paradoxal, mommification et decomposition: observations et hypothèses. *Bulletins et Mémoires de la Société d'Anthropologie de Paris*, n.s. 8 (3-4): 313-327.

Pereira, G. 1996. *Potrero de Guadalupe: anthropologie funéraire d'une communauté prétarasque du nord du Michoacán, Mexique.* Unpublished PhD thesis, Université Paris 1 – la Sorbonne: Paris.

# Mortuary Practices at Aztalan: A Reappraisal of an Elite Burial at a Middle Mississippian Site in the Western Great Lakes Region of the Midwestern United States

Norman C. Sullivan[1*] and Roland Rodell[2]

[1] Anthropology/Department of Social and Cultural Sciences
Marquette University, Milwaukee, WI, USA 53233

[2] Anthropology/Department of Anthropology and Sociology
University of Wisconsin – Rock County, Janesville, WI, USA 53546

*Email for correspondence: norman.sullivan@marquette.edu

**Abstract**

The mortuary practices of the Middle Mississippian site at Cahokia are briefly compared with the practices at Aztalan, an affiliated site near the periphery of the Mississippian cultural region. There are some parallels in the treatment of the dead at both sites and the similarity of pattern may be tied to a participation in the Southeastern Ceremonial Complex. The complex included a spirit force known as Birdman (or Morningstar) who had a regenerative capacity. A high status burial in Mound 72 at Cahokia has been thought, by many archaeologists, to demonstrate a spiritual link between the elite of the community and cosmic forces. A very similar program is observed in an elite burial at Aztalan. At both sites, the high status individual was buried with numerous cut and drilled beads. Beyond this, at Cahokia there were four decapitated males buried in the vicinity of the high status individual while at Aztalan there was one decapitated male although not in direct proximity to the high status individual. Nonetheless, it is suggested that the Aztalan elite burial also represents the cosmic link with Birdman.

**Keywords**: Middle Mississippian, Cahokia, Aztalan, Mortuary Practices, Birdman

## Introduction

Mortuary practices are of significant interest to anthropologists since the practices of burial reflect social attributes of the deceased (Fletcher 1978; Joyce 2001) as well as community rituals and beliefs (Parker Pearson 1999). The aim of this study is to investigate the linkage of social status and belief in two elite interments from two Middle Mississippian sites. Both sites are foci of the Middle Mississippian Culture (hereafter Mississippian). The Mississippian was distributed in regions adjacent to major tributaries of the Mississippi River. Sites of the Mississippian are found from the Gulf Coast to the western Great Lakes and from the southeast United States to the eastern Great Plains (Emerson 1997; Pauketat 2004). The economies of Mississippian communities varied to some degree although food production, primarily eastern flint corn, played a fundamental role (Scarry 1993). Mississippian sites have the recurrent attributes of distinct ceramic forms, ritual precincts comprised of flat-topped mounds arranged around plazas and wooden stockades surrounding elite areas (Pauketat 2004).

Cahokia was a very large Mississippian centre situated in the area of St. Louis, Missouri and East Saint Louis, Illinois (Figure 1). The Mississippian component at Cahokia dates from about 1200 BP to 600 BP (Young and Fowler 2000). At its peak, during the Lohman Phase (950-900 BP) and Stirling Phase (900 to 800 BP), the community encompassed an area of approximately 13 km$^2$ (Pauketat 2004). The population of the city is estimated to have been between 10,000 (Pauketat 2004) and 15,000 people (Young and Fowler 2000) although it has been estimated as high as 25,000 (Gregg 1975). Cahokia included at least 120 mounds. The central precinct of Cahokia includes mounds of different forms as well as Mound 38 (Monks Mound) which is a rectangular, flat topped platform 30.4m high covering a total area of 6.47 hectares. Adjacent to the Monks Mound plaza was a structure of wooden posts aligned to mark the equinoctes and solstices (Wittry 1969).

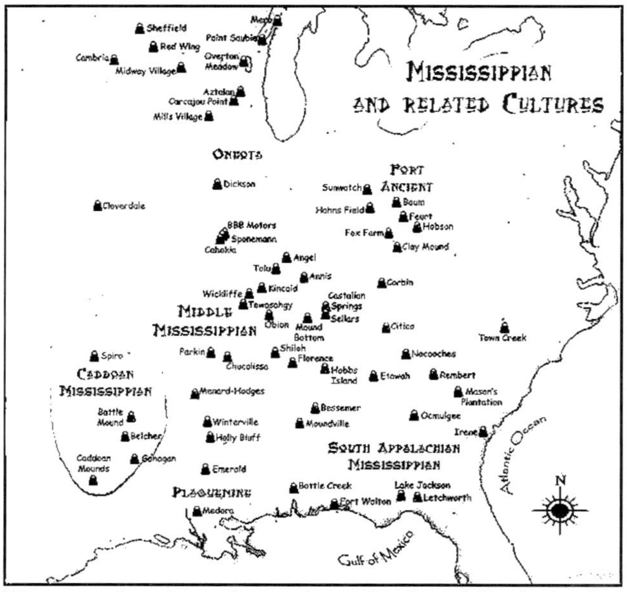


**Figure 1**: A schematic of the Mississippian heartland and regional variants. Cahokia is situated on the east and west banks of the Mississippi River in the area of central Missouri. Aztalan is in south central Wisconsin in the western Great Lakes region.

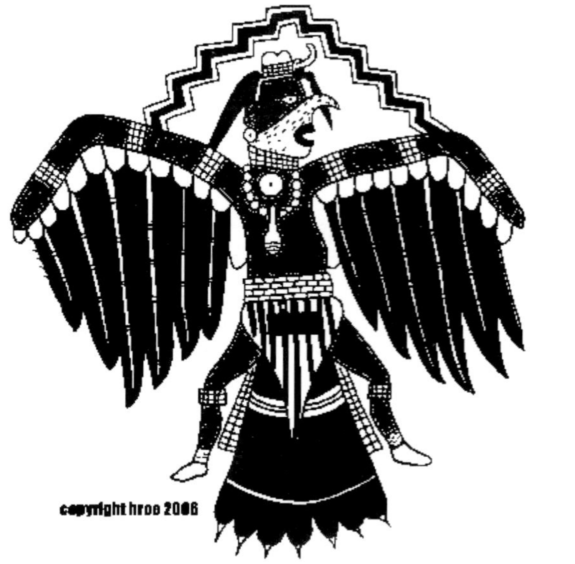

**Figure 2**: A rendering of the Birdman. In some Mississippian depictions, the Birdman is also shown holding a severed head as well as a war mace and wearing prosopic ear pieces.

A significant component of the religious life of Mississippian peoples was the Southeast Ceremonial Complex which was a cosmological construct linking human experience and the supernatural realm (Waring and Holder 1945). An important element of the supernatural realm was Morningstar who embodied the idea of resurrection and was one of the spiritual parents of humans. Brown and Dye (2007) have convincingly demonstrated the link between Morningstar and Birdman (Figure 2). Birdman is a recurring motif in the Southeast Ceremonial Complex. He is typically depicted holding a severed head and an 'apronlike' accoutrement hung from the belt which Brown and Dye (2007) interpret to be a scalplock.

Aztalan is the second site of interest here and is located in south central Wisconsin on a waterway that is a minor tributary of the Mississippi (Figure 1). The site covers an area of approximately 7.28 hectares and includes a central plaza and two flat top mounds and one conical mound enclosed by a wood palisade. In addition, there is a series of small conical mounds northwest of the palisade. At the closest point, the series of conical mounds are approximately 91m west of the northwest corner of the site and they continue for at least 345m. The actual number and extent of the mounds is uncertain since they were significantly damaged by early Euroamerican settlers.

The site has long been of interest to archaeologists as it was thought to represent a Mississippian intrusion into a region already occupied by local indigenous populations (Goldstein and Richards 2000). The Mississippian occupation at Aztalan approximately coincides with the Stirling Phase at Cahokia and dates to approximately 900 to 800 BP (Hall 2000). The cultural affiliation of the population at Aztalan remains a matter of debate although recent research is helping to achieve some clarification. Hall (2000) points out that approximately three-quarters of the ceramics found at the site can be attributed to local traditions and, from this, infers that Aztalan represents a local population acculturated into Mississippian lifeways. The biological data may help clarify this. Sullivan (1985) identified the sequela of tuberculosis in a non-Mississippian skeletal series from a southwest Wisconsin site that is coeval with Aztalan and suggests that the disease was introduced by Mississippian peoples from Cahokia. This follows from the argument that Cahokia was the most likely place of origin for tuberculosis in pre-Columbian Midwest populations since it was the only community sufficiently large to have served as a reservoir for the disease (Buikstra and Cook 1981; Buikstra and Williams 1991, cf. also Roberts and Buikstra 2003). A more compelling argument can be made from the documentation that three Aztalan burials have a strontium isotope signal that coincides with the levels identified from human remains at Cahokia (Price *et al.* 2007). Price cautiously refrains from arguing that Cahokia was the place of origin of the Aztalan burials. It is proposed here that some elements of the mortuary practices Aztalan parallel the practices observed at Cahokia which may be further indication that part of the population at Aztalan originated from Cahokia.

**Mississippian Mortuary Practices**

At Cahokia there are different burial programs that likely reflect status and persona of the dead. Milner (1984) has described the manner of burials for non-elite members of the society in which cemeteries are located in outlying areas. Pauketat and colleagues (2002) have described the disposal of isolated human skeletal elements found in borrow pits adjacent to the central plaza and Monks Mound. Postmortem alterations were observed in this disarticulated skeletal sample and these included polish, cut marks and greenstick fractures (Pauketat *et al.* 2002).

Of particular interest here is the treatment of the dead observed in Mound 72. This was a ridge type mound located approximately 850m south of Monks Mound and was excavated between 1967 and 1971 by crews from the University of Wisconsin-Milwaukee under the direction of Melvin Fowler (1997). The mound was constructed in four or more episodes and the separate mounds were united into the final size of 42.6m by 21.9m. The high status individual in Mound 72 was an adult male extended on a bed of cut shell beads that were formed in the shape of a bird (Figure 3). Adjacent to the burial were the interments of six individuals interpreted to be 'retainers' as well as grave offerings of projectile point caches, sheet copper and mica, and ground stone artifacts. To the northwest of the elite individual was a subfloor burial pit with the remains of at least 54 females aged between about 15 and 40 years and adjacent to that was a separate pit containing four males whose heads and hands had been cut off. Along the west margin of the mound were two linear burial pits with additional 'retainer' burials. A few burials in these groups were slightly flexed at the knees but most were fully extended. Finally, at the northernmost part of the mound there were an additional three pits each with multiple extended burials. Unfortunately, the burials from all parts of the mound were poorly preserved and have never been fully analyzed and described.

Brown and Dye (2007) caution against seeking facile links between imagery and physical evidence since this could lead to superficial explanations and miss the real messages being conveyed. Nonetheless, it is widely accepted that essential iconographic elements of Birdman are represented in the elite burial in Mound 72 (Fowler *et al.*1999; Pauketat and Bernard 2004). The avimorphic form of the cape and the associated burials without heads suggest an identification of the Birdman. The identification of the elite burial with the Birdman allows the Mound 72 mortuary program to be interpreted as an enactment of a rite ensuring regeneration rather than a simple demonstration of social status differentials or warfare.

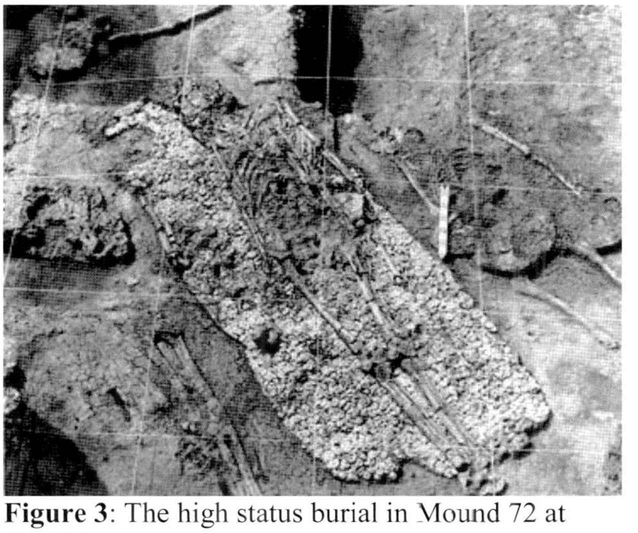

**Figure 3**: The high status burial in Mound 72 at Cahokia.

**Aztalan Mortuary Practices**

The programs for the treatment of the dead observed at Cahokia are, in some ways paralleled, at Aztalan. Disarticulated human remains, some with postmortem alterations (cutmarks, spiral fractures and burning), were found scattered in many areas of the plaza as well as in features (Sullivan 1990; Anderson 1994). The recovery of disarticulated human skeletal remains scattered in the plaza distinguishes Aztalan from Cahokia. However, it is possible that the human remains from the plaza were originally in features that were disturbed by subsequent activities at the site, including farming by Euroamerican settlers in the late nineteenth and early twentieth centuries. Using the data from Sullivan (1990) and Anderson (1994), the frequencies of upper limb *versus* lower limb elements found in features *versus* elements found in village fill were tested with a four cell chi square and the value of .18 fails to document a significant difference (df = 3, $p<.01$). The relative frequencies of human skeletal elements with post mortem alterations *versus* those without were also compared for the samples from the features and the sample from the village fill. Again, a four cell crossbreak was used and the value of 8.18 does not achieve significance at $p<.01$ but does at $p<.05$ (df=3)

Given the low statistical power of the chi-square, the more stringent probability is given preference here. Therefore, it is suggested that the human remains excavated from the plaza area may have originally been deposited in features which were subsequently disturbed in activities of the original inhabitants of the site or by more recent agricultural activities.

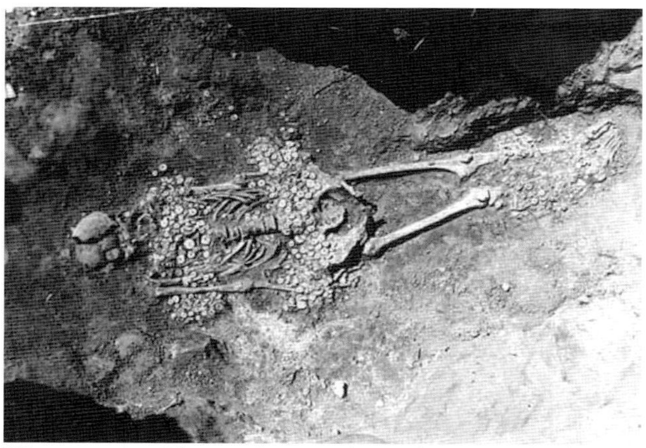

**Figure 4**: The misnamed 'Princess' burial at Aztalan.

There are also primary, extended inhumations with indications of differences in the status of the deceased (Maher 1958), the cremated remains of at least ten individuals excavated from a flat top mound in the northwest corner of the enclosure (Rowe 1958) and one high status burial outside the enclosure. The high status individual was excavated in 1920 and was referred to as 'The Princess Burial' (Barrett 1933). Even though the individual might be appropriately described as gracile, there was no further examination of the skeletal remains to confirm the sex determination. During accessioning, the skeletal remains of the burial were mixed in with the rest of the skeletal collection, without appropriate identification, and the sex of the individual is likely to remain uncertain. The burial was extended in a subfloor pit at the centre of a mound which was estimated to have been 13m in diameter and was located approximately 320m north of the northwest corner of the enclosure wall. The burial included 1,996 beads most of which were discoidal in form and made from river clam shells. Additionally, there were some tubular beads (the actual number was unspecified in the report) which Barrett thought were made from a Gulf Coast clam species (Figure 4). The beads were concentrated in three 'belts', one at the shoulders, a second above the innominates and the third covering most of the lower leg. This is the only burial every excavated in Wisconsin with dense clusters of beads and represents the most elaborate treatment for a burial ever found in the state.

Maher (1958) noted the excavation of another extended burial of interest which was found at the northwest margin of the enclosure (Figure 5). This individual was available for examination and was well preserved. Based on observations of the innominate, the individual was determined to have been a male with an estimated age at death in his late twenties (Breathnach 1965). There are no perimortem or postmortem alterations in the skeletal remains of the burial. This individual is of particular interest because the cranium and mandible as well as the right forearm were absent. The missing forearm may have been the result of the construction of a new palisade wall adjacent to the right side of the body (Figure 5) although this is uncertain and the excavation notes did not address this. The remainder of the burial, however, was undisturbed. The burial also differs from most others at the site in that there are neither grave goods nor any preparation of a burial chamber made from lenses of sand or gravel.

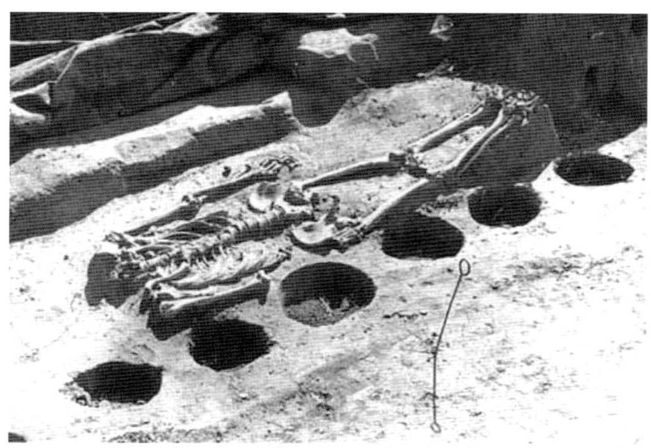

**Figure 5**: The headless male burial along the northwest enclosure at Aztalan.

No certain meaning can be ascribed to either of the unusual burials at Aztalan. However, it is suggested here that the elite at Aztalan were re-enacting a form of the regenerative ritual practiced by adherents of the Southeast Ceremonial Complex. There is no test that can verify this. However, there is a robust body of archaeological and ethnographic evidence that attests to the importance of the Birdman concept for late pre-Columbian peoples in the western Great Lakes area. Brown (2004) has suggested that Birdman is often characterized by long nosed, prosopic (∏ρόσωΠον meaning face) ear decorations. These small mask-like accoutrements are found at numerous sites in the states of Illinois and Wisconsin, including Aztalan (Duncan and

Diaz-Granados 2000). Brown (2004) also links the Birdman with the cosmology of First Nations people of the western Great Lakes region including the Ho-Chunk (Winnebago). Among indigenous peoples of the upper Midwest the Birdman is known as Red Horn or 'Who Wears Man Faces on His Ears'. Radin (1948) also observes features of Red Horn that parallel the Birdman, particularly in the practice of taking heads and in his regenerative capacity.

## Conclusion

It would probably be too much to expect finding a precise linkage between the elite burial practices at both Cahokia and Aztalan. Nonetheless, there is a parallel and it accords with widespread religious beliefs and practices from the pre-Columbian and contact eras. This might assist in strengthening the argument for the actual movement of at least a coterie of people from Cahokia to distant locations in the Mississippian sphere of interaction. Even if the population at Aztalan was comprised mostly of an acculturated indigenous people, as adduced by ceramic forms, the biological data and the evidence from complex religious beliefs attests to an actual migration rather than just the transport of ideas.

## Acknowledgements

Carter Lupton, Director of the History Program at the Milwaukee Public Museum was of invaluable assistance in the preparation of this paper. We also very much appreciate the assistance of several individuals in making the illustrations available. Figures 1 and 2 are open source Wikicommons schematics. The use of Figure 3 was generously permitted by Dr. Bonnie Styles, Director, Illinois State Museum. Figure 4 is used with the permission of Susan Otto of the Milwaukee Public Museum and Figure 5 with the permission of Jennifer Kolb, Director of the Museum, Wisconsin Historical Society.

## Literature Cited

Anderson, K.L. 1994. The Aztalan site: a human skeletal inventory and excavation history. Unpublished MA thesis, The University of Chicago.

Barrett, S.A. 1933. *Ancient Aztalan*. Bulletin of the Public Museum of the City of Milwaukee, No. 13. Milwaukee Public Museum: Milwaukee.

Breathnach, A.S. 1965. *Frazer's anatomy of the human skeleton* (6th edition). Little, Brown and Company: Boston.

Brown, J.A. 2004. On the identity of Birdman within Mississippian period art and iconography. In: Reilly, F.K.III and Garber, J. (eds.) *Ancient objects and sacred realms*. University of Texas Press: Austin. 56-106.

Brown, J.A. and Dye, D.H. 2007. Severed heads and sacred scalplocks. In: Chacon, R.J. and Dye, D.H. (eds.) *The taking and displaying of human body parts by Amerindians*. Springer Verlag: Berlin. 278-298.

Buikstra, J.E. and Cook, D.C. 1981. Pre-Columbian tuberculosis in west-central Illinois: prehistoric disease in biocultural perspective. In: Buikstra, J E. (ed.) *Prehistoric tuberculosis in the Americas*. Scientific Papers No. 5, Northwestern University Archaeological Program. Department of Anthropology, Northwestern University: Evanston. 115-139.

Buikstra, J.E. and Williams, S. 1991. Tuberculosis in the Americas: current perspectives. In: Aufderheide, A.C. and Ortner, D.J. (eds.) *Human paleopathology: current syntheses and future options*. Smithsonian Institution Press: Washington, D.C. 161-172.

Duncan, J.R. and Diaz-Granados, C. 2000. Of masks and myths. *Midcontinental Journal of Archaeology* 25:1-26.

Emerson, T.E. 1997. *Cahokia and the archaeology of power*. University of Alabama Press: Tuscaloosa.

Fletcher, R. 1978. *In a country churchyard*. Granada Publishing: London.

Fowler, M. 1997. *The Cahokia atlas. A historical atlas of Cahokia archaeology*. Revised edition. University of Illinois Studies in Archaeology, Number 2. University of Illinois Press: Urbana.

Fowler, M.L., Rose, J., Vander Leest, B. and Ahler, S.R. 1999. *The Mound 72 area: dedicated and sacred space in early Cahokia* Reports of Investigation, Number 54. Illinois State Museum: Springfield.

Goldstein, L.G. and Richards, J.D. 2000. Ancient Aztalan: the cultural and ecological context of a late prehistoric site in the Midwest. In: Emerson, T.E. and Lewis, R.B. (eds.) *Cahokia and the hinterlands: middle Mississippian cultures of the Midwest*. University of Illinois Press. Urbana. 193-206.

Gregg, M.L. 1975. A population estimate for Cahokia. In: Brown, J.A. (ed.) *Perspectives in Cahokia archaeology*. Illinois Archaeological Survey Bulletin 10. Illinois Archaeological Survey: Urbana. 126-136.

Hall, R.L. 2000. Cahokia identity and interaction models of Cahokia Mississippian. In: Emerson, T.E. and Lewis, R.B. (eds.) *Cahokia and the hinterlands. middle Mississippian cultures of the Midwest*. University of Illinois Press: Urbana. 3-34.

Joyce, R.A. 2001. Burying the dead at Tlatilco: social memory and social identities. In: Chesson, M.S. (ed.) *Social memory, identity and death: anthropological perspectives on mortuary rituals*. Archaeological Papers of the American Anthropological Association Number 10. American Anthropological Association: Washington D.C. 12-26.

Maher, R.F. 1958. The excavation and reconstruction of the southwest pyramidal mound at Aztalan. *The Wisconsin Archeologist* 39: 77-101.

Milner, G.R. 1984. Social and temporal implications of variation among American bottom Mississippian cemeteries. *American Antiquity* 49: 468-488.

Parker Pearson, M. 1999. *The archaeology of death and burial*. Texas A&M University Press: College Station.

Pauketat, T.R. 2004. *Ancient Cahokia and the Mississippians*. Cambridge University Press: Cambridge.

Pauketat, T.R. and Bernard, N.S. 2004. *Cahokia mounds*. Oxford University Press: Oxford.

Pauketat, T.R., Kelly, L.S. Fritz, G.J. Lopinot, N.H. Elias, S. and Hargrave, E. 2002. The residues of feasting and public ritual at early Cahokia. *American Antiquity* 67: 257-279.

Price, T.D., Burton, J.H. and Stoltman, J.B. 2007. Place of origin of prehistoric inhabitants of Aztalan, Jefferson County, Wisconsin. *American Antiquity* 72: 524-538.

Radin, P. 1948. *Winnebago hero cycles: a study in Aboriginal literature*. Indiana University Press: Bloomington.

Roberts, C.A. and Buikstra, J.E. 2003. *The Bioarchaeology of tuberculosis: a global view on a reemerging disease*. University of Florida Press: Gainesville.

Rowe, C. 1958. A crematorium at Aztalan. *The Wisconsin Archeologist* 39: 101-110.

Scarry, C.M. 1993. Variability in Mississippian crop production strategies. In: Scarry, M.C. (ed.) *Farmers and foragers in the eastern Woodlands*. University of Florida Press: Gainesville. 78-90.

Sullivan, N.C. 1985. Tuberculosis in a late Woodland effigy mound population. *The Wisconsin Archeologist* 66: 71-76.

Sullivan, N.C. 1990. The biological consequences of the Mississippian expansion into the western Great Lakes region: a study of prehistoric culture contact. In: Nelson, S.M. and Kehoe, A.B. (eds.) *Powers of observation: alternative views in archeology*. Archeological Papers of the American Anthropological Association, Number 2. American Anthropological Association: Washington D.C. 73-87.

Waring, A.J. and Holder, P. 1945. A prehistoric ceremonial complex in the Southeastern United States. *American Anthropologist* 47: 1-34.

Wittry, W. 1969. Discovering and interpreting the Cahokia woodhenges. *The Wisconsin Archeologist* 77: 26-35.

Young, B.W. and Fowler, M.L. 2000. *Cahokia: the great American metropolis*. University of Illinois Press: Urbana.

# Stature of Males Interred with Weapons in Early Medieval England

Simon Mays

English Heritage
Fort Cumberland, Eastney
Portsmouth, PO4 9LD

Email for correspondence: simon.mays@english-heritage.org.uk

**Abstract**
In the early 5th century AD, Britain ceased to be part of the Roman Empire. This led to profound changes in social, economic and cultural life. These changes were mediated by an influx of Germanic migrants from continental Europe, although the scale and nature of this migration are unclear. In the 1990s, Heinrich Härke argued that, in 5th-7th century burials from England, stature was greater in males interred with weapons, and this was likely due to them being of continental Germanic, as opposed to native British descent. Although innovative in approach, Härke's work has been criticised for its lack of statistical analysis and for its uncritical use of osteological data culled from bone reports. The current work reanalyses skeletal remains from early medieval burials with weapons. The aim is to determine whether they do have a significantly higher than average stature, and if so whether this could be due to them being of continental Germanic descent or whether other explanations are more likely. Stature and stress indicators are recorded in 70 skeletons from 16 English 5th-7th century cemeteries. Results confirm that males with weapons are taller than average stature in England for the period, but they are also taller than mean stature for continental early medieval populations. They do not show any indication of reduced levels of childhood stress, as might be expected if their taller stature reflected favourable growth conditions. If males with weapons are of continental Germanic descent, then they were not drawn randomly from their parent populations as regards stature.

**Keywords**: Anglo-Saxon, Palaeopathology, Osteometry, Stress Indicators, Germanic

## Introduction

The withdrawal of the Roman presence in Britain in the early 5th century AD precipitated profound changes in social, economic and cultural life. These changes were mediated by an influx of migrants from mainland Europe, principally from what is now north Germany, into England, although the nature and scale of this migration continue to be debated (Higham 1992; Hammerow 1997; Hooke 1997; Weale *et al.* 2002; Hills 2003; Thomas *et al.* 2006; Härke 2007). Among these changes were the way in which the dead were buried. In the late Romano-British period, the normative rite was extended unaccompanied inhumation. In the succeeding early medieval period, from the 5th century onward, in most of England burial practices changed to resemble those in continental north-west Europe. Both cremation and inhumation were used, and people were often buried with grave goods, practices which continued until the 7th or 8th century. The number and type of grave goods varies widely from burial to burial, presumably reflecting, at least to some extent, the social position of the deceased. In addition, deposition of many of the more elaborate metalwork items appears to be linked to the sex of the individual. Weapons of war are normally found with males, jewellery and items of personal adornment, such as brooches, are normally found with females (Lucy 2000).

In a series of papers, Härke (1990; 1992; 1997; 2005) investigated the male weapon burial rite at English cemetery sites using both artifactual and osteological data, the latter culled from site osteological reports. The weapons in these burials comprise (in descending order of frequency) spear, shield, sword, seax (a short, single-edged sword), axe and arrows. These are found in a minority of male burials, so aspects other than simply the sex of the deceased must have affected decisions concerning their deposition in the grave. One factor appears to be social status, as burials with weapons are also generally richer in other grave goods than those without. However, Härke felt it unlikely that they signified a warrior elite. Weapons are sometimes found with juvenile individuals too young to have been warriors. Härke also found that neither the prevalence of healed fractures, nor weapon trauma, were elevated in burials with weapons. He argued that interment with weapons more likely symbolised some other aspect of male social persona. Looking at burials from seven English cemetery sites dating to the 5th-7th century AD, Härke found that mean stature was about 2cm greater in males with weapons. A 7th-8th century site failed to show a difference, leading Härke to suggest that the stature differential broke down during the 7th century. Chiefly because rates of dental enamel hypoplasias appeared similar in males interred with and without weapons, he felt that the higher stature in the former probably did not reflect more favourable conditions in the growth period. Noting that the weapon rite in England follows existing Germanic burial styles in continental Europe, and that English 5th-7th century males are taller than their Romano-British predecessors, Härke suggested that the higher stature in burials with weapons is indicative of ethnic Germanic (as opposed to native British) descent. Burial with weapons of war was thus inferred to be a signifier of affilitation to a foreign, culturally dominant group in multi-ethnic Dark Age England.

A number of criticisms may be levelled at Härke's analysis. It is unclear whether the stature differences he observed are statistically valid. There are also problems with his use of osteological data taken from site reports. For example, due to the high degree of subjectivity in scoring of gross dental enamel hypoplasias, it is not possible to compare data on their frequencies between different authors. His analysis of traumatic lesions takes no account of confounding factors such as differential skeletal survival. Nevertheless, the biocultural approach used was innovative for its time, and is directed at a compelling aspect of early medieval burial archaeology.

The aims of the current work are to shed further light on the relationship between early medieval male burials with weapons and stature. Specifically, attempts will be made to determine whether males with weapons have significantly higher estimated statures than the male mean for the period, and systematic analysis of some childhood stress indicators and skeletal trauma will be undertaken to determine their relative levels in burials with weapons. The overall aim is to determine whether Anglo-Saxon males buried with weapons were tall for the period, and if so to try and shed light on whether this is more likely due to differences in nutrition during childhood or whether they are likely to reflect Germanic ethnicity as suggested by Härke. Analysis of richly furnished female burials will also be conducted to investigate whether there is any patterning that resembles that seen in the male burials.

**Materials and Methods**

The study material comprises 70 burials from 16 cemeteries from England dating from the late 5th-late 7th century AD (Fig. 1). Numbers range from 1 to 12 burials from each site. This data set is different to that which formed the basis for Härke's work. The burials used were selected for a study whose aim was to evaluate artifact-based burial chronologies using high-precision radiocarbon dating (Scull and Bayliss 1999; Bayliss *et al.* in press), as well as investigating biocultural aspects of early medieval populations. The burials were selected on the basis of the artifacts they contain: weapons for males, items of personal adornment (principally brooches and beads) for females. This material is well-suited to the purposes of the current study. Firstly, it is unselected on the basis of osteological criteria. Secondly, the rich grave goods of the burials mean that they are likely to represent higher status members of early medieval society; this enables comparison between high status males and females. Thirdly, the existence of radiocarbon dates for each burial enables tight chronological control.

All burials were adult (aged approximately 18+ years). Sex was determined using dimorphic aspects of the pelvis and skull (Brothwell 1981). Stature was estimated from long-bone lengths, using the formulae of Trotter and Gleser (1952, 1958, 1977). In order to evaluate evidence for nutritional stress and disease during the growth period, dental enamel hypoplasias and porotic hyperostosis of the orbital roofs (cribra orbitalia) were recorded. The presence of skeletal injuries was also noted.

Dental enamel hypoplasias most often present as depressed transverse bands on the enamel tooth crown. They represent disturbances of enamel formation, generally as a result of disease or poor nutrition (Goodman and Rose 1990). Dental enamel hypoplasias are more often seen on anterior teeth than on premolars or molars (Goodman and Armelagos 1985). In the current material they were recorded, on a presence-absence basis, in the anterior dentition only. Teeth were examined visually, no attempt was made to study microscopic defects. The anterior dentition potentially records defects which formed when the individual was between about 1 and 6 years old (Reid and Dean 2006).

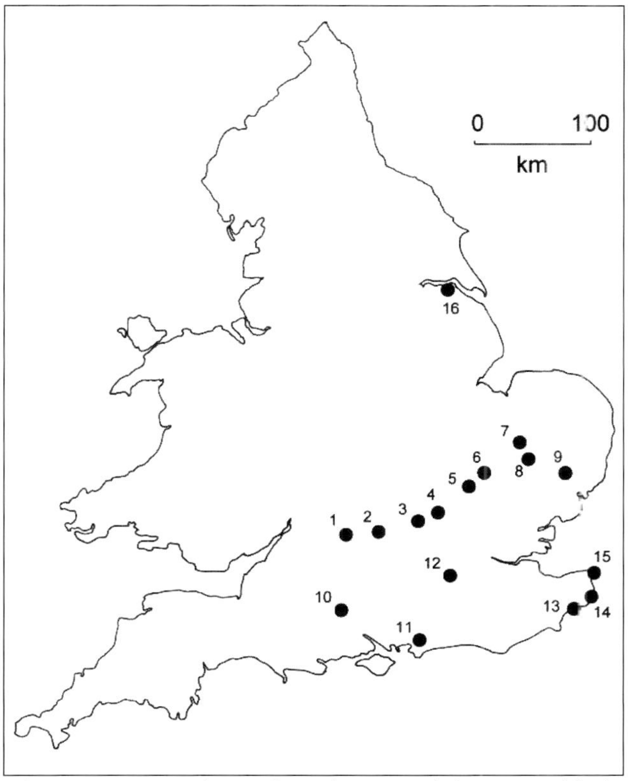


**Figure 1**: Location of study material. 1, Lechlade Butler's Field; 2, Berinsfield; 3, Tring Hill Aston Clinton; 4, Dunstable Marina Drive; 5, Melbourn Water Lane; 6, Barrington Edix Hill; 7, Lakenheath Eriswell; 8, Westgarth Gardens; 9, Coddenham; 10, Ford Laverstock; 11, Apple Down Compton; 12, Gally Hills Banstead Down; 13, Dover Buckland; 14, Mill Hill Deal; 15, St Peter's Tip Broadstairs; 16, Castledyke South.

Porotic hyperostosis may arise due to a number of conditions, but when there is overgrowth of the diploe with thinning of the outer table it appears to represent a response to anaemia, most probably megaloblastic (Walker *et al.* 2009) or iron deficiency (Moseley 1965; Stuart-Macadam 1989) anaemia, the diploic hyperplasia being an effort to combat anaemia by raising erythrocyte production. Potential causes of anaemia include parasitic or other gut infections, and dietary deficiencies (Moseley 1965; Stuart-Macadam 1989). In adulthood, a need for increased erythropoiesis is usually met by reconversion of yellow to red marrow so there is normally no hyperplasia of the marrow space. Hence lesions indicative of anaemia seen in adult skeletons are usually thought to be relics of childhood disease (Stuart-Macadam 1985). The precise period of childhood during which an individual is most likely to sustain lesions that persist into adult life is unclear. However, given the rapid growth in the orbital region characteristic of the early years of life (Humphrey 1998), lesions occurring during this period would likely be obliterated by remodelling, so that those changes present in adult skeletons may mainly represent disease occurring in later childhood. Care was taken to distinguish lesions due to anaemia from those due to other conditions, such as scurvy, which do not cause diploic hypertrophy (Ortner 2003: 275). Porotic hyperostosis in the orbital roofs was scored on a presence – absence basis in individuals with one or both orbital roofs preserved.

**Results**

In the study material there are a total of 33 males with weapons and 37 female burials. The summary statistics for stature are presented in Table 1.

The mean stature for the females in the current study (161.3cm) closely resembles the mean stature for the period (Table 1), suggesting that females buried with rich items of personal adornment were not taller than average. However, the male figure (176.7cm) differs significantly (t=3.88, p=0.001) from the overall male mean for the period of 172cm (Table 1). One possible explanation for the high male stature observed is that the males measured for stature in the current group simply happened to come from communities where male stature was greater than average for the period. Ten of the male burials measured for stature come from sites with large numbers of burials and for which the extant osteological report provides mean male stature values estimated using identical methods to those in the current work: Barrington Edix Hill (Duhig 1998), Berinsfield (Harman 1995), Castledyke South (Boylston *et al.* 1998) and Lechlade Butler's Field (Harman 1998). Of these 10 individuals, 9 show stature figures greater than the male mean for the site from which they come, a statistically significant imbalance (chi-square=6.4, p<0.02). This would seem to suggest that the burials with weapons in the current work are not only tall compared with the average stature for the period but also in comparison with the average for their communities.

The median radiocarbon dates for the male burials range from 499-659 AD (Bayliss *et al.* in press). There was no significant correlation between median radiocarbon date and male stature (r=0.004).

**Table 1**: Estimated stature (cm) of males and females in the current study material, with comparative data.

| | | Current data | | Comparative data | |
|---|---|---|---|---|---|
| | N | Mean | Sd | Pooled 5th-7th century English mean stature[1] | Pooled 5th-11th century British mean stature[2] |
| Males | 17 | 176.7 | 5.0 | 172.1 | 172 |
| Females | 26 | 161.3 | 6.3 | 160.8 | 161 |

[1]Data from Hirst and Clark (2009: Table 55); comprises osteological reports on 51 sites, 11 of which also yielded skeletal material examined for the current work. Sites are cemeteries with Germanic style grave goods, N=548 males, 481 females.

[2]Data from Roberts and Cox (2003: Table 8.1); comprises burials from an unspecified number of British sites dating from 5th-11th century AD, N=996 males, 751 females.

The data for dental enamel hypoplasias and cribra orbitalia are given in Table 2. If the males in the current study group were taller than average because of favourable conditions during childhood then one might expect them to show lower levels of dental enamel hypoplasias and porotic hyperostosis than the females, who were not taller than average for the period. Although the frequencies of these stress indicators is somewhat higher in the females than the males, there is no statistically valid difference between them (dental enamel hypoplasia, chi-square (Yates' continuity correction) = 0.84, p=0.36; porotic hyperostosis chi-square=0.64, p=0.43).

**Table 2**: Prevalence of dental enamel hypoplasia and porotic hyperostosis in the current study material

| | Dental enamel hypoplasia | Porotic hyperostosis |
|---|---|---|
| Males | 2/28 (7%) | 4/23 (17%) |
| Females | 5/26 (19%) | 7/26 (27%) |

The overall prevalence of healed fractures among the burials with weapons was similar to that in the female burials (4/33 (12%) of burials with weapons showed a fracture (5/2105 bones examined) compared to 6/37 (16%) of women (7/3363 bones examined)). With the possible exception of one male burial from Barrington Edix Hill (Duhig 1998: 182-183), none of the current study sample shows evidence for blade injury, and none of the other injuries can be clearly attributed to interpersonal violence rather than accidental trauma.

## Discussion

The current results offer statistical support for Härke's contention that male burials with weapons have higher than average stature. The dating evidence provides no support for Härke's suggestion that stature differential of burials with weapons broke down in the 7th century.

At a population level, adult stature is an indicator of conditions during the growth period, favourable conditions being associated with increased stature (Tanner 1989: 161). It seems likely that the presence of weapons as grave goods indicates an elevated social status because burials with weapons are generally richer in grave goods than burials without weapons (Härke 1990). If this social status was ascribed at birth, then the social subgroup signified by burial with weapons may have had better living conditions in infancy and childhood and hence have attained higher than average stature. However, the data on dental enamel hypoplasias and cribra orbitalia offer no evidence that childhood conditions were more favourable for the male burials with weapons than in a group of females who were not taller than average for the period. The current work therefore provides no evidence that the tall stature of the males accompanied by weapons was due to particularly favourable conditions during the growth period.

A second possibility is that, if the presence of weapons as grave goods indicated a warrior, or some other social role for which an imposing physique might be advantageous, then taller adults might be selected for this social position or may more often have achieved this, or taller juveniles might preferentially be selected as candidates for such a role in future. These taller members of society may be so because of genetic factors (they came from tall families) and / or because they enjoyed better conditions during childhood. It is difficult to evaluate this hypothesis fully using the current data, however it is worth noting that the data on trauma suggest that whatever male role is signified by burial with weapons, there is no evidence that it exposed individuals to an elevated risk of skeletal injury. This may be consistent with Härke's idea that burial with weapons did not normally signify active warrior status.

There remains the hypothesis that the inclusion of weapons as grave furnishings served as identifiers of individuals of Germanic origin and that is the reason for their tall stature. For this explanation to be viable, the Germanic migrants would need to have been taller than the native British. Drawing on data presented by Harman *et al.* (1981) and Wells (1969), Härke (1990) suggested that there was a stature increase between the Romano-British and the early medieval periods, which might be consistent with this. Subsequent larger-scale surveys of stature in early British populations seem to confirm this pattern. For example, Roberts and Cox (2003: Table 8.1), using data from 2292 males and 1793 females, document a stature increase from the Roman to the early medieval period in both sexes. However, Roberts and Cox also demonstrate fluctuations in mean values between other archaeological periods when it would be naive to ascribe them to arrival of taller or shorter invaders. The stature increase between Romano-British and early medieval periods in Britain is not therefore compelling evidence of an influx from a taller foreign population, and indeed Roberts and Cox (2003: 396) suggest that it may reflect health benefits of a more dispersed settlement pattern in the latter period.

Another approach to investigating whether continental migrants to England were of greater stature would be to compare them with interments from 'native British' burial grounds of similar date. Some 5$^{th}$-8$^{th}$ century cemeteries in western England lack distinctive Germanic burial practices and grave goods. They may arguably represent indigenous communities outside the apparent core area of Anglo-Saxon settlement. Pooled stature data from three such sites with large numbers of burials (Ulwell, Dorset (Waldron 1988) and Cannington (Brothwell *et al.* 2000) and Henley Wood, Yatton (Bayley 1974), both Somerset, giving a total of 102 males, 117 females) yields a male mean of 168.3cm and a female mean of 162.8cm. The male stature from these west of England sites is less than that of the burials with weapons examined in the current work ($t=6.95$, $p<0.0001$); there is no significant difference in female stature between these sites and the current work. The stature of the males in these western England sites is approximately 4cm less than the mean given for males from early medieval English cemeteries with Germanic grave goods by Hirst and Clark (2009), but as standard deviations are not available for the pooled data, the statistical significance of this difference cannot be assessed. These results may support the idea of taller immigrant males coming into England during the early medieval period. However this interpretation is dependent upon the assumption that the western England cemeteries lacking typical Germanic grave goods and burial practices represent indigenous British communities. Given the complex array of factors that may influence mortuary treatment, of which ethnicity is but one, this assumption may be simplistic.

It is unclear whether mean male stature was greater in continental Germanic populations than those from England during the early medieval period. Collation of osteological data from ten 5$^{th}$-8$^{th}$ century cemeteries from western Germany (Hauschild 1925; Bach 1986; Altmann 2006), gives pooled stature figures of 171.0cm for males (N=546) and 161.1cm for females (N=384). These are similar to figures cited above from early medieval England. Reviewing the osteological evidence up to 1968, Huber (1968) concluded that early medieval populations from northern Europe should be regarded as a homogenous group as far as stature was concerned; there seems little reason to revise that conclusion. The stature of the male burials with weapons in the current study is significantly greater than that of the mean male figure for the continental Germanic cemeteries in the above studies ($t=4.71$, $p<0.001$). Therefore, if the English burials with weapons were of Germanic stock, this would imply that migrants were not randomly drawn from continental populations with regard to stature, but that they were taller than average for continental communities.

Some studies of skeletal material from early medieval Germany also appear to show differences in stature among males according to whether they were buried with weapons, or otherwise according to social rank. Straub (1956) and Czarnetzki *et al.* (1985) found stature differences by social rank in some cemeteries in south-west Germany, those of inferred higher rank being taller. Also looking at south-west German material, Huber (1968) divided male burials into 'heavily armed', 'lightly armed' and 'unarmed', and found that the heavily armed group were the tallest, the unarmed the shortest, with the lightly armed occupying an intermediate position. However, it is unclear whether the patterns identified by these authors were statistically significant.

One scenario that has been suggested for the coming of the Germanic migrants is that it was elite male social groups that migrated from their continental homelands to England (discussion in Higham 1992 and Hills 2003). If, as Härke claimed, the English burials with weapons were of Germanic stock, then the tall stature of the burials with weapons relative to both continental and other English burials might be consistent with a model of elite migration. We would still need to explain why elite females are not taller than average as well (even if migrants were mainly males, they would have passed their genes onto offspring of both sexes) but perhaps females' ethnic status was not identified by deposition of rich grave goods. Alternatively, it may be that in continental Europe and in Britain, wealthier social groups (or at least their male members) simply had better living conditions and tended to be taller for that reason rather than any ethnic difference. Against this, the current work provided no evidence for reduced levels of stress markers in male burials with weapons, as might be expected if their tall stature reflected favourable conditions in the growth period. However, the statistical power to detect patterning in this data was limited by small sample sizes.

## Conclusions

The current work provides statistical support for the idea that, in England, early medieval males buried with weapons of war were taller than average for the period. Härke (1990) has previously suggested that burials with weapons are of ethnic Germanic stock, and were taller for this reason. The current work suggests that they are also taller than average for continental Germanic groups, so if they were of Germanic descent it would appear that migrants were not randomly drawn from their parent populations as regards stature. If Härke's (1990) contention that the burials with weapons are of migrant stock is correct, then the migration to England may have been mainly of those of elite social status. Whatever roles were signified by interment with weapons, there is no evidence that they were connected with increased risk of physical injury.

Due to the limited sample size, the current work should be considered a pilot study. It would be useful to assess more fully the osteological status of burials with weapons in early medieval England using larger sample sizes. In particular, it would be useful to obtain systematic data on stress indicators and on cranial and post-cranial skeletal morphology in order to determine whether burials with weapons differ from other burials in health and nutrition during childhood, activity patterns, and in aspects of skeletal morphology that might imply genetic distinctiveness. Comparison with skeletal material from continental Germanic populations, and perhaps with that from British early medieval cemeteries lacking Germanic-style grave goods, would also be useful. This work would require re-analysis of skeletal remains; data in osteological site reports is unsuited to such a purpose as they have not been gathered to address these specific questions, and there are difficulties in pooling data which has been gathered by different authors using different methodologies.

## Acknowledgements

Thanks are due to Alex Bayliss for permitting access to the radiocarbon dates for the burials in the current work in advance of their full dissemination. I am also grateful to delegates at the 2010 BABAO meeting for useful discussion. Thanks also due to Chris Knüsel and to two anonymous reviewers whose insightful comments have improved this manuscript.

## Literature Cited

Altmann, S. 2006. Das merowingerzeitliche Gräberfeld von Dachwig, Lkr Gotha. *Alt-Thüringen* 39: 145-176.

Bach, A. 1986. *Germanen-Slawen-Deutche. Anthropologische bearbeitung des frühmittelalterlichen Gräberfeldes von Rohrstedt, Kreis Sonderhausen.* Weimar Monographien zur ur- und frühgeschichte. Museum für ur- und frühgeschichte Thüringens: Weimar.

Bayley, J. 1974. *Henley Wood, Yatton, Somerset, human bone*. AML Report 1635. English Heritage: Portsmouth.

Bayliss, A., Hines, J., Nielsen, K.H., McCormac, G. and Scull, C. in press. *Anglo-Saxon graves and grave goods of the sixth and seventh centuries AD: a chronological framework*. Society for Medieval Archaeology Monograph. Maney: Leeds.

Boylston, A., Wiggins, R. and Roberts, C. 1998. Human skeletal remains. In: Drinkall, G. and Foreman, M. (eds.) *The Anglo-Saxon cemetery at Castledyke South, Barton-on-Humber*. Sheffield Academic Press: Sheffield. Sheffield Excavation Reports No. 6. 221-236.

Brothwell, D.R. 1981. *Digging up bones* (3rd edition). Oxford University Press/British Museum (Natural History): Oxford.

Brothwell, D.R., Powers, R., Hirst, S.M., Wright, S.M. and Gauthier, S. 2000. The human biology. In: Rahtz, P., Hirst, S. and Wright, SM. (eds.) *Cannington cemetery. Excavations 1962-3 of Prehistoric, Roman, Post-Roman and later features at Cannington Park Quarry, Near Bridgwater, Somerset*. Society for the Promotion of Roman Studies: London. Britannia Monograph Series No. 17. 131-256.

Czarnetzki, A., Uhlig, C. and Wolf, R. 1985. *Menschen des frühen Mittelalters im Spiegel der Anthropologie und Medizin*. Speyer: Munich.

Duhig, C. 1998. The human skeletal material. In: Malim, T. and Hines, J. (eds.) *The Anglo-Saxon cemetery at Edix Hill (Barrington A), Cambridgeshire*. Council for British Archaeology: York. Council for British Archaeology Research Report 112. 154-199.

Goodman, A.H. and Armelagos, G.J. 1985. Factors affecting the distribution of enamel hypoplasias within the human permanent dentition. *American Journal of Physical Anthropology* 68: 479–493.

Goodman, A.H. and Rose, J.C. 1990. Assessment of systemic physiological perturbations from dental enamel hypoplasias and associated histological structures. *Yearbook of Physical Anthropology* 33: 59–110.

Hammerow, H. 1997. Migration theory and the Anglo-Saxon 'identity crisis'. In: Chapman, J. and Hammerow, H. (eds.) *Migrations and invasions in archaeological explanation*. Archaeopress, Oxford. British Archaeological Reports, International Series No. 664. 33-44.

Härke, H. 1990. "Warrior graves"? The background of the Anglo-Saxon weapon burial rite. *Past and Present* 126: 22-43.

Härke, H. 1992. Changing symbols in a changing society: the Anglo-Saxon weapon burial rite in the 7th century. In: Carver, M.O.H. (ed.) *The Age of Sutton Hoo*. Boydell: Woodbridge. 149-165.

Härke, H. 1997. Early Anglo-Saxon social structure. In: Hines, J. (ed.) *The Anglo-Saxons from the migration period to the eighth century*. Boydell: Woodbridge. 125-170.

Härke, H. 2005. The Anglo-Saxon weapon burial rite: an interdisciplinary analysis. *Opus* 3: 197-207

Härke, H. 2007. Ethnicity, race and migration in mortuary archaeology: an attempt at a short answer. In: Semple, S. and Williams, H. (eds) *Early medieval mortuary practices*. University of Oxford School of Archaeology: Oxford. Anglo-Saxon Studies in Archaeology and History No. 14. 12-18.

Harman, M. 1995. The human bones. In: Boyle, A., Dodd, A., Miles, D. and Mudd, A. (ed.) *Two Oxfordshire Anglo-Saxon cemeteries: Berinsfield and Didcot*. Oxford Archaeological Unit: Oxford. Thames Valley Landscapes Monograph No. 8. 106-108.

Harman, M. 1998. The human remains. In: Boyle, A., Jennings, D., Miles, D. and Palmer, S. (ed.) *The Anglo-Saxon cemetery at Butler's Field, Lechlade, Gloucestershire*. Oxford Archaeological Unit: Oxford. Thames Valley Landscapes Monograph No. 10. 43-52.

Harman, M., Molleson, T.I. and Price, J.L. 1981. Burials, bodies and beheadings in Romano-British and Anglo-Saxon cemeteries. *Bulletin of the British Museum of Natural History* 35: 145–188.

Hauschild, M.W. 1925. Die menschlichen Skelettfunde des Gräberfeldes von Anderten, bei Hannover. *Zeitschrift für Morphologie und Anthropologie* 25: 221-241.

Higham, N. 1992. *Rome, Britain and the Anglo-Saxons*. Seaby: London.

Hills, C. 2003. *Origins of the English*. Duckworth: London.

Hirst, S. and Clark, D. 2009. *Excavations at Mucking. Volume 3: the Anglo-Saxon cemeteries*. Museum of London Archaeology: London.

Hooke, D. 1997. The Anglo-Saxons in England in the seventh and eighth centuries: aspects of location in space. In: Hines, J. (ed.) *The Anglo-Saxons from the migration period to the eighth century*. Boydell: Woodbridge. 65-99.

Huber, N.M. 1968. The problem of stature increase: looking from the past to the present. In: Brothwell, D.R. (ed) *The Skeletal Biology of Earlier Human Populations*. Pergamon: Oxford. 67-102.

Humphrey, L.T. 1998. Growth patterns in the modern human skeleton. *American Journal of Physical Anthropology* 105: 57-72.

Lucy, S. 2000. *The Anglo-Saxon way of death.* Sutton: Stroud.

Moseley, J.E. 1965. The paleopathological riddle of "symmetrical osteoporosis". *American Journal of Roentgenology* 95: 135-142.

Ortner, D.J. 2003. *Identification of pathological conditions in human skeletal remains.* Academic Press: London.

Reid, D.J. and Dean, M.C. 2006. Variation in modern human enamel formation times. *Journal of Human Evolution* 50: 329-346.

Roberts, C. and Cox, M. 2003. *Health and disease in Britain from prehistory to the present day.* Sutton: Stroud.

Scull, C. and Bayliss, A. 1999. Radiocarbon dating and Anglo-Saxon graves. In: von Freeden, U., Koch, U. and Wieczorek, A. (eds.) *Völker an Nord- und Ostsee und die Franken: Akten des 48 Sachsensymposiums in Mannheim vom 7 bis 11 September 1997.* Manheimer Geschichtsblätter, Beiheft 2, Neue Folge. Rudolf Habelt: Berlin. 39-50.

Straub, R. 1956. Zur Kontinuität der voralamannischen Bevölkerungen. *Badische Fundberichte* 20: 127-137.

Stuart-Macadam, P. 1985. Porotic hyperostosis: representative of a childhood condition. *American Journal of Physical Anthropology* 66: 391–398.

Stuart-Macadam, P. 1989. Porotic hyperostosis: relationship between orbital and vault lesions. *American Journal of Physical Anthropology* 80: 187-193.

Tanner JM. 1989. *Foetus into man* (2nd edition). Castlemead: Ware.

Thomas, M.G., Stumpf, M.P.H. and Härke, H. 2006. Evidence for an apartheid-like social structure in Anglo-Saxon England. *Proceedings of the Royal Society of London Series B* 273: 2651-2657.

Trotter, M. and Gleser, G.C. 1952. Estimation of stature from long-bones of American Whites and Negroes. *American Journal of Physical Anthropology* 10: 463–514.

Trotter, M. and Gleser, G.C. 1958. A re-evaluation of estimation of stature based on measurements of stature taken during life and of long-bones after death. *American Journal of Physical Anthropology* 16: 79–123.

Trotter, M. and Gleser, G.C. 1977. Corrigenda to "estimation of stature from long-bones of American Whites and Negroes", American Journal of Physical Anthropology (1952). *American Journal of Physical Anthropology* 47: 355-356.

Waldron, T. 1988. The human bone. In: Cox, P.W. (ed.) A seventh-century inhumation cemetery at Shepherd's Farm, Ulwell, near Swanage, Dorset. *Proceedings of the Dorset Natural History and Archaeology Society* 110: 37-48.

Walker, P.L., Bathurst, R.R., Richman, R., Gjerdrum, T. and Andrushko, V.A. 2009. The causes of porotic hyperostosis and cribra orbitalia: a reappraisal of the iron-deficiency-anemia hypothesis. *American Journal of Physical Anthropology* 139: 109-125.

Weale, M.E, Weiss, D.A., Jager, R.F., Bradman, N. and Thomas, M.G. 2002. Y chromosome evidence for Anglo-Saxon mass migration. *Molecular Biology and Evolution* 19: 1008-1021.

Wells, L.H. 1969. Stature in earlier races of mankind. In: Brothwell, D. and Higgs, E. (eds.) *Science in Archaeology* (2nd edition). Thames and Hudson: London. 453-467.

# The Uses of Field Anthropology on the Excavation of the St-Rumbold Cemetery, Mechelen, Belgium

Katrien Van de Vijver

Physical Anthropologist, St. Rumbold Cemetery
City Council of Mechelen
Department of Archaeology
Pitzemburgstraat 8
2800 Mechelen
Belgium

Email for correspondence: katvdv83@hotmail.com

**Abstract**

With the increasing trend of rescue excavations and the limited time provided for archaeological excavations it is even more important that as much information as possible can be ascertained on the field. On the excavation of the cemetery of St.Rumbold in Mechelen, Belgium, it was attempted to reconcile the severe deadline with rigorous registration of the bones and their burial context. The principles of *Field Anthropology*, developed by Henri Duday in the 1970's, teaches us that the position and orientation of the different bones can tell us about the original position of the body and its context, which are subject to taphonomy. Since more than 4000 individuals were excavated on this site, this will hopefully provide us with a large, provenanced research collection, with information on the dynamics of Medieval and post-Medieval cemeteries, mortuary ritual and society. The methods provide an important contribution to the study of burials, even when the time provided is limited.

**Keywords**: Archaeothanatology, Medieval, Post Medieval, Taphonomy, Decomposition

## Introduction

As more and more excavations, including those of cemeteries, become rescue excavations with limited time-frames, it is important to develop methods that allow for a maximum of information to be collected on site. In November 2009 the city council of Mechelen ordered the rescue excavation of the North Cemetery of the St-Rumbold Cathedral, due to building plans for underground parking, which lasted 16 months. Based on preliminary research, 4000 burials were estimated to have been preserved within the limits of the construction pit. Because this was a unique opportunity to excavate a large amount of burials, dating from a period spanning over 800 years, *archaeothanatology,* the study of biological and social death, was used as an instrument to contribute to the study of the burials. Human remains are often merely collected on site, more attention is paid to the overall body position, grave inclusions and the architecture of the burial. The study of human remains should however begin *in situ*, and *l'antropologie du terrain* or *archaeothanatology,* was developed by Henri Duday in the 1970's, to offer new perspectives and methods (Duday 1990; Willis and Tayles 2009: 547). Through the meticulous determination and study of the exact position and orientation of the different bones, grave inclusions and architecture, and their spatial relation to each other, we can interpret their movement as the body decomposed, the original position of the bones and the characteristics of the burial context for mortuary analysis and taphonomic processes (Boddington 1987: 27-42; Brothwell 1987: 22-26; Duday 1990; Nillson Stuts 1998: 5-17; Duday 2006: 30-56; Nillson Stuts 2006: 217-233; Willis and Tayles 2009: 547).

The aim here is to demonstrate the use and potential of these principles and methods on any archaeological excavation with human remains, through examples from the rescue excavation of the St.Rumbold Cemetery, to deduce important additional information on original context and taphonomic history.

**Archaeothanatology**

The study of *l'antropologie du terrain* requires considerable knowledge of anatomy and the decomposition process. The different tissues in the body decompose at different rates and ligaments are of the last soft tissues to decompose. In the study of burials the preservation or loss of articulations of bones indicates the potential for movement. A distinction is made between labile and persistent articulations. Labile articulations, e.g. between hand bones, are rapidly lost and their preservation is often used to determine a primary deposit. Persistent articulations last longer and are present in joints which carry most biomechanical stress. There is no fixed schedule of the loss of the different articulations and their conservation depends, and can inform us, on the type and shape of the burial environment, soil matrix, original position, treatment of the body and later interaction (Duday 1990: 31-33; Maureille and Sellier 1996: 313-315; Duday 2006: 33-34; 2009: 25-30; Duday and Guillon 2006: 126-128). Boddington and Brothwell also commented on the uses for mortuary studies. The position of the different bones, their linearity or parallel-sided effect and their movements (bone tumble) can inform us on the original body position, information on the original burial context and possible later handling of the remains (Boddington 1987: 27-42; Brothwell 1987: 22-26).

Once articulations are lost, bones can move under the influence of gravity, sediment pressure, bioturbation, flotation by ground water or later interaction. Gravity can affect bones in existing open spaces or because new spaces appear through the decomposition of soft tissue, as and when articulations are lost. When the body is covered by sediment, the influx of soil will encapsulate the bones in their place (Duday 1990: 34-39; 2006: 34-35 and 40-43; Duday and Guillon 2006: 137-144; Duday 2009: 34-40 and 52-57). This depends on the soil matrix, in fine dry grained soil there is what Duday describes as the 'hour-glass effect', wherein open spaces are progressively filled in, inhibiting bone movement. The effect of all the bones held in place can only be achieved when the soil is in direct contact with the body and is therefore demonstration of a deposit made in plain earth. In clay or granular sediment, open spaces are longer preserved, allowing bones to fall within the internal space of the body. Some movement is however always evident and the current situation is a result of sediment pressure and the laws of gravity (Duday 2006: 41-42; Willis and Tayles 2009: 548-549).

The location and particular movements of the bones and the preservation or loss of articulations will indicate the original position of the body when gravity is the cause of movement. The type of context plays an important role, in a coffin or crypt there will be an open space in which gravity will cause unstable bones to move, such as hand or foot bones. In a plain earth burial bone movement will be prevented by the influx of soil. The shape of the pit or container will allow or inhibit movement, the so-called 'wall effect'. In a tight shroud or coffin, the strong lateral pressure will cause medial movement of the bones, with a strong linearity. The durability of the container is important, if it decomposes before all articulations are lost, sediment will enter the context and cause obstruction (Duday 1990: 39-42; 2006: 43-44; Duday and Guillon 2006: 131-133 and 137-146). The objects associated with the body will move in accordance to the same laws. Any objects or structures present in the burial which decompose at a later time than the soft tissues will cause particular movements of the disarticulated bones (Duday 2006: 40-43; Duday and Guillon 2006: 146).

Multiple burial in the same grave over a long period will lead to the disturbance of bones in older depositions, as opposed to when the time inbetween is too short or when there are layers of soil inbetween. Synchronous decomposition of bodies, placed on and next to each other, will lead to the formation of new open spaces in which the bones will fall (Duday 1990: 44-47; 2006: 48-52).

In secondary depositions the recording of the bones, their determination and position, will provide information on the deposition dynamic of the contexts, for example some ossuaries in the St. Rumbold cemetery consisted of stacked, ordered and selected long bones and crania (Fig.1), others were random depositions. In secondary depositions it is impossible to use the articulations to determine individuals. Bones are linked to an individual by fitting fragments, occasionally joints, age, pathological identification and pairing (Duday 2006: 51).

The application of field anthropological methods relies on anatomical and anthropological knowledge and meticulous recording. In an ideal situation every single element found on a site is recorded, with a large number of cleaning and recording phases, to record every element and object in 3D, with a description of identification, preservation, orientation, slope, side, anatomical

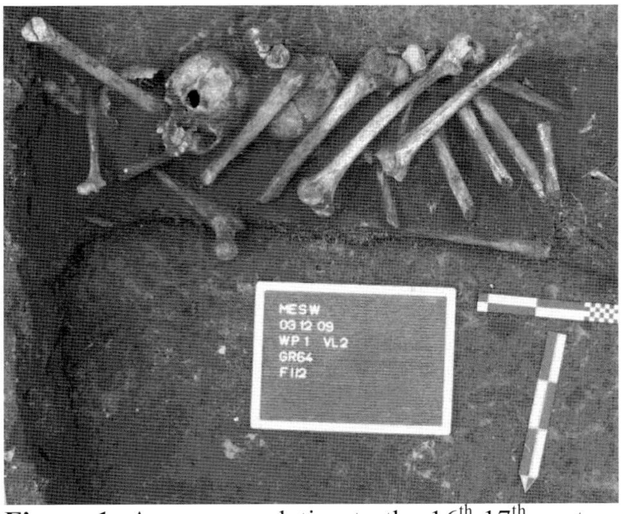

**Figure 1:** An ossuary dating to the 16th-17th century AD, with stacked and ordered long bones and crania, which suggest selection and deliberate deposition.

plane and level after removal (Duday and Guillon 2006: 120-125). Naturally the determination of the burial context also depends on the observation on site of the shape and nature of stratigraphical units, the presence of a linear association of coffin nails, traces of wood from the coffins, etc., but the osteological information may offer an important contribution to this research (Duday 1990: 30-31). The preservation or absence of anatomical articulations between bones, and their movement depends on the original body position, the burial context, whether plain earth burial, coffin or shroud, shape and size of the pit or container, the soil matrix, later intrusions and taphonomic processes (Boddington 1987: 27-42; Brothwell 1987: 22-26; Duday 1990; Nillson Stuts 1998: 5-17; Duday 2006: 30-56; Nillson Stuts 2006: 217-233; Willis and Tayles 2009: 547).

**St. Rumbold's Cemetery**

According to historical sources the cemetery of the Cathedral of St. Rumbold was in use as early as 1000 AD and was discontinued in 1785, as the result of an edict by the Holy Roman Emperor Joseph II banning *intramural* cemeteries. The site is also supposed to be the location of the 9th-century Merovingian Abbey and the 10th-century Chapter, the origins of the foundation of Mechelen. The discovery of several Karolingian (late 8th-10th century AD) objects in the oldest layers suggests that burial in this location could go as far back as the 9th century. These burials would have been located around the chapel that held the relics of St. Rumbold, also believed to have been near this location (Kinnaer unpublished; Goetstouwers 1956: 47-48; Installé 1996: 7-24; Van de Vijver *et al.* 2011: 120-122).

The site is located in what is now the city centre, at the north side of the Cathedral. The burials, which were relatively well preserved, were excavated in five arbitrary layers, which start at *c.* 6.30-6.20 metres above sea level, with the original soil at *c.* 4.60-4.50 metres. Although these are only preliminary dates, the upper layers (1 and 2) are dated in the 17th and 18th centuries AD, based on the material found in the layer and the grave cuts, and consist of dark brown, greyish sandy soil. Underneath these layers was a brownish soil of light loamy sand, dating to the 15th to 16th centuries AD. The layer immediately above the original soil consisted of a yellow-brown sand, with the original soil a yellow sand. The burials in these layers are preliminarily dated to the 12th to 14th century, although it is possible that radiocarbon-dating will provide older dates (Van de Vijver *et al.* 2011: 120-122).

The time provided for the excavation was extremely limited, but as this was an important opportunity to excavate burials with information on their context, a compromise between time constraints and scientific methods was made to retrieve as much information as possible. The team consisted of three archaeologists, one physical anthropologist and eight field technicians. The site was divided in four trenches which were excavated consecutively. Burials were excavated within the observable soil features to the level of the bones. A photograph was made in zenith, i.e. perpendicular to the context, to limit distortions, with geographical reference points to make up for the lack of detailed drawings. The outlines were plotted on a general plan of the site, to study spatial relations. The burials were recorded on a burial form, including information on orientation, position of the body, burial context, a preliminary inventory, age, sex, preservation, measurements, finds, levels and position and movement of the bones according to field anthropology. The methods of field anthropology described earlier represent an ideal situation, but archaeologists and anthropologists often deal with rescue excavations. Although it was impossible to excavate each individual burial in layers and each single bone separately, the position of the majority of the bones within an individual burial was recorded, with their identification and anatomical view and a preliminary interpretation and notes. This recording is useful as fragments can often not be determined on photographs and there was not enough time to clean the burials comprehensively. In the multiple burials, individuals were excavated in layers, so that each deposition is recorded separately. Ossuaries were excavated in layers, with identification and location of each element, to interpret the deposition dynamic.

Only the first trench, with 689 burials, could be sampled for abdominal content and on-site collection of aDNA samples. From the third trench onwards, it was unfortunately no longer possible to excavate the area comprehensively. More than 3600 burials were excavated, which as yet need to be studied more closely, but it was already clear on the field that using the principles of *archaeothanatology* provides much additional information, which will be demonstrated by examples.

## Application of the Methods of Archaeothanatology

Based on observations on site, preliminary distinctions can be made. The majority of the burials are single, primary depositions, buried in plain earth or in a coffin. For the burials in plain earth we can distinguish those buried without any wrapping, for example in burial GR920 (17$^{th}$-18$^{th}$ century AD), in which almost all articulations, including the hand bones, had been preserved (Fig.2). None of the bones seems to have encountered an obstruction. The ribs are in their original anatomical position, preserving the thoracic volume. No grave cut could be observed, but the particular preservation of the articulations indicates that soil entered the burial very soon and that the bones were in direct contact with the soil, while the lack of obstruction suggests a wide grave cut. The presence of wrapping can be indicated by strong lateral pressure and a delayed incursion of sediment. In burial GR3086, dating to the 15$^{th}$-16$^{th}$ century (Fig.3), which had no traces of a coffin delineation, this is clearly evident in the extreme lateral pressure on the bones, with the humeri almost touching. The bones of the axial skeleton were very eroded, but still in their anatomical position. This is an intriguing context, one possibility is that lateral pressure was already present at the time of deposition, with hyper medial rotation of the limbs and increased when the bones started to disarticulate. Another possibility is that the medial longitudinal part of the body caved in as the result of collapse of lower contexts in combination with the strong lateral pressure, although other theories should also be considered. Based on comparisons of a large number of data, it must be possible to deduce whether and in which burials the body was wrapped.

A very clear example of a coffin burial, is burial GR595, dating to the 12$^{th}$-13$^{th}$ century AD, in which a clear delineation could be observed on site (Fig.4).

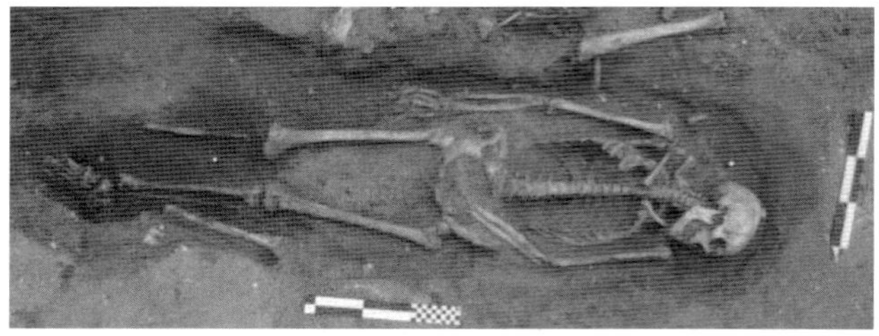

**Figure 2:** Burial GR920. Study of the bones indicated that almost all articulations had been preserved, including those of the labile joints, suggesting that this was a plain earth burial.

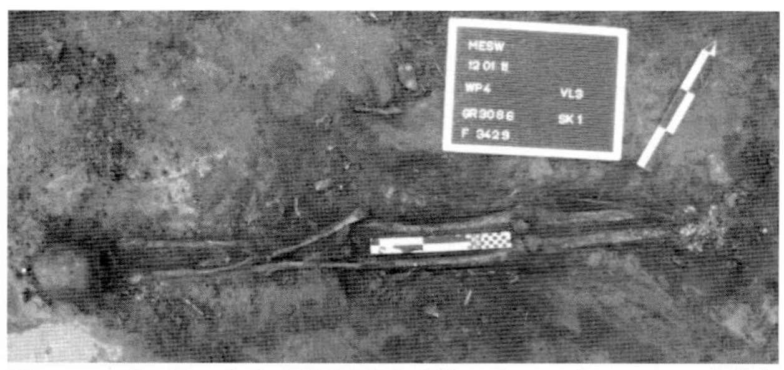

**Figure 3:** Burial GR3086. The long bones exhibit strong medial movement, suggesting severe lateral pressure. This could indicate a close wrapping of the body.

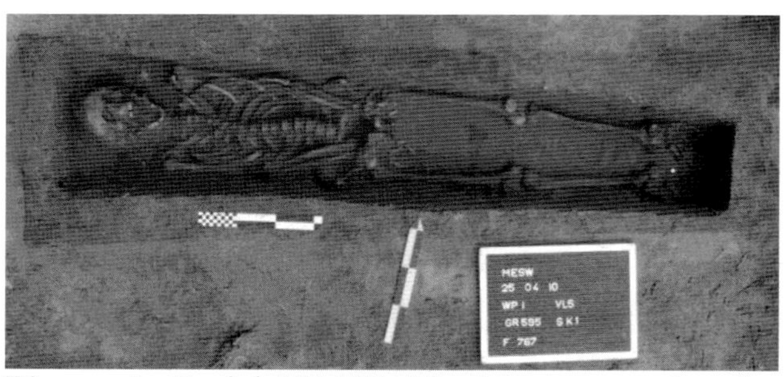

**Figure 4:** Burial GR595. The bones moved under the influence of gravity, evident in the loss of articulation in the hand and feet bones, the forward movement of the ribs, indicating a coffin burial. The coffin wall is indicated by the position of the lower limbs and the patellae.

The bones clearly responded to the influence of gravity, the mandible fell at the loss of the temporo-mandibular articulation, the labile articulations of hand and feet were lost, while the ribs fell forward. The coffin walls prevented the patellae from falling as the result of the lateral rotation of the lower limbs. Another burial GR634, dating to the same period, of which a coffin delineation could be observed on site, shows preservation of the labile articulations in the hand, indicating that sediment entered sooner (Fig.5). Besides an indication of the type of burial context, the location and position of the bones also suggest the confines of the context. Although the right coffin wall was no longer visible, the medial rotation of the right humerus, the inhibited fall of the right innominate bone and patella clearly indicate the context limit.

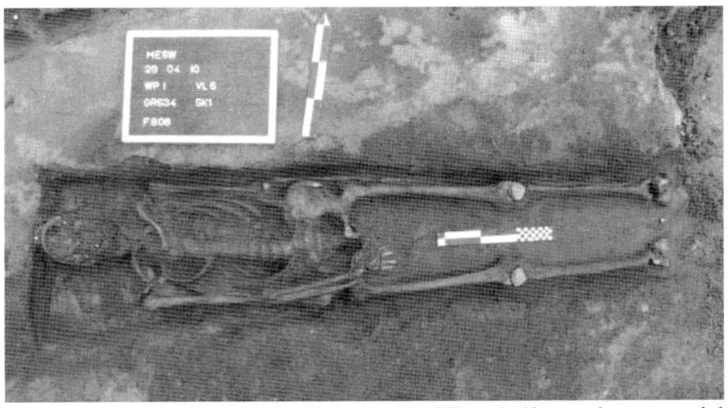

**Figure 5:** Burial GR634. A coffin delineation could be observed on site, the preservation of the labile articulations in the hand however indicates that sediment entered the burial before complete decomposition of the ligaments.

In burial GR985, in which there were only vague traces of a coffin delineation around the bones, the loss of the articulations in the hand bones and ribs that fell forward, confirm that it concerns a coffin burial (Fig.6). The strong linearity in the long bones suggests lateral pressure, also suggested by the verticalisation of the clavicles, and indicates the location of the coffin walls.

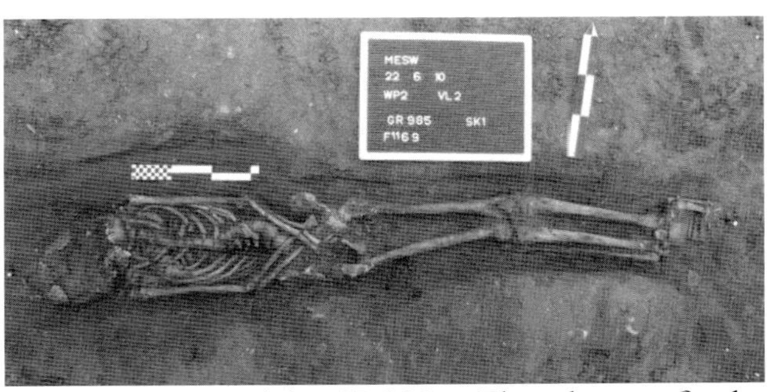

**Figure 6:** Burial GR985. The loss of the articulations in the hand bones and the forward movement of the ribs suggest that it concerns a coffin burial, although there was no coffin delineation. The strong linearity in the long bones suggests lateral pressure, also indicated by the verticalisation of the clavicles, and indicates the location of the coffin walls.

Burial GR617 is a small neonate coffin, the feature of which lies within a larger coffin delineation of an adult female (Fig.7). The burial was excavated in three stages, first within the smaller coffin, to record the relation of the bones to this context, and then enlarged to the larger coffin, to record the association between the two individuals, and finally removing the neonate to expose the entire adult individual. It was found that the neonatal bones rested between the adult's spine and ribs, restricted by its coffin walls, on a thin layer of dark organic soil. The neonate was buried in a separate coffin on top, as the adult bones were undisturbed and bone movements were in accordance with single burial in open space. On the right side of the neonate, some bones became disarticulated, among others the right femur and ribs, which would correspond with a fall into the cavity against the adult spine. Unfortunately it can not be determined whether the deposition of the two coffins was simultaneous.

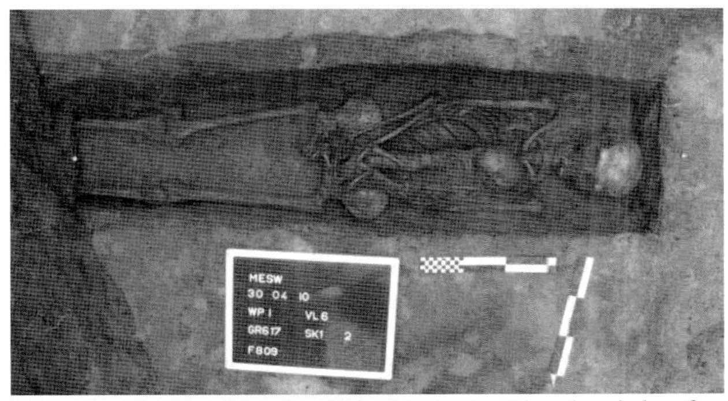

**Figure 7**: Double burial GR617. The burial of a neonate in a small coffin, within the coffin lines of an adult female. The movement and position of the different bones suggests the small coffin was located over the larger one and that decomposition occurred separately.

**Discussion**

The dark-brown colour of the upper made it impossible to distinguish grave cuts and coffin delineations in the upper post-Medieval layers. Disturbances, both human and natural, also obscured many features. The use of the principles of *archaeothanatology* often provided clues on site for the nature of the context and aided in the excavation of the multiple burials. However, a comprehensive study of the collected data will be needed to confidently distinguish the different types. There is significant variation in the position and movement, since the position of hands and feet affect the potential for gravity as would the presence of any wrapping or clothing, and it is the combination of different observations and comparisons within a large collection of data that is important for the study of body position, burial context and taphonomic processes. There were also a number of more noticeable variations, in which no immediately clear explanation or cause could be discerned. One of these variations concerns the burials which were completely compressed and for which there is as yet no clear explanation. Outward movement of the ribs in combination with medial rotation of the upper limbs was sometimes observed. A possible suggestion is that differences in body mass affect the potential movement of the bones after decomposition of the soft tissues. Occasionally close wrapping of the body was observed with coffin delineation, allowing room between the bones and the coffin wall.

Although in depth study is required to answer for the many variations and types that could be observed on site, some preliminary categories can be distinguished. Both primary and secondary deposition occurred, with both deliberate, ordered and selected deposition of disturbed bone, and random depositions in pits. Single and multiple burials were found, with simultaneous as well as consecutive depositions. Remains were deposited in plain earth burials or coffins, wrapped in a shroud or clothed. Study of the data, statistical and spatial analysis of the burials will hopefully distinguish more groups and determine differences over time. No obvious differences between periods were observed on site, apart from a much higher degree of intercutting of burials in the post-Medieval periods and a more consistent orientation in the Medieval burials.

## Conclusion

Considering the nature of the site, with in the younger layers a very low visibility of features in the soil, the methods provided by the principles of *archaeothanatology* have provided us with a means to record characteristics of the burial context no longer visible on site. The recording of the preservation or loss of anatomical articulations between bones and their movement indicates the original position of the body, the burial context, whether plain earth burial, coffin or shroud, shape and size of the pit or container. This will make it possible to deduce the different types of burial used, with further distinctions between coffin and plain earth burials, associated with size, type and quality of burial container, burial in clothes, type of wrapping, etc., and whether there are chronological trends or groups that may be recognized. Even on an emergency excavation it is clearly worth the small effort on site to record these traits, particularly since they can not be retrieved later. The use of field anthropology on this excavation has greatly complemented the information that could be retrieved from the burials and can be used on rescue excavations as well as research excavations with more time. The principles may be applied to the information from all the burials on this cemetery and compared, to provide a large and comprehensive reference collection. This will provide information on the dynamics of Medieval and post-Medieval cemeteries, with chronological and spatial trends and social groups and mortuary ritual.

## Acknowledgements

I would like to thank the Department of Archaeology of the city of Mechelen and the archaeologists working with me on site, Silvia Depuydt, Clara Boffin, Ben Terryn and Frederik Wuyts, for using the methods described above and contributing to this research, with the aid of the field technicians. The excavation was funded by the City Council of Mechelen, with the support of the European Union (EFRO), the Flemish Government and the Province of Antwerp.

## Literature Cited

Boddington, A. 1987. Chaos, disturbance and decay in an Anglo-Saxon cemetery. In: Boddington A., Garland A.N. and Janaway R.C. (eds.) *Death, decay and reconstruction: approaches to archaeology and forensic science*. Manchester University Press: Manchester. 27-42.

Brothwell, D. 1987. Decay and disorder in the York Jewbury skeletons. In: Boddington, A., Garland, A.N., Janaway, R.C. (eds.) *Death, decay and reconstruction: approaches to archaeological and forensic science.* Manchester University Press: Manchester. 22–26.

Duday, H. 1990. L'anthropologie "de terrain": reconnaissance et interpretation des gestes funeraires. *Bulletins et Mémoires de la Societé d'Anthropologie de Paris* 3-4: 29-50.

Duday, H. 2006. *Archaeothanatology* or the archaeology of death. In: Gowland, R. and Knüsel, C. (eds.) *Social archaeology of funerary remains*. Oxbow: Oxford. 30-56.

Duday, H. 2009. *The archaeology of the dead. Lectures in archaeothanatology*. Oxbow: Oxford.

Duday, H. and Guillon, M. 2006. Understanding the circumstances of decomposition when the body is skeletonised. In: Schmitt, A., Cunha, E. and Pinheiro, J. (eds.) *Forensic anthropology and medicine. Complementary sciences from recovery to cause of death.* Human Press: Totowa NJ. 117–157.

Goetstouwers, A. 1956. *De oorkonden der Abdij Rozendaal der orde van Cîteaux, I. Tongerlo, 1956, XIX,* 47-48, nr.46. Commissie voor geschiedkundige en Folkloristische opzoekingen der provincie Antwerpen: Westerlo.

Installé, H. 1996 (id est 1997). De Sint-Romboutskerk. In: Installé, H. (ed.) *Historische stedenatlas van België, Mechelen, II., Handelingen van de koninklijke kring voor oudheidkunde, letteren en kunst van Mechelen, dl. C aflevering II.* Koninklijke Kring voor Oudheidkunde, Letteren en Kunst: Mechelen. 7-24.

Kinnaer, F. n.d. *Het belang van de Wollemarkt/Sint-Romboutskerkhof.* Unpublished text.

Maureille, B. and Sellier, P. 1996. Dislocation en ordre paradoxal, momification et décomposition: observations et hypotheses. *Bulletins et Mémoires de la Societé d'Anthropologie de Paris* Nouvelle Série. Tome 8 N°3-4: 313-327.

Nilsonn Stutz, L. 1998. Dynamic cadavers. A "field anthropological" analysis of the Skateholm II burials. *Lund Archaeological Review (LAR)* 1998: 5-17.

Nilsson Stutz, L. 2006. Unwrapping the dead: searching for evidence of wrappings in the mortuary practices at Zvejnieki. In: Larsson, L. and Zagorska, I. (eds.) *Back to the origin. New research in the Mesolithic Neolithic Zvejnieki cemetery and environment, northern Latvia.* Acta Archaeologica Lundensia, Series in 8, no.52. Almqvist & Wiksell International: Stockholm. 217–233.

Van de Vijver, K., Depuydt, S., Boffin, C., Terryn, B. and Wuyts, F. 2011. De eerste bevindingen van de opgraving van het St.Romboutskerkhof, Mechelen (Antw.). *Archaeologia Mediaevalis* 34: 120-126.

Willis, A. and Tayles, N. 2009. Field anthropology: application to burial contexts in prehistoric south-east Asia. *Journal of Archaeological Science* 36: 547-554.